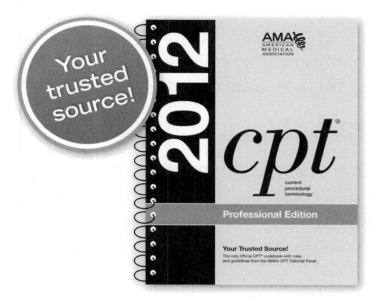
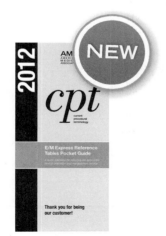
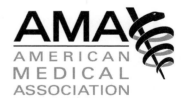

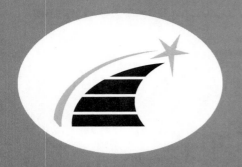

Stay up to date!
Access the latest ICD-9-CM and HCPCS code updates throughout the year

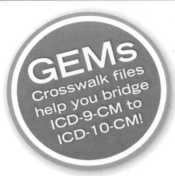

GEMs
Crosswalk files help you bridge ICD-9-CM to ICD-10-CM!

- Access the mid-year code updates as soon as they are published by the government
- Sign up now for email alerts that let you know when new codes are posted

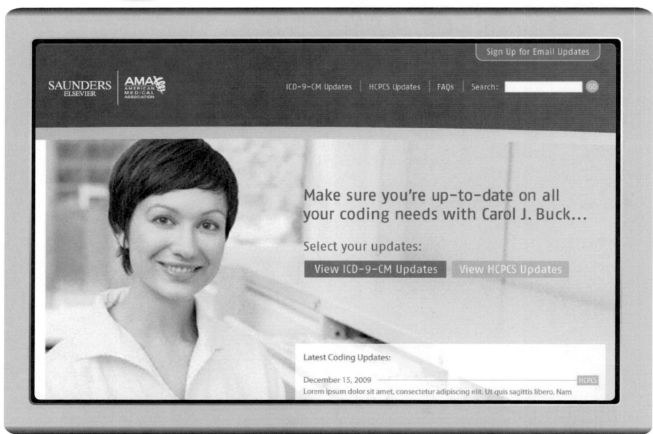

Trust Carol J. Buck, the AMA, and Elsevier to give you quick access to the most up-to-date codes!

www.codingupdates.com

2012
HCPCS Level II

STANDARD EDITION

2012
HCPCS Level II

Carol J. Buck
MS, CPC, CPC-H, CCS-P

Former Program Director; Medical Secretary Programs
Northwest Technical College; East Grand Forks, Minnesota

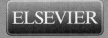

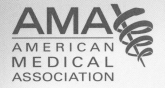

AMERICAN
MEDICAL
ASSOCIATION

ELSEVIER
SAUNDERS

3251 Riverport Lane
St. Louis, Missouri 63043

ISSN: 2211-9485

2012 HCPCS LEVEL II STANDARD EDITION

ISBN: 978-1-4557-0771-3

Notices

Knowledge and best practice in this field are constantly changing. As new research and experience broaden our understanding, changes in research methods, professional practices, or medical treatment may become necessary.

Practitioners and researchers must always rely on their own experience and knowledge in evaluating and using any information, methods, compounds, or experiments described herein. In using such information or methods they should be mindful of their own safety and the safety of others, including parties for whom they have a professional responsibility.

With respect to any drug or pharmaceutical products identified, readers are advised to check the most current information provided (i) on procedures featured or (ii) by the manufacturer of each product to be administered, to verify the recommended dose or formula, the method and duration of administration, and contraindications. It is the responsibility of practitioners, relying on their own experience and knowledge of their patients, to make diagnoses, to determine dosages and the best treatment for each individual patient, and to take all appropriate safety precautions.

To the fullest extent of the law, neither the Publisher nor the authors, contributors, or editors, assume any liability for any injury and/or damage to persons or property as a matter of products liability, negligence or otherwise, or from any use or operation of any methods, products, instructions, or ideas contained in the material herein.

ISBN: 978-1-4557-0771-3

Publisher: Jeanne Olson
Senior Developmental Editor: Jenna Johnson
Publishing Services Manager: Pat Joiner-Myers
Senior Designer: Amy Buxton

Printed in the United States of America

Last digit is the print number: 9 8 7 6 5 4 3 2 1

TECHNICAL COLLABORATORS

Jacqueline Klitz Grass, MA, CPC
Coding Specialist
Grand Forks, North Dakota

Nancy Maguire, ACS, CRT, PCS, FCS, HCS-D, APC, AFC
Physician Consultant for Auditing and Education
University City, Texas

CONTENTS

GUIDE TO USING THE 2012 HCPCS LEVEL II CODES   x

SYMBOLS AND CONVENTIONS   xi

2012 HCPCS UPDATES   xiii

2012 HCPCS INDEX   1

2012 HCPCS TABLE OF DRUGS   25

2012 HCPCS: LEVEL II NATIONAL CODES

Introduction   78

CMS Healthcare Common Procedure Coding System (HCPCS)   87

Updates will be posted on http://codingupdates.com when available.

Check the Centers for Medicare and Medicaid Services (http://www.cms.gov/Manuals/IOM/list.asp) website and http:codingupdates.com for IOMs.

GUIDE TO USING THE 2012 HCPCS LEVEL II CODES

Medical coding has long been a part of the health care profession. Through the years medical coding systems have become more complex and extensive. Today, medical coding is an intricate and immense process that is present in every health care setting. The increased use of electronic submissions for health care services only increases the need for coders who understand the coding process.

2012 HCPCS Level II was developed to help meet the needs of today's coder.

All material adheres to the latest government versions available at the time of printing.

Annotated

Throughout this text, revisions and additions are indicated by the following symbols:

◄ **New:** Additions to the previous edition are indicated by the color triangle.

← **Revised:** Revisions within the line or code from the previous edition are indicated by the color arrow.

✔ **Reinstated** indicates a code that was previously deleted and has now been reactivated.

✖ ~~deleted~~ words have been removed from this year's edition.

HCPCS Symbols

⊗ **Special coverage instructions** apply to these codes. Usually these special coverage instructions are included in the Internet Only Manuals (IOM) select references at http: codingupdates.com.

◆ **Not covered or valid by Medicare** is indicated by the diamond. Usually the reason for the exclusion is included in the Internet Only Manuals (IOM) select references at http:codingupdates.com.

✳ **Carrier discretion** is an indication that you must contact the individual third-party payers to find out the coverage available for codes identified by this symbol.

NDC Drugs approved for Medicare Part B are listed as NDC (National Drug Code). All other FDA-approved drugs are listed as Other.

Color and/or *italic* typeface is added by the publisher and does not appear in the official code set.

SYMBOLS AND CONVENTIONS

HCPCS Symbols

Special coverage instructions apply to these codes. Usually these instructions are included in the Internet Only Manuals (IOM) select references located at http:codingupdates.com.

⊗ **L3540** Miscellaneous shoe additions, sole, full
IOM: 100-2, 15, 290

The Internet Only Manuals (IOM) give instructions regarding use of the code. IOM select references are located at http: codingupdates.com.

Not covered or valid by Medicare is indicated by the diamond. Usually the reason for the exclusion is included in the IOM references located at http: codingupdates.com.

◆ **A6533** Gradient compression stocking, thigh length, 18–30 mm Hg, each
IOM: 100-02, 15, 130; 100-03, 4, 280.1

Carrier discretion is an indication that you must contact the individual third-party payers for the coverage for these codes.

✳ **A6154** Wound pouch, each

Codes shown are for illustration purposes only and may not be current codes.

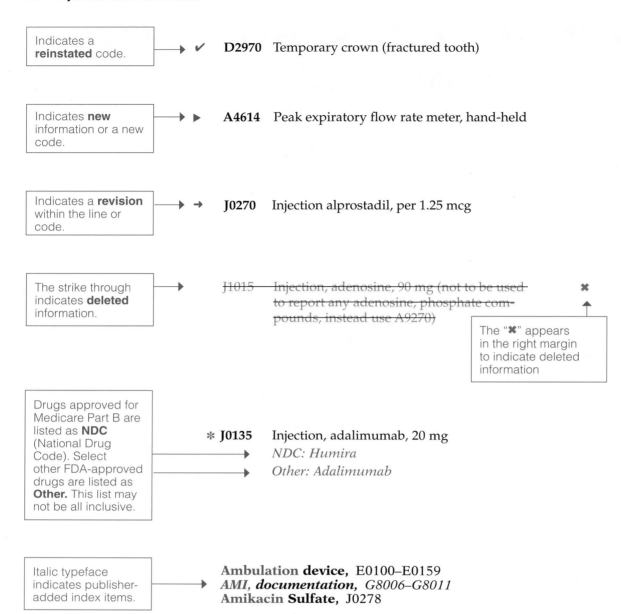

Indicates a **reinstated** code.

✔ **D2970**   Temporary crown (fractured tooth)

Indicates **new** information or a new code.

▶ **A4614**   Peak expiratory flow rate meter, hand-held

Indicates a **revision** within the line or code.

→ **J0270**   Injection alprostadil, per 1.25 mcg

The strike through indicates **deleted** information.

▶ ~~J1015~~   ~~Injection, adenosine, 90 mg (not to be used to report any adenosine, phosphate compounds, instead use A9270)~~   ✖

The "✖" appears in the right margin to indicate deleted information

Drugs approved for Medicare Part B are listed as **NDC** (National Drug Code). Select other FDA-approved drugs are listed as **Other.** This list may not be all inclusive.

✳ **J0135**   Injection, adalimumab, 20 mg
          NDC: Humira
          Other: Adalimumab

Italic typeface indicates publisher-added index items.

Ambulation device, E0100–E0159
AMI, documentation, G8006–G8011
Amikacin Sulfate, J0278

Codes shown are for illustration purposes only and may not be current codes.

2012 HCPCS New/Revised/Deleted Codes and Modifiers

HCPCS quarterly updates are posted on the companion website (http://www.codingupdates.com) when available.

NEW CODES/MODIFIERS

AY	E0988	G0448	G8653	G8706	G8745	G8783	G8821	G8858	G8895	J2358	L6715
AZ	E1831	G0449	G8654	G8707	G8746	G8784	G8822	G8859	G8896	J2426	L6880
CS	E2358	G0450	G8655	G8708	G8747	G8785	G8823	G8860	G8897	J2507	L8693
DA	E2359	G0451	G8656	G8709	G8748	G8786	G8824	G8861	G8898	J3095	Q0162
GU	E2622	G0908	G8657	G8710	G8749	G8787	G8825	G8862	G8899	J3262	Q0478
GX	E2623	G0909	G8658	G8711	G8750	G8788	G8826	G8863	G8900	J3357	Q0479
NB	E2624	G0910	G8659	G8712	G8751	G8789	G8827	G8864	G8901	J3385	Q2026
PD	E2625	G0911	G8660	G8713	G8752	G8790	G8828	G8865	G8902	J7131	Q2027
PT	E2626	G0912	G8661	G8714	G8753	G8791	G8829	G8866	G8903	J7180	Q2035
A4566	E2627	G0913	G8662	G8715	G8754	G8792	G8830	G8867	G8904	J7183	Q2036
A5056	E2628	G0914	G8663	G8716	G8755	G8793	G8831	G8868	G8905	J7196	Q2037
A5057	E2629	G0915	G8664	G8717	G8756	G8794	G8832	G8869	G8906	J7309	Q2038
A7020	E2630	G0916	G8665	G8718	G8757	G8795	G8833	G8870	G9147	J7312	Q2039
A9272	E2631	G0917	G8666	G8720	G8758	G8796	G8834	G8871	G9156	J7326	Q2043
A9273	E2632	G0918	G8667	G8721	G8759	G8797	G8835	G8872	J0131	J7335	Q4117
A9584	E2633	G0919	G8668	G8722	G8760	G8798	G8836	G8873	J0171	J7665	Q4118
A9585	G0157	G0920	G8669	G8723	G8761	G8799	G8837	G8874	J0221	J7686	Q4119
C1749	G0158	G0921	G8670	G8724	G8762	G8800	G8838	G8875	J0257	J8561	Q4120
C1830	G0159	G0922	G8671	G8725	G8763	G8801	G8839	G8876	J0490	J8562	Q4121
C1840	G0160	G8629	G8672	G8726	G8764	G8802	G8840	G8877	J0558	J9043	Q4122
C1886	G0161	G8630	G8673	G8727	G8765	G8803	G8841	G8878	J0561	J9179	Q4123
C8931	G0162	G8631	G8674	G8728	G8767	G8805	G8842	G8879	J0588	J9228	Q4124
C8932	G0163	G8632	G8682	G8730	G8768	G8806	G8843	G8880	J0597	J9302	Q4125
C8933	G0164	G8633	G8683	G8731	G8769	G8807	G8844	G8881	J0638	J9307	Q4126
C8934	G0428	G8634	G8685	G8732	G8770	G8808	G8845	G8882	J0712	J9315	Q4127
C8935	G0429	G8635	G8694	G8733	G8771	G8809	G8846	G8883	J0775	J9351	Q4128
C8936	G0434	G8642	G8695	G8734	G8772	G8810	G8847	G8884	J0840	K0741	Q4129
C9275	G0436	G8643	G8696	G8735	G8773	G8811	G8848	G8885	J0897	K0742	Q4130
C9279	G0437	G8644	G8697	G8736	G8774	G8812	G8849	G8886	J1290	K0743	Q5010
C9285	G0438	G8645	G8698	G8737	G8775	G8813	G8850	G8887	J1557	K0744	S0119
C9286	G0439	G8646	G8699	G8738	G8776	G8814	G8851	G8888	J1559	K0745	S0148
C9287	G0442	G8647	G8700	G8739	G8777	G8815	G8852	G8889	J1599	K0746	S0169
C9366	G0443	G8648	G8701	G8740	G8778	G8816	G8853	G8890	J1725	L3674	S3722
C9367	G0444	G8649	G8702	G8741	G8779	G8817	G8854	G8891	J1786	L4631	S8130
C9732	G0445	G8650	G8703	G8742	G8780	G8818	G8855	G8892	J1826	L5312	S8131
C9800	G0446	G8651	G8704	G8743	G8781	G8819	G8856	G8893	J2265	L5961	T1505
E0446	G0447	G8652	G8705	G8744	G8782	G8820	G8857	G8894			

REVISED CODES/MODIFIERS

Change in Short Description	E0637	G8427	G8578	L3671	Q4115	A6549
	E0638	G8428	G8580	L3677	Q4116	E0765
GA	E0641	G8431	G8583	L6000	S9900	E0978
RA	E0642	G8432	G8586	L6010		E1161
RB	E0691	G8433	G8605	L6020	**Change in**	G0306
V5	G0151	G8447	G8608	L7368	**Administration**	G0307
V6	G0152	G8448	G8611	Q0499	SC	G0339
V7	G0153	G8482	G8614	Q4101	A6530	G0340
A4399	G0154	G8509	G8617	Q4102	A6533	K0730
A5112	G0406	G8510	G8620	Q4103	A6534	
A6011	G0407	G8511	G8623	Q4104	A6535	**Change in Short**
A6248	G0408	G8539	G8626	Q4105	A6536	**Description**
A6260	G0425	G8542	J0129	Q4106	A6537	J9208
A6261	G0426	G8553	J0220	Q4107	A6538	K0669
A6262	G0427	G8573	J0256	Q4108	A6539	K0899
A7013	G0431	G8574	J0598	Q4110	A6540	
B4034	G0432	G8575	J1561	Q4111	A6541	**Miscellaneous**
B4035	G0433	G8576	J9060	Q4112	A6544	**Change**
B4036	G0435	G8577	L2005	Q4113	A6545	A4619

DELETED CODES/MODIFIERS

C9255	G0430	G8040	G8114	G8223	G8322	G8403	G8534	J1390	L1500
C9256	G0440	G8041	G8115	G8226	G8326	G8407	G8537	J1470	L1510
C9258	G0441	G8051	G8116	G8231	G8330	G8408	G8538	J1480	L1520
C9259	G8006	G8052	G8117	G8234	G8334	G8409	G8636	J1490	L3672
C9260	G8007	G8053	G8129	G8238	G8338	G8423	G8637	J1500	L3673
C9261	G8008	G8054	G8130	G8240	G8341	G8424	G8638	J1510	L3964
C9262	G8009	G8055	G8131	G8243	G8345	G8425	G8639	J1520	L3965
C9263	G8010	G8056	G8152	G8246	G8351	G8426	G8640	J1530	L3966
C9264	G8011	G8057	G8153	G8248	G8354	G8429	G8641	J1540	L3968
C9265	G8012	G8058	G8154	G8251	G8357	G8434	G8675	J1550	L3969
C9266	G8013	G8059	G8155	G8254	G8360	G8435	G8676	J1785	L3970
C9267	G8014	G8060	G8156	G8257	G8362	G8436	G8677	J1825	L3972
C9268	G8015	G8061	G8157	G8260	G8365	G8437	G8678	J2321	L3974
C9269	G8016	G8062	G8159	G8263	G8367	G8438	G8679	J2322	L4380
C9270	G8017	G8075	G8162	G8266	G8370	G8439	G8680	J7130	L5311
C9271	G8018	G8076	G8164	G8268	G8371	G8440	G8681	J7184	L7266
C9272	G8019	G8077	G8165	G8271	G8372	G8441	G8684	J9062	L7272
C9273	G8020	G8078	G8166	G8274	G8373	G8443	G8686	J9080	L7274
C9274	G8021	G8079	G8167	G8276	G8374	G8445	G8687	J9090	L7500
C9276	G8022	G8080	G8170	G8279	G8375	G8446	G8688	J9091	Q0179
C9277	G8023	G8081	G8171	G8282	G8376	G8449	G8689	J9092	Q1003
C9278	G8024	G8082	G8172	G8285	G8377	G8453	G8690	J9093	Q2025
C9280	G8025	G8085	G8182	G8289	G8378	G8454	G8691	J9094	Q2040
C9281	G8026	G8093	G8183	G8293	G8379	G8455	G8692	J9095	Q2041
C9282	G8027	G8094	G8184	G8296	G8380	G8456	G8693	J9096	Q2042
C9283	G8028	G8099	G8185	G8298	G8381	G8457	G9041	J9097	Q2044
C9284	G8029	G8100	G8186	G8299	G8382	G8466	G9042	J9110	Q4109
C9365	G8030	G8103	G8193	G8302	G8383	G8467	G9043	J9140	S0146
C9406	G8031	G8104	G8196	G8303	G8384	G8479	G9044	J9290	S0161
C9729	G8032	G8106	G8200	G8304	G8385	G8480	J0128	J9291	S0181
C9730	G8033	G8107	G8204	G8305	G8386	G8481	J0170	J9350	S0196
C9731	G8034	G8108	G8209	G8306	G8387	G8488	J0559	J9375	S0625
C9801	G8035	G8109	G8214	G8307	G8388	G8507	J0560	J9380	S2270
C9802	G8036	G8110	G8217	G8308	G8389	G8508	J0570	K0734	S2344
E0220	G8037	G8111	G8219	G8310	G8390	G8518	J0580	K0735	S3628
E0230	G8038	G8112	G8220	G8314	G8391	G8519	J0704	K0736	S3905
E0238	G8039	G8113	G8221	G8318	G8402	G8520	J0970	K0737	S9075
E0571									

HCPCS 2012 INDEX

A

Abatacept, J0129
Abciximab, J0130
Abdomen
   dressing holder/binder, A4462
   pad, low profile, L1270
Abduction **control, each,** L2624
Abduction restrainer, A4566
Abduction **rotation bar, foot,** L3140–L3170
AbobotulinumtypeA, J0586
Absorption **dressing,** A6251–A6256
Access, site, occlusive, device, G0269
Access **system,** A4301
Accessories
   ambulation devices, E0153–E0159
   artificial kidney and machine (*see also* ESRD), E1510–E1699
   beds, E0271–E0280, E0300–E0326
   wheelchairs, E0950–E1030, E1050–E1298, *E2201–E2295*, E2300–2399, K0001–K0109
ACE/ARB therapy, G8468–G8475
Acetaminophen, J0131 ◄
Acetazolamide **sodium,** J1120
Acetylcysteine
   inhalation solution, J7604, J7608
   injection, J0132
Activity, therapy, G0176
Acyclovir, J0133
Adalimumab, J0135
Adenosine, J0150, J0152
Adhesive, A4364
   bandage, A6413
   disc or foam pad, A5126
   remover, A4455, A4456
   support, breast prosthesis, A4280
   wound, closure, G0168
Administration, **Part D**
   supply, tositumomab, G3001
   vaccine, hepatitis B, G0010
   vaccine, influenza, G0008
   vaccine, pneumococcal, G0009
Admission, observation, G0379
Administrative, **Miscellaneous and Investigational,** A9000–A9999
Adrenalin, J0171
Advanced life support, A0390, A0426, A0427, A0433
Aerosol
   compressor, ~~E0571~~, E0572
   compressor filter, K0178–K0179
   mask, K0180
AFO, E1815, E1830, L1900–L1990, L4392, L4396
Agalsidase **beta,** J0180
Aggrastat, J3245
A-hydroCort, J1710
Aide, **home, health,** *G0156, S9122, T1021*
   bath/toilet, E0160–E0162, E0235, E0240–E0249

Aide (Continued)
   services, G0151–G0156, G0179–G0181, S5180, S5181, S9122, T1021, T1022
Air **bubble detector, dialysis,** *E1530*
Air **fluidized bed,** E0194
Air **pressure pad/mattress,** E0186, E0197
Air **travel and nonemergency transportation,** A0140
Alarm
   not otherwise classified, A9280
   pressure, dialysis, E1540
Alatrofloxacin **mesylate,** J0200
Albumin, **human,** P9041, P9042
Albuterol
   all formulations, inhalation solution, concentrated, J7610, J7611
   all formulations, inhalation solution, unit dose, J7609, J7613
   all formulations, inhalation solution, J7620
Alcohol/substance, **assessment,** *G0396, G0397, H0001, H0003, H0049*
Alcohol, A4244
Alcohol **wipes,** A4245
Aldesleukin **(IL2),** J9015
Alefacept, J0215
Alemtuzumab, J9010
Alert **device,** A9280
Alginate **dressing,** A6196–A6199
Alglucerase, J0205
Alglucosidase, J0220
Alglucosidase **alfa,** J0221 ◄
Alphanate, J7186
Alpha-1-proteinase **inhibitor, human,** J0256, J0257 ←
Alprostadil
   injection, J0270
   urethral suppository, J0275
ALS mileage, A0390
Alteplase **recombinant,** J2997
Alternating **pressure mattress/pad,** A4640, E0180, E0181, E0277
Ambulance, A0021–A0999
   air, A0430, A0431, A0435, A0436
   disposable supplies, A0382–A0398
   oxygen, A0422
Ambulation **device,** E0100–E0159
Amikacin **Sulfate,** J0278
Aminolevulinate, J7309
Aminolevulinic **acid HCl,** J7308
Aminophylline, J0280
Amiodarone **HCl,** J0282
Amitriptyline **HCl,** J1320
Ammonia **N-13,** A9526
Ammonia **test paper,** A4774
Amniotic **membrane,** V2790
Amobarbital, J0300
Amphotericin **B,** J0285
   Lipid Complex, J0287–J0289

Ampicillin
  sodium, J0290
  sodium/sulbactam sodium, J0295
Amputee
  adapter, wheelchair, E0959
  prosthesis, L5000–L7510, L7520, L7900, L8400–L8465
  stump sock, L8470–L8485
  wheelchair, E1170–E1190, E1200, K0100
Amygdalin, J3570
Anadulafungin, J0348
Analysis
  semen, G0027
Angiography, iliac, artery, G0278
  reconstruction, G0288
  renal, artery, G0275
Anistreplase, J0350
Ankle splint, recumbent, K0126–K0130
Ankle-foot orthosis (AFO), L1900–L1990, L2106–
    L2116, L4361, L4392, L4396
Anterior-posterior-lateral orthosis, L0700, L0710
Antidepressant, documentation, G8126–G8128
Anti-emetic, oral, Q0163–Q0181, J8498, J8597
Anti-hemophilic factor (Factor VIII), J7190–J7192
Anti-inhibitors, per I.U., J7198
Antimicrobial, prophylaxis, documentation,
  G8201
Anti-neoplastic drug, NOC, J9999
Antithrombin III, J7197
Antithrombin recombinant, J7196
Apomorphine, J0364
Appliance
  cleaner, A5131
  pneumatic, E0655–E0673
Application, heat, cold, E0200–E0239
Aprotinin, J0365
Aqueous
  shunt, L8612
  sterile, J7051
ARB/ACE therapy, G8468–G8475
Arbutamine HCl, J0395
Arch support, L3040–L3100
  intralesional, J3302
Arformoterol, J7605
Aripiprazole, J0400
Arm, wheelchair, E0973
Arsenic trioxide, J9017
Artificial
  cornea, L8609
  kidney machines and accessories (*see also* Dialysis),
    E1510–E1699
  larynx, L8500
  saliva, A9155
Arthrography, injection, sacroiliac, joint, G0259,
  G0260
Arthroscopy, knee, surgical, G0289, S2112, S2300
Asparaginase, J9020
Aspiration, bone marrow, G0364
Aspirator, VABRA, A4480

Assessment
  alcohol/substance, G0396, G0397, H0001, H0003,
    H0049
  audiologic, V5008–V5020
  cardiac output, M0302
  speech, V5362–V5364
Attachment, walker, E0154–E0159
Astramorph, J2275
Atropine
  inhalation solution, concentrated, J7635
  inhalation solution, unit dose, J7636
Atropine sulfate, J0461
Audiologic assessment, V5008–V5020
Auditory osseointegrated device, L8690–L8693
Aurothioglucose, J2910
Azacitidine, J9025
Azathioprine, J7500, J7501
Azithromycin injection, J0456

B

Back supports, L0621–L0861, L0960
Baclofen, J0475, J0476
Bacterial sensitivity study, P7001
Bag
  drainage, A4357
  enema, A4458
  irrigation supply, A4398
  urinary, A4358, A5112
Basiliximab, J0480
Bath, aid, E0160–E0162, E0235, E0240–E0249
Bathtub
  chair, E0240
  stool or bench, E0245, E0247–E0248
  transfer rail, E0246
  wall rail, E0241, E0242
Battery, L7360, L7364–L7368
  charger, E1066, L7362, L7366
  replacement for blood glucose monitor,
    A4233–A4234
  replacement for cochlear implant device,
    L8623–L8624
  replacement for TENS, A4630
  ventilator, A4611–A4613
BCG live, intravesical, J9031
Beclomethasone inhalation solution, J7622
Bed
  accessories, E0271–E0280, E0300–E0326
  air fluidized, E0194
  cradle, any type, E0280
  drainage bag, bottle, A4357, A5102
  hospital, E0250–E0270, E0300–E0329
  pan, E0275, E0276
  rail, E0305, E0310
  safety enclosure frame/canopy, E0316
Behavioral, health, treatment services, H0002–H2037
Belimumab, J0490 ◄

◄ New   ← Revised   ✔ Reinstated   ~~deleted~~ Deleted

Belt
  extremity, E0945
  ostomy, A4367
  pelvic, E0944
  safety, K0031
  wheelchair, E0978, E0979
Bench, bathtub (*see also* Bathtub), E0245
Bendamustine HCl, J9033
Benesch boot, L3212–L3214
Benztropine, J0515
Betadine, A4246, A4247
Betamethasone
  acetate and betamethasone sodium phosphate, J0702
  inhalation solution, J7624
Bethanechol chloride, J0520
Bevacizumab, J9035, Q2024
Bifocal, glass or plastic, V2200–V2299
Bilirubin (phototherapy) light, E0202
Binder, A4465
Biofeedback device, E0746
Bioimpedance, electrical, cardiac output, M0302
Biperiden lactate, J0190
Bitolterol mesylate, inhalation solution
  concentrated, J7628
  unit dose, J7629
Bivalirudin, J0583
Bladder calculi irrigation solution, Q2004
Bleomycin sulfate, J9040
Blood
  count, G0306, G0307, S3630
  fresh frozen plasma, P9017
  glucose monitor, E0607, E2100, E2101, *S1030, S1031*
  glucose test, A4253
  granulocytes, pheresis, P9050
  ketone test, A4252
  leak detector, dialysis, E1560
  leukocyte poor, P9016
  mucoprotein, P2038
  platelets, P9019
  platelets, irradiated, P9032
  platelets, leukocytes reduced, P9031
  platelets, leukocytes reduced, irradiated, P9033
  platelets, pheresis, P9034
  platelets, pheresis, irradiated, P9036
  platelets, pheresis, leukocytes reduced, P9035
  platelets, pheresis, leukocytes reduced, irradiated, P9037
  pressure monitor, A4660, A4663, A4670
  pump, dialysis, E1620
  red blood cells, deglycerolized, P9039
  red blood cells, irradiated, P9038
  red blood cells, leukocytes reduced, P9016
  red blood cells, leukocytes reduced, irradiated, P9040
  red blood cells, washed, P9022
  strips, A4253
  supply, P9010 P9022
  testing supplies, A4770
  tubing, A4750, A4755

Blood collection devices accessory, A4257, E0620
BMI, G8417–G8422
Body jacket
  scoliosis, L1300, L1310
Body sock, L0984
Body, mass, index, G8417–G8422
Bond or adhesive, ostomy skin, A4364
Bone
  density, study, G0130
  marrow, aspiration, G0364
Boot
  pelvic, E0944
  surgical, ambulatory, L3260
Bortezomib, J9041
Brachytherapy radioelements, Q3001
Breast prosthesis, L8000–L8035, L8600
  adhesive skin support, A4280
Breast pump
  accessories, A4281–A4286
  electric, any type, E0603
  heavy duty, hospital grade, E0604
  manual, any type, E0602
Breathing circuit, A4618
Brompheniramine maleate, J0945
Budesonide inhalation solution, J7626, J7627, J7633, J7634
Bulking agent, L8604
Buprenorphine hydrochloride, J0592
Bus, nonemergency transportation, A0110
Busulfan, J0594, J8510
Butorphanol tartrate, J0595
Bypass, graft, coronary, artery
  documentation, G8160–G8163
  surgery, S2205–S2209

C

C-1 Esterase Inhibitor, J0597–J0598
Cabazitaxel, J9043 ◀
Cabergoline, oral, J8515
Caffeine citrate, J0706
CABG, documentation, G8160–G8163
Cabinet/System, ultraviolet, E0691–E0694
CAD documentation, G8160–G8163
Calcitriol, J0636
Calcitonin-salmon, J0630
Calcitrol, S0169
Calcium
  disodium edetate, J0600
  gluconate, J0610
  glycerophosphate and calcium lactate, J0620
  lactate and calcium glycerophosphate, J0620
  leucovorin, J0640
Calibrator solution, A4256
Canakinumab, J0638

Cancer, screening
  cervical or vaginal, G0101
  colorectal, G0104–G0106, G0120–G0122,
    G0328, S3890
  prostate, G0102, G0103
Cane, E0100, E0105
  accessory, A4636, A4637
Canister
  disposable, used with suction pump, A7000
  non-disposable, used with suction pump, A7001
Cannula, **nasal,** A4615
Capecitabine, **oral,** J8520, J8521
Capsaicin **patch,** J7335
Carbon **filter,** A4680
Carboplatin, J9045
Cardia **Event, recorder, implantable,** E0616
Cardiokymography, Q0035
Cardiovascular **services,** M0300–M0301
Carmustine, J9050
Care, coordinated, G9001–G9011, H1002
Case **management,** T1016, T1017
Care plan, G0162
Caspofungin **acetate,** J0637
Cast
  hand restoration, L6900–L6915
  materials, special, A4590
  supplies, A4580, A4590, Q4001–Q4051
  thermoplastic, L2106, L2126
Caster
  front, for power wheelchair, K0099
  wheelchair, E0997, E0998
Catheter, A4300–A4355
  anchoring device, A5200, A4333, A4334
  cap, disposable (dialysis), A4860
  external collection device, A4327–A4330, A4347
  implanted, A7042, A7043
  indwelling, A4338–A4346
  insertion tray, A4354
  intermittent with insertion supplies, A4353
  irrigation supplies, A4355
  male external, A4324, A4325, A4348
  oropharyngeal suction, A4628
  starter set, A4329
  trachea (suction), A4609, A4610, A4624
  transtracheal oxygen, A4608
  vascular, A4300, A4301
Catheterization, **specimen collection,** P9612, P9615
CBC, G0306, G0307
Cefazolin **sodium,** J0690
Cefepime **HCl,** J0692
Cefotaxime **sodium,** J0698
Ceftaroline **fosamil,** J0712 ◀
Ceftazidime, J0713
Ceftizoxime **sodium,** J0715
Ceftriaxone **sodium,** J0696
Cefuroxime **sodium,** J0697
CellCept, K0412
Cellular **therapy,** M0075

Cement, **ostomy,** A4364
Centrifuge, A4650
Cephalin **Floculation, blood,** P2028
Cephalothin **sodium,** J1890
Cephapirin **sodium,** J0710
Certification, physician, home, health, G0179–G0182
Certolizumab **pegol,** J0718
Cerumen, removal, G0268
Cervical
  cancer, screening, G0101
  cytopathology, G0123, G0124, G0141–G0148
  halo, L0810–L0830
  head harness/halter, E0942
  orthosis, L0100–L0200
  traction, E0855, E0856
Cervical **cap contraceptive,** A4261
Cervical-thoracic-lumbar-sacral **orthosis (CTLSO),**
  L0700, L0710
Cetuximab, J9055
Chair
  adjustable, dialysis, E1570
  lift, E0627
  rollabout, E1031
  sitz bath, E0160–E0162
  transport, E1035–E1039
Chelation **therapy,** M0300
Chemical **endarterectomy,** M0300
Chemistry **and toxicology tests,** P2028–P3001
Chemotherapy
  administration, Q0083–Q0085 (hospital reporting
    only)
  drug, oral, not otherwise classified, J8999
  drugs (*see also* drug by name), J9000–J9999
Chest **shell (cuirass),** E0457
Chest **Wall Oscillation System,** E0483
  hose, replacement, A7026
  vest, replacement, A7025
Chest **wrap,** E0459
Chin **cup, cervical,** L0150
Chloramphenicol **sodium succinate,** J0720
Chlordiazepoxide **HCl,** J1990
Chloromycetin **Sodium Succinate,** J0720
Chloroprocaine **HCl,** J2400
Chloroquine **HCl,** J0390
Chlorothiazide **sodium,** J1205
Chlorpromazine **HCl,** J3230
Choroid, lesion, destruction, G0186
Chorionic **gonadotropin,** J0725
Chromic **phosphate P32 suspension,** A9564
Chromium **CR-51 sodium chromate,** A9553
Cidofovir, J0740
Cilastatin **sodium, imipenem,** J0743
Ciprofloxacin, **for intravenous infusion,** J0744
Cisplatin, J9060
Cladribine, J9065
Clamp
  dialysis, A4910, A4918, A4920
  external urethral, A4356

◀ New   ← Revised   ✔ Reinstated   ~~deleted~~ Deleted

Cleanser, wound, A6260
Cleansing agent, dialysis equipment, A4790
Clofarabine, J9027
Clonidine, J0735
Closure, wound, adhesive, tissue, G0168
Clotting time tube, A4771
Clubfoot wedge, L3380
Cochlear prosthetic implant, L8614
    accessories, L8615–L8617
    batteries, L8621–L8624
    replacement, L8619, L8627–L8629
Codeine phosphate, J0745
Colchicine, J0760
Cold/Heat, application, E0200–E0240
Colistimethate sodium, J0770
Collagen
    meniscus implant procedure, G0428
    skin test, G0025
    urinary tract implant, L8603
    wound dressing, A6020–A6024
Collagenase, Clostridium Histolyticum, J0775
Collar, cervical
    multiple post, L0180–L0200
    nonadjust (foam), L0120
Colorectal, screening, cancer, G0104–G0106,
    G0120–G0122, G0328, S3890
Coly-Mycin M, J0770
Comfort items, A9190
Complete, blood, count, G0306, G0307
Commode, E0160–E0175
    chair, E0170–E0171
    lift, E0625, E0172
    pail, E0167
    seat, wheelchair, E0968
Composite dressing, A6203–A6205
Compressed gas system, E0424–E0480
Compressor
    aerosol, E0572, E0575
    air, E0565
    nebulizer, E0570–E0585
    pneumatic, E0650–E0676
Compression
    bandage, A4460
    burn garment, A6501–A6512
    stockings, A6530–A6549
Compressor, E0565, E0570, ~~E0571~~, E0572,
    E0650–E0652
Conductive gel/paste, A4558
Conductivity meter, bath, dialysis, E1550
Conference, team, G0175, G9007, S0220, S0221
Congo red, blood, P2029
Contact layer, A6206–A6208
Contact lens, V2500–V2599
Continent device, A5081, A5082, A5083
Continuous glucose monitoring system
    receiver, A9278
    sensor, A9276
    transmitter, A9277

Continuous passive motion exercise device, E0936
Continuous positive airway pressure (CPAP)
    device, E0601
    compressor, K0269
Contraceptive
    cervical cap, A4261
    condoms, A4267, A4268
    diaphragm, A4266
    intratubal occlusion device, A4264
    intrauterine, copper, J7300
    intrauterine, levonorgestrel releasing, J7302
    levonorgestrel, implants and supplies, A4260
    patch, J7304
    spermicide, A4269
    supply, A4267–A4269
    vaginal ring, J7303
Contracts, maintenance, ESRD, A4890
Contrast material
    injection during MRI, A4643
    low osmolar, A4644–A4646
Coordinated, care, G9001–G9011
Corneal tissue processing, V2785
Corset, spinal orthosis, L0970–L0976
Corticorelin ovine triflutate, J0795
Corticotropin, J0800
Corvert, *see* Ibutilide fumarate
Cosyntropin, J0833, J0834
Cough stimulating device, A7020, E0482
Counseling, smoking and tobacco cessation, G0436,
    G0437
Count, blood, G0306, G0307, S3636
Counterpulsation, external, G0166
Cover, wound
    alginate dressing, A6196–A6198
    foam dressing, A6209–A6214
    hydrogel dressing, A6242–A6248
    non-contact wound warming cover, and accessory,
        A6000, E0231, E0232
    specialty absorptive dressing, A6251–A6256
CPAP (continuous positive airway pressure)
    device, E0601
    headgear, K0185
    humidifier, A7046
    intermittent assist, E0452
Cradle, bed, E0280
Crib, E0300
Cromolyn sodium, inhalation solution, unit
    dose, J7631, J7632
Crotalidae, polyvalent immune fab, J0840 ◄
Crutches, E0110–E0118
    accessories, A4635–A4637, K0102
Cryoprecipitate, each unit, P9012
CTLSO, L1000–L1120, L0700, L0710
Cuirass, E0457
Culture sensitivity study, P7001
Cushion, wheelchair, E0977
Cyanocobalamin Cobalt C057, A9559
Cycler dialysis machine, E1594

◄ New   ← Revised   ✔ Reinstated   ~~deleted~~ Deleted

Cyclophosphamide, J9070
  oral, J8530
Cyclosporine, J7502, J7515, J7516
Cytarabine, J9100
  liposome, J9098
Cytomegalovirus **immune globulin (human),**
  J0850
Cytopathology, cervical or vaginal, G0123, G0124,
* G0141–G0148*

D

Dacarbazine, J9130
Daclizumab, J7513
Dactinomycin, J9120
Dalalone, J1100
Dalteparin **sodium,** J1645
Daptomycin, J0878
Darbepoetin **Alfa,** J0881–J0882
Daunorubicin
  Citrate, J9151
  HCl, J9150
DaunoXome, *see* **Daunorubicin citrate**
Decitabine, J0894
Decubitus **care equipment,** E0180–E0199
Deferoxamine **mesylate,** J0895
Defibrillator, **external,** E0617, K0606
  battery, K0607
  electrode, K0609
  garment, K0608
Degarelix, J9155
Deionizer, **water purification system,** E1615
Delivery/set-up/dispensing, A9901
Denileukin **diftitox,** J9160
Denosumab, J0897 ◄
Density, bone, study, G0130
Depo-estradiol **cypionate,** J1000
Dermal filler injection, G0429
Desmopressin **acetate,** J2597
Destruction, lesion, choroid, G0186
Detector, **blood leak, dialysis,** E1560
Dexamethasone
  acetate, J1094
  inhalation solution, concentrated, J7637
  inhalation solution, unit dose, J7638
  intravitreal implant, J7312
  oral, J8540
  sodium phosphate, J1100
Dextran, J7100
Dextrose
  saline (normal), J7042
  water, J7060, J7070
Dextrostick, A4772
Diabetes
  evaluation, G0245, G0246
  shoes, A5500–A5508
  training, outpatient, G0108, G0109

Diagnostic
  radiology services, R0070–R0076
Dialysate
  concentrate additives, A4765
  solution, A4728
  testing solution, A4760
Dialysis
  air bubble detector, E1530
  bath conductivity, meter, E1550
  chemicals/antiseptics solution, A4674
  disposable cycler set, A4671
  emergency, G0257
  equipment, E1510–E1702
  extension line, A4672–A4673
  filter, A4680
  fluid barrier, E1575
  forceps, A4910
  home, S9335, S9339
  kit, A4820
  pressure alarm, E1540
  shunt, A4740
  supplies, A4650–A4927
  thermometer, A4910
  tourniquet, A4910
  unipuncture control system, E1580
  unscheduled, G0257
  venous pressure clamp, A4918
Dialyzer, A4690
Diaper, T1500, T4521–T4540
  adult incontinence garment, A4520
Diazepam, J3360
Diazoxide, J1730
Dicyclomine **HCl,** J0500
Diethylstilbestrol **diphosphate,** J9165
Digoxin, J1160
Digoxin **immune fab (ovine),** J1162
Dihydroergotamine **mesylate,** J1110
Dimenhydrinate, J1240
Dimercaprol, J0470
Dimethyl **sulfoxide (DMSO),** J1212
Diphenhydramine **HCl,** J1200
Dipyridamole, J1245
Disarticulation
  lower extremities, prosthesis,
    L5000–L5999
  upper extremities, prosthesis,
    L6000–L6692
Disease
  status, oncology, G9063–G9139
Disposable **supplies, ambulance,** A0382, A0384,
  A0392–A0398
Dispensing, fee, pharmacy, G0333, Q0510–Q0514,
* S9430*
DME
  miscellaneous, A9900–A9999
DMSO, J1212
Dobutamine **HCl,** J1250
Docetaxel, J9171

Documentation
antidepressant, G8126–G8128
blood pressure, G8476–G8478
bypass, graft, coronary, artery, documentation, G8160–G8163
CABG, G8160–G8163
dysphagia, G8232
dysphagia, screening, G8232, V5364
eye, functions, G8315–G8333
influenza, immunization, G8482–G8484
osteoporosis, G8401
pharmacologic therapy for osteoporosis, G8634, G8635
prophylaxis, DVT, G8218
prophylactic parenteral antibiotic, G8629–G8632
prophylaxis, thrombosis, deep, vein, G8218
urinary, incontinence, G8063, G8267
Dolasetron mesylate, J1260
Dome and mouthpiece (for nebulizer), A7016
Dopamine HCl, J1265
Doripenem, J1267
Dornase alpha, inhalation solution, unit dose form, J7639
Doxercalciferol, J1270
Doxil, J9001
Doxorubicin HCl, J9000, J9001
Drainage
bag, A4357, A4358
board, postural, E0606
bottle, A5102
Dressing (see also Bandage), A6020–A6406
alginate, A6196–A6199
collagen, A6020–A6024
composite, A6203–A6205
contact layer, A6206–A6208
foam, A6209–A6215
gauze, A6216–A6230, A6402–A6406
holder/binder, A4462
hydrocolloid, A6234–A6241
hydrogel, A6242–A6248
specialty absorptive, A6251–A6256
transparent film, A6257–A6259
tubular, A6457
Droperidol, J1790
and fentanyl citrate, J1810
Dropper, A4649
Drug screen, G0434
Drugs (see also Table of Drugs)
administered through a metered dose inhaler, J3535
antiemetic, J8489, J8597, Q0163–Q0181
chemotherapy, J8500–J9999
disposable delivery system, 5 ml or less per hour, A4306
disposable delivery system, 50 ml or greater per hour, A4305
immunosuppressive, J7500–J7599
infusion supplies, A4230–A4232, A4221, A4222
inhalation solutions, J7608–J7699
non-prescription, A9150

Drugs *(Continued)*
not otherwise classified, J3490, J7599, J7699, J7799, J8499, J8999, J9999
oral, NOS, J8499
prescription, oral, J8499, J8999
Dry pressure pad/mattress, E0179, E0184, E0199
Durable medical equipment (DME), E0100–E1830, K Codes
Duraclon, *see* **Clonidine**
Dyphylline, J1180
Dysphagia, screening, documentation, G8232, V5364
Dystrophic, nails, trimming, G0127

E

Ear mold, V5264
Ecallantide, J1290
Echocardiography injectable contrast material, A9700
Eculizumab, J1300
ED, visit, G0380–G0384
Edetate
calcium disodium, J0600
disodium, J3520
Eggcrate dry pressure pad/mattress, E0184, E0199
Elastic garments, A4466
Elbow
disarticulation, endoskeletal, L6450
orthosis (EO), E1800, L3700–L3740, L3760
protector, E0191
Electric, nerve, stimulator, transcutaneous, A4595, E0720–E0749
Electrical work, dialysis equipment, A4870
Electromagnetic, therapy, G0295, G0329
Electronic medication compliance, T1505
Electrodes, per pair, A4556
Elevating leg rest, K0195
Elliotts b solution, J9175
Emergency department, visit, G0380–G0384
EMG, E0746
Eminase, J0350
Endarterectomy, chemical, M0300
Endoscope sheath, A4270
Endoskeletal system, addition, L5848, L5856–L5857, L5925, *L5961*
Enfuvirtide, J1324
Enoxaparin sodium, J1650
Enema, bag, A4458
Enteral
feeding supply kit (syringe) (pump) (gravity), B4034–B4036
formulae, B4149–B4156
nutrition infusion pump (with alarm) (without), B9000, B9002
therapy, supplies, B4000–B9999
Epinephrine, J0171
Epirubicin HCl, J9178

Epoetin **alpha,** J0885–J0886, Q4081
Epoprostenol, J1325
Equipment
  decubitus, E0181–E0199
  exercise, A9300, E0935, E0936
  orthopedic, E0910–E0948, E1800–E8002
  oxygen, E0424–E0486, E1353–E1406
  pump, E0781, E0784, E0791
  respiratory, E0424–E0601
  safety, E0700, E0705
  traction, E0830–E0900
  transfer, E0705
  trapeze, E0910–E0912, E0940
  whirlpool, E1300, E1310
Ergonovine **maleate,** J1330
Eribulin **mesylate,** J9179 ◄
Ertapenem **sodium,** J1335
Erythromycin **lactobionate,** J1364
ESRD (End-Stage Renal Disease; *see also* **Dialysis)**
  machines and accessories, E1500–E1699
  plumbing, A4870
  supplies, A4651–A4929
Estrogen **conjugated,** J1410
Estrone **(5, Aqueous),** J1435
Ethanolamine **oleate,** J1430
Etidronate **disodium,** J1436
Etonogestrel **implant system,** J7307
Etoposide, J9181
  oral, J8560
Euflexxa, J7323
Evaluation
  conformity, V5020
  contact lens, S0592
  diabetic, G0245, G0246
  footwear, G8410–G8416
  fundus, G8325–G8328
  hearing, S0618, V5008, V5010
  hospice, G0337
  multidisciplinary, H2000
  nursing, T1001
  ocularist, S9150
  performance measurement, S3005
  resident, T2011
  speech, S9152
  team, T1024
  treatment response, G0254
Everolimus, J8561 ◄
Examination
  gynecological, S0610–S0613
  ophthalmological, S0620, S0621
  pinworm, Q0113
  ringworm, S0605
Exercise
  class, S9451
  equipment, A9300, *E0935, E0936*
External
  ambulatory infusion pump, E0781, E0784
  ambulatory insulin delivery system, A9274

External *(Continued)*
  power, battery components, L7360–L7368
  power, elbow, L7160–L7191
  urinary supplies, A4356-A4359
Extremity
  belt/harness, E0945
  traction, E0870–E0880
Eye
  case, V2756
  functions, documentation, G8315–G8333
  lens (contact) (spectacle), V2100–V2615
  prosthetic, V2623, V2629
  service (miscellaneous), V2700–V2799

F

Faceplate, **ostomy,** A4361
Face **tent, oxygen,** A4619
Factor **VIIA coagulation factor, recombinant,** J7189
Factor **VIII, anti-hemophilic factor,** J7185, J7190–J7192
Factor **IX,** J7193, J7194, J7195
Factor **XIII, anti-hemophilic factor,** J7180 ◄
Family **Planning Education,** H1010
Fee
  coordinated care, G9001–G9011
  dispensing, pharmacy, G0333, Q0510–Q0514, S9430
Fentanyl **citrate,** J3010
  and droperidol, J1810
Fern **test,** Q0114
Ferumoxytol, Q0138, Q0139
Filgrastim **(G-CSF),** J1440, J1441
Filler, **wound**
  alginate dressing, A6199
  foam dressing, A6215
  hydrocolloid dressing, A6240, A6241
  hydrogel dressing, A6248
  not elsewhere classified, A6261, A6262
Film, **transparent (for dressing),** A6257–A6259
Filter
  aerosol compressor, A7014
  dialysis carbon, A4680
  ostomy, A4368
  tracheostoma, A4481
  ultrasonic generator, A7014
Fistula **cannulation set,** A4730
Flebogamma, J1572
Flowmeter, E0440, E0555, E0580
Floxuridine, J9200
Fluconazole, **injection,** J1450
Fludarabine **phosphate,** J8562, J9185
Fluid **barrier, dialysis,** E1575
Flunisolide **inhalation solution,** J7641
Fluocinolone, J7311
Fluorodeoxyglucose **F-18 FDG,** A9552
Fluorouracil, J9190

◄ New   ← Revised   ✔ Reinstated   ~~deleted~~ Deleted

Foam
    dressing, A6209–A6215
    pad adhesive, A5126
Folding walker, E0135, E0143
Foley catheter, A4312–A4316, A4338–A4346
Fomepizole, J1451
Fomivirsen sodium intraocular, J1452
Fondaparinux sodium, J1652
Footdrop splint, L4398
Footplate, E0175, E0970, L3031
Footwear, orthopedic, L3201–L3265
Forearm crutches, E0110, E0111
Formoterol, J7640
    fumarate, J7606
Fosaprepitant, J1453
Foscarnet sodium, J1455
Fosphenytoin, Q2009
Fracture
    bedpan, E0276
    frame, E0920, E0930, E0946–E0948
    orthosis, L2106–L2136, L3980–L3986
    orthotic additions, L2180–L2192, L3995
Fragmin, *see* **Dalteparin sodium**
Frames (spectacles), V2020, V2025
Fulvestrant, J9395
Furosemide, J1940

G

Gadobutrol, A9585 ◄
Gadofosveset trisodium, A9583
Gadoxetate disodium, A9581
Gait trainer, E8000–E8002
Gallium Ga67, A9556
Gallium nitrate, J1457
Galsulfase, J1458
Gammagard liquid, J1569
Gamma globulin, J1460, J1560
Gammaplex, J1557 ◄
Gamunex, J1561
Ganciclovir
    implant, J7310
    sodium, J1570
Garamycin, J1580
Gas system
    compressed, E0424, E0425
    gaseous, E0430, E0431, E0441, E0443
    liquid, E0434–E0440, E0442, E0444
Gatifloxacin, J1590
Gauze (see also Bandage)
    impregnated, A6222–A6233, A6266
    non-impregnated, A6402–A6404
Gefitinib, J8565
Gel
    conductive, A4558
    pressure pad, E0185, E0196
Gemcitabine HCl, J9201

Gemtuzumab ozogamicin, J9300
Generator
    ultrasonic with nebulizer, E0574
Gentamicin (Sulfate), J1580
Glasses
    air conduction, V5070
    binaural, V5120–V5150
    bone conduction, V5080
    frames, V2020, V2025
    hearing aid, V5230
Glaucoma
    screening, G0117, G0118
Gloves, A4927
Glucagon HCl, J1610
Glucose
    monitor with integrated lancing/blood sample
        collection, E2101
    monitor with integrated voice synthesizer, E2100
    test strips, A4253, A4772
Gluteal pad, L2650
Glycopyrrolate, inhalation solution, concentrated, J7642
Glycopyrrolate, inhalation solution, unit dose, J7643
Gold
    sodium thiomalate, J1600
Gomco drain bottle, A4912
Gonadorelin HCl, J1620
Goserelin acetate implant (see also Implant), J9202
Grab bar, trapeze, E0910, E0940
Gradient, compression stockings, A6530–A6549
Grade-aid, wheelchair, E0974
Granisetron HCl, J1626
Gravity traction device, E0941
Gravlee jet washer, A4470
Guaiac, stool, G0394
Guidelines, practice, oncology, G9056–G9062

H

Hair analysis (excluding arsenic), P2031
Hallus-Valgus dynamic splint, L3100
Hallux prosthetic implant, L8642
Haloperidol, J1630
    decanoate, J1631
Halo procedures, L0810–L0860
Halter, cervical head, E0942
Hand finger orthosis, prefabricated, L3923
Hand restoration, L6900–L6915
    partial prosthesis, L6000–L6020
    orthosis (WHFO), E1805, E1825, L3800–L3805, L3900-L3954
    rims, wheelchair, E0967
Handgrip (cane, crutch, walker), A4636
Harness, E0942, E0944, E0945
Headgear (for positive airway pressure device), K0185

◄ New	← Revised	✔ Reinstated	~~deleted~~ Deleted

Hearing
  assessment, S0618, V5008, V5010
  devices, V5000–V5299, L8614
  services, V5000–V5999
Heat
  application, E0200–E0239
  lamp, E0200, E0205
  infrared heating pad system, A4639, E0221
  pad, A9273, E0210, E0215, E0237, E0249
Heater **(nebulizer),** E1372
Heavy duty, wheelchair, E1280–E1298, K0006,
    K0007, K0801–K0886
Heel
  elevator, air, E0370
  protector, E0191
  shoe, L3430–L3485
  stabilizer, L3170
Helicopter, **ambulance (***see also* **Ambulance)**
Helmet
  cervical, L0100, L0110
  head, A8000–A8004
Hemin, J1640
Hemi-wheelchair, E1083–E1086
Hemipelvectomy **prosthesis,** L5280
Hemodialysis **machine,** E1590
Hemodialyzer, **portable,** E1635
Hemofil **M,** J7190
Hemophilia **clotting factor,** J7190–J7198
  NOC, J7199
Hemostats, A4850
Hemostix, A4773
Hepagam B
  IM, J1571
  IV, J1573
Heparin
  infusion pump, dialysis, E1520
  lock flush, J1642
  sodium, J1644
Hepatitis B, vaccine, administration, G0010
Hep-Lock **(U/P),** J1642
Hexalite, A4590
High **osmolar contrast material,** Q9958–Q9964
Hip
  disarticulation prosthesis, L5250, L5270
  orthosis (HO), L1600–L1690
Hip-knee-ankle-foot **orthosis (HKAFO),**
    L2040–L2090
Histrelin
  acetate, J1675
  implant, J9225
HKAFO, L2040–L2090
Home
  glucose, monitor, E0607, E2100, E2101, S1030, S1031
  health, aide, G0156, S9122, T1021
  health, clinical, social worker, G0155
  health, nursing, skilled, G0154
  health, occupational, therapist, G0152
  health, physical therapist, G0151

Home (Continued)
  health, physician, certification, G0179–G0182
  health, respiratory therapy, S5180, S5181
  therapist, speech, S9128
Home **Health Agency Services,** T0221
HOPPS, **C1000–C9999**
Hospice home care, Q5010
Hospital
  bed, E0250–E0304, E0328, E0329
  observation, G0378, G0379
Hospital **Outpatient Payment System,** *C1000–C9999*
Hot **water bottle,** A9273
Human **fibrinogen concentrate,** J1680
Humidifier, A7046, E0550–E0563
Hyalgan, J7321
Hyalomatrix, Q4117
Hyaluronan, **J7326**◄
Hyaluronate, **sodium,** J7317
Hyaluronidase, J3470
  ovine, J3471–J3473
Hydralazine **HCl,** J0360
Hydraulic **patient lift,** E0630
Hydrocollator, E0225, E0239
Hydrocolloid **dressing,** A6234–A6241
Hydrocortisone
  acetate, J1700
  sodium phosphate, J1710
  sodium succinate, J1720
Hydrogel **dressing,** A6242–A6248, A6231–A6233
Hydromorphone, J1170
Hydroprogesterone, **caproate,** J1725◄
Hydroxyzine **HCl,** J3410
Hylan **G-F 20,** J7325
Hyoscyamine **Sulfate,** J1980
Hyperbaric **oxygen chamber, topical,** A4575
~~Hypertonic saline solution, J7130~~

I

Ibandronate **sodium,** J1740
Ibutilide **Fumarate,** J1742
Ice
  cap, E0230
  collar, E0230
Idarubicin **HCl,** J9211
Idursulfase, J1743
Ifosfamide, J9208
Iliac, artery, angiography, G0278
Iloprost, Q4074
Imiglucerase, J1786
Immune **globulin**
  Flebogamma, J1572
  Gammagard liquid, J1569
  Gammaplex, J1557◄
  Gamunex, J1561
  HepaGam B, J1571
  Hizentra, J1559

◄ **New**   ← **Revised**   ✔ **Reinstated**   ~~deleted~~ **Deleted**

Immune globulin *(Continued)*
  NOS, J1566
  Octagam, J1568
  Privigen, J1459
  Rho(D), J2788, J2790
  Rhophylac, J2791
  Subcutaneous, J1562
Immunosuppressive drug, not otherwise classified, J7599
Implant
  access system, A4301
  aqueous shunt, L8612
  breast, L8600
  cochlear, L8614, L8619
  collagen, urinary tract, L8603
  dextranomer/hyaluronic acid copolymer, L8604
  ganciclovir, J7310
  hallux, L8642
  urinary tract, L8603, L8606
  infusion pump, programmable, E0783, E0786
  joint, L8630, L8641, L8658
  lacrimal duct, A4262, A4263
  metacarpophalangeal joint, L8630
  metatarsal joint, L8641
  neurostimulator pulse generator, L8681–L8688
  not otherwise specified, L8699
  ocular, L8610
  ossicular, L8613
  osteogenesis stimulator, E0749
  percutaneous access system, A4301
  replacement implantable intraspinal catheter, E0785
  synthetic, urinary, L8606
  vascular graft, L8670
Implantable radiation dosimeter, A4650
Impregnated gauze dressing, A6222–A6230
Incobotulinumtoxin a, J0588◄
Incontinence
  appliances and supplies, A4310, A4360, A5071–A5075, A5102–A5114, K0280, K0281
  garment, A4520, T4521–T4543
  supply, A4335, A4356–A4358
  treatment system, E0740
  urinary, documentation, G8063, G8067
Indium IN-111
  carpromab pendetide, A9507
  ibritumomab tiuxetan, A9542
  labeled autologous white blood cells, A9570
  labeled autologous platelets, A9571
  oxyquinoline, A9547
  pentetate, A9548
  pentetreotide, A9572
  satumomab, A4642
Infliximab injection, J1745
Influenza
  immunization, documentation, G8482–G8484
  vaccine, administration, G0008
  virus vaccine, Q2035–Q2039

Infusion
  pump, ambulatory, with administrative equipment, E0781
  pump, heparin, dialysis, E1520
  pump, implantable, E0782, E0783
  pump, implantable, refill kit, A4220
  pump, insulin, E0784
  pump, mechanical, reusable, E0779, E0780
  pump, uninterrupted infusion of Epiprostenol, K0455
  saline, J7030–J7060
  supplies, A4219, A4221, A4222, A4230–A4232, E0776–E0791
  therapy, other than chemotherapeutic drugs, Q0081
Inhalation solution *(see also* **drug name),** J7608–J7699, Q4074
Injection device, needle-free, A4210
Injections *(see also* **drug name),** J0120–J7320
  arthrography, sacroiliac, joint, G0259, G0260
  supplies for self-administered, A4211
INR, monitoring, G0248–G0250
Insertion tray, A4310–A4316
Insulin, J1815, J1817, S5550–S5571
  ambulatory, external, system, A9274
  treatment, outpatient, G9147
Integra flowable wound matrix, Q4114
Interferon
  Alpha, J9212–J9215
  Beta-1 a, J1826, Q3025–Q3026
  Beta-1 b, J1830
  Gamma, J9216
Intermittent
  assist device with continuous positive airway pressure device, E0470–E0472
  limb compression device, E0676
  peritoneal dialysis system, E1592
  positive pressure breathing (IPPB) machine, E0500
Interphalangeal joint, prosthetic implant, L8658, L8659
Interscapular thoracic prosthesis
  endoskeletal, L6570
  upper limb, L6350–L6370
Intervention, tobacco, G9016
Intraconazole, J1835
Intraocular
  lenses, V2630–V2632
Intrapulmonary percussive ventilation system, E0481
Intrauterine copper contraceptive, J7300
Iodine Iobenguane sulfate I-131, A9508
Iodine I-123 iobenguane, A9582
Iodine I-123 ioflupane, A9584◄
Iodine I-123 sodium iodide, A9509, A9516
Iodine I-125 serum albumin, A9532
  sodium iodide, A9527
  sodium iothalamate, A9554
Iodine I-131 iodinated serum albumin, A9524
  sodium iodide capsule, A9517, A9528
  sodium iodide solution, A9529–A9531
  tositumomab, A9544–A9545

◄ New   ← Revised   ✔ Reinstated   ~~deleted~~ Deleted

Iodine swabs/wipes, A4247
IPD
  system, E1592
Ipilimumab, J9228◄
IPPB machine, E0500
Ipratropium bromide, inhalation solution, unit dose, J7644, J7645
Irinotecan, J9206
Iron
  Dextran, J1750
  sucrose, J1756
Irrigation/evacuation system, bowel
  control unit, E0350
  disposable supplies for, E0352
Irrigation solution for bladder calculi, Q2004
Irrigation supplies, A4320–A4322, A4355, A4397–A4400
Islet, transplant, G0341–G0343, S2102
Isoetharine HCl, inhalation solution
  concentrated, J7647, J7648
  unit dose, J7649, J7650
Isolates, B4150, B4152
Isoproterenol HCl, inhalation solution
  concentrated, J7657, J7658
  unit dose, J7659, J7660
Isosulfan blue, Q9968
Item, non-covered, A9270
IUD, J7300, S4989
IV pole, each, E0776, K0105
Ixabepilone, J9207

J

Jacket
  scoliosis, L1300, L1310
Jaw, motion, rehabilitation system, E1700–E1702
Jenamicin, J1580

K

Kanamycin sulfate, J1840, J1850
Kartop patient lift, toilet or bathroom (*see also* Lift), E0625
Ketorolac thomethamine, J1885
Kidney
  ESRD supply, A4650–A4927
  machine, accessories, E1500–E1699
  machine, E1500–E1699
  system, E1510
  wearable artificial, E1632
Kits
  enteral feeding supply (syringe) (pump) (gravity), B4034–B4036
  fistula cannulation (set), A4730
  parenteral nutrition, B4220–B4224
  surgical dressing (tray), A4550
  tracheostomy, A4625

Knee
  arthroscopy, surgical, G0289, S2112, S2300
  disarticulation, prosthesis, L5150, L5160
  joint, miniature, L5826
  orthosis (KO), E1810, L1800–L1885
Knee-ankle-foot orthosis (KAFO), L2000–L2039, L2126–L2136
  addition, high strength, lightweight material, L2755
Kyphosis pad, L1020, L1025

L

Laboratory
  services, P0000–P9999
Laboratory tests
  chemistry, P2028–P2038
  microbiology, P7001
  miscellaneous, P9010–P9615, Q0111–Q0115
  toxicology, P3000–P3001, Q0091
Lacrimal duct implant
  permanent, A4263
  temporary, A4262
Lactated Ringer's infusion, J7120
Laetrile, J3570
Lancet, A4258, A4259
Lanreotide, J1930
Laronidase, J1931
Larynx, artificial, L8500
Laser blood collection device and accessory, E0620, A4257
Lead investigation, T1029
Lead wires, per pair, A4557
Leg
  bag, A4358, A5105, A5112
  extensions for walker, E0158
  rest, elevating, K0195
  rest, wheelchair, E0990
  strap, replacement, A5113–A5114
Legg Perthes orthosis, L1700–L1755
Lens
  aniseikonic, V2118, V2318
  contact, V2500–V2599
  eye, V2100–V2615, V2700–V2799
  intraocular, V2630–V2632
  low vision, V2600–V2615
  progressive, V2781
Lepirudin, J1945
Lesion, destruction, choroid, G0186
Leucovorin calcium, J0640
Leukocyte poor blood, each unit, P9016
Leuprolide acetate, J9217, J9218, J9219, J1950
Levalbuterol, all formulations, inhalation solution
  concentrated, J7607, J7612
  unit dose, J7614, J7615
Levetiracetam, J1953
Levocarnitine, J1955
Levofloxacin, J1956

◄ New   ← Revised   ✔ Reinstated   ~~deleted~~ Deleted

Levoleucovorin, J0641
Levonorgestrel, **(contraceptive), implants and supplies,** J7306
Levorphanol **tartrate,** J1960
Lexidronam, A9604
Lidocaine **HCl,** J2001
Lift
  patient (includes seat lift), E0621–E0635
  shoe, L3300–L3334
Lightweight, wheelchair, E1087–E1090, E1240–E1270, E2618
Lincomycin **HCl,** J2010
Linezolid, J2020
Liquid **barrier, ostomy,** A4363
Lodging, **recipient, escort nonemergency transport,** A0180, A0200
LOPS, G0245–G0247
Lorazepam, J2060
Loss of protective sensation, G0245–G0247
Low **osmolar contrast material,** Q9965–Q9967
LSO, L0621–L0640
Lubricant, A4402, A4332
Lumbar **flexion,** L0540
Lumbar-sacral **orthosis (LSO),** L0621–L0640
LVRS, services, G0302–G0305
Lymphocyte **immune globulin,** J7504, J7511

M

Machine
  IPPB, E0500
  kidney, E1500–E1699
Magnesium **sulphate,** J3475
Maintenance **contract,** ESRD, A4890
Mammography, screening, G0202
Mannitol, J2150, J7665 ←
Mapping, vessel, for hemodialysis access, G0365
Marker, tissue, A4648
Mask
  aerosol, K0180
  oxygen, A4620
Mastectomy
  bra, L8000
  form, L8020
  prosthesis, L8030, L8600
  sleeve, L8010
Matristem, Q4118–Q4120
Mattress
  air pressure, E0186
  alternating pressure, E0277
  dry pressure, E0184
  gel pressure, E0196
  hospital bed, E0271, E0272
  non-powered, pressure reducing, E0373
  overlay, E0371–E0372
  powered, pressure reducing, E0277
  water pressure, E0187

*Measurement **period***
  left ventricular function testing, G8682
  not an eligible candidate for left ventricular function testing, G8683
  left ventricular function testing not performed, NOS, G8685
Mecasermin, J2170
Mechlorethamine **HCl,** J9230
Medicaid, codes, T1000–T9999
Medical **and surgical supplies,** A4206–A8999
*Medical **nutritional therapy,** G0270, G0271*
*Medical **services, other,** M0000–M9999*
Medroxyprogesterone **acetate,** J1051, J1055
Medroxyprogesterone **acetate/estradiol cypionate,** J1056
Melphalan
  HCl, J9245
  oral, J8600
*Mental, **health, training services,** G0177*
Meperidine, J2175
  and promethazine, J2180
Mepivacaine **HCl,** J0670
Meropenem, J2185
Mesna, J9209
Metacarpophalangeal **joint, prosthetic implant,** L8630, L8631
Metaproterenol **sulfate, inhalation solution**
  concentrated, J7667, J7668
  unit dose, J7669, J7670
Metaraminol **bitartrate,** J0380
Metatarsal **joint, prosthetic implant,** L8641
Meter, **bath conductivity, dialysis,** E1550
Methacholine **chloride,** J7674
Methadone **HCl,** J1230
Methocarbamol, J2800
Methotrexate
  oral, J8610
  sodium, J9250, J9260
Methyldopate **HCl,** J0210
Methylene **blue,** Q9968
Methylprednisolone
  acetate, J1020–J1040
  oral, J7509
  sodium succinate, J2920, J2930
Metoclopramide **HCl,** J2765
Micafungin **sodium,** J2248
Microbiology **test,** P7001
Midazolam **HCl,** J2250
Mileage
  ALS, A0390
  ambulance, A0380, A0390
Milrinone **lactate,** J2260
Mini-bus, **nonemergency transportation,** A0120
Minocycline **hydrochloride,** J2265 ◀
Mitomycin, J9280
Mitoxantrone **HCl,** J9293
MNT, G0270, G0271
*Mobility **device, physician, service,** G0372*

◀ New   ← Revised   ✔ Reinstated   ~~deleted~~ Deleted

Modalities, with office visit, M0005–M0008
Moisture exchanger for use with invasive mechanical ventilation, A4483
Moisturizer, skin, A6250
Monitor
    blood glucose, E0607
    blood pressure, A4670
    pacemaker, E0610, E0615
Monitoring feature/device, A9279
Monitoring, INR, G0248–G0250
Monoclonal antibodies, J7505
Morphine sulfate, J2270, J2271
    sterile, preservative-free, J2275
Motion, jaw, rehabilitation system, E1700–E1702
Mouthpiece (for respiratory equipment), A4617
Moxifloxacin, J2280
Mucoprotein, blood, P2038
Multiaxial ankle, L5986
Multidisciplinary services, H2000–H2001, T1023–T1028
Multiple post collar, cervical, L0180–L0200
Multi-Podus type AFO, L4396
Muromonab-CD3, J7505
Mycophenolate mofetil, J7517
Mycophenolic acid, J7518

N

Nabilone, J8650
Nails, trimming, dystrophic, G0127
Nalbuphine HCl, J2300
Naloxone HCl, J2310
Naltrexone, J2315
Nandrolone
    decanoate, J2320
    narrowing device, wheelchair, E0969
Nasal
    application device, K0183
    pillows/seals (for nasal application device), K0184
    vaccine inhalation, J3530
Nasogastric tubing, B4081, B4082
Natalizumab, J2323
Nebulizer, E0570–E0585
    ~~aerosol compressor, E0571~~
    aerosol mask, A7015
    corrugated tubing, disposable, A7010
    corrugated tubing, non-disposable, A7011
    filter, disposable, A7013
    filter, non-disposable, A7014
    heater, E1372
    large volume, disposable, prefilled, A7008
    large volume, disposable, unfilled, A7007
    not used with oxygen, durable, glass, A7017
    pneumatic, administration set, A7003, A7005, A7006
    pneumatic, nonfiltered, A7004
    portable, E0570
    small volume, A7003–A7005

Nebulizer *(Continued)*
    ultrasonic, E0575
    ultrasonic, dome and mouthpiece, A7016
    ultrasonic, reservoir bottle, non-disposable, A7009
    water collection device, large volume nebulizer, A7012
Needle, A4215
    non-coring, A4212
    with syringe, A4206–A4209
Negative pressure wound therapy pump, E2402
    accessories, A6550
Nelarabine, J9261
Neonatal transport, ambulance, base rate, A0225
Neostigmine methylsulfate, J2710
Nerve, conduction, sensory, test, G0255
Nerve stimulator with batteries, E0765
Nesiritide injection, J2324
Neuromuscular stimulator, E0745
Neurostimulator
    battery recharging system, L8695
    pulse generator, L8681–L8688
Nitrogen N-13 ammonia, A9526
NMES, E0720–E0749
Nonchemotherapy drug, oral, NOS, J8499
Noncovered services, A9270
Nonemergency transportation, A0080–A0210
Nonimpregnated gauze dressing, A6216–A6221, A6402–A6404
Nonprescription drug, A9150
Not otherwise classified drug, J3490, J7599, J7699, J7799, J8499, J8999, J9999, Q0181
NPH, J1820
NPWT, pump, E2402
NTIOL category 3, Q1003
NTIOL category 4, Q1004
NTIOL category 5, Q1005
Nursing care, T1030–T1031
Nursing service, direct, skilled, outpatient, G0128
Nursing, skilled, home, health, G0154
Nutrition
    enteral infusion pump, B9000, B9002
    parenteral infusion pump, B9004, B9006
    parenteral solution, B4164–B5200
    therapy, medical, G0270, G0271

O

Observation
    admission, G0379
    hospital, G0378
    LPN or RN, G0163
Occipital/mandibular support, cervical, L0160
Occult, blood, G0394
Occupational, therapy, G0129, S9129
Octafluoropropane, Q9956
Octagam, J1568
Octreotide acetate, J2353, J2354
Ocular prosthetic implant, L8610

◄ New   ← Revised   ✔ Reinstated   ~~deleted~~ Deleted

Ofatumumab, J9302
Olanzapine, J2358
Omalizumab, J2357
OnabotulinumtoxinA, J0585
Oncology
  disease status, G9063–G9139
  practice guidelines, G9056–G9062
  visit, G9050–G9055
Ondansetron **HCl,** J2405
Ondansetron **oral,** Q0162
One arm, drive attachment, K0101
Oprelvekin, J2355
O & P supply/accessory/service, L9900
Oral device/appliance, E0485–E0486
Oral/nasal mask, A7027
  nasal pillows, A7029
  oral cushion, A7028
*Oral, **NOS, drug,** J8499*
Oropharyngeal suction catheter, A4628
Orphenadrine, J2360
Orthopedic shoes
  arch support, L3040–L3100
  footwear, L3201–L3265, *L3000–L3649*
  insert, L3000–L3030
  lift, L3300–L3334
  miscellaneous additions, L3500–L3595
  positioning device, L3140–L3170
  transfer, L3600–L3649
  wedge, L3340–L3420
Orthotic additions
  carbon graphite lamination, L2755
  fracture, L2180–L2192, L3995
  halo, L0860
  lower extremity, L2200–L2999, L4320
  ratchet lock, L2430
  scoliosis, L1010–L1120, L1210–L1290
  shoe, L3300–L3595, L3649
  spinal, L0970–L0984
  upper limb, L3810–L3890, *L3900, L3901,*
    ~~L3810–L3890~~, L3995
Orthotic devices
  ankle-foot (AFO; *see also* Orthopedic shoes), E1815,
    E1816, E1830, L1900–L1990, L2102–L2116,
    L3160, L4361
  anterior-posterior-lateral, L0700, L0710
  cervical, L0100–L0200
  cervical-thoracic-lumbar-sacral (CTLSO), L0700,
    L0710
  elbow (EO), E1800, E1801, L3700–L3740
  fracture, L2102–L2136, L3980–L3986
  halo, L0810–L0830
  hand, finger, prefabricated, L3923
  hand, (WHFO), E1805, E1825, L3807,
    L3900–L3954
  hip (HO), L1600–L1690
  hip-knee-ankle-foot (HKAFO), L2040–L2090
  interface material, E1820
  knee (KO), E1810, E1811, L1800–L1885

Orthotic devices *(Continued)*
  knee-ankle-foot (KAFO; *see also* Orthopedic shoes),
    L2000–L2038, L2126–L2136
  Legg Perthes, L1700–L1755
  lumbar, L0625–L0640
  multiple post collar, L0180–L0200
  not otherwise specified, L0999, L1499, L2999,
    L3999, L5999, L7499, L8039, L8239
  pneumatic splint, L4350–L4379
  pronation/supination, E1818
  repair or replacement, L4000–L4210
  replace soft interface material, L4390–L4394
  sacroiliac, L0600–L0620
  scoliosis, L1000–L1499
  shoe, *see* Orthopedic shoes
  shoulder (SO), L1840, L3650, L3674
  shoulder-elbow-wrist-hand (SEWHO),
    L3960–L3978
  side bar disconnect, L2768
  spinal, cervical, L0100–L0200
  spinal, DME, K0112–K0116
  thoracic, L0210
  ~~thoracic-hip-knee-ankle (THKO), L1500–L1520~~
  toe, E1830
  wrist-hand-finger (WHFO), E1805, E1806, E1825,
    L3900–L3954
Orthovisc, J7324
Ossicula prosthetic implant, L8613
Osteogenesis stimulator, E0747–E0749, E0760
Osteoporosis
  documentation, G8401
Ostomy
  accessories, A5093
  belt, A4396
  pouches, A4416–A4434
  skin barrier, A4401–A4449
  supplies, A4361–A4421, A5051–A5149
*Overdoor, **traction,** E0860*
Oxacillin sodium, J2700
Oxaliplatin, J9263
Oxygen
  ambulance, A0422
  battery charger, E1357
  battery pack/cartridge, E1356
  catheter, transtracheal, A7018
  chamber, hyperbaric, topical, A4575
  concentrator, E1390–E1391
  DC power adapter, E1358
  delivery system, topical NOS, E0446
  equipment, E0424–E0486, E1353–E1406
  liquid oxygen system, E0433
  mask, A4620
  medication supplies, A4611–A4627
  rack/stand, E1355
  regulator, E1353
  respiratory equipment/supplies, A4611–A4627,
    E0424–E0480
  supplies and equipment, E0425–E0444, E0455

◄ New   ← Revised   ✔ Reinstated   ~~deleted~~ Deleted

Oxygen *(Continued)*
  tent, E0455
  tubing, A4616
  water vapor enriching system, E1405, E1406
  wheeled cart, E1354
Oxymorphone **HCl,** J2410
Oxytetracycline **HCl,** J2460
Oxytocin, J2590

P

Pacemaker **monitor,** E0610, E0615
Paclitaxel, J9265
Paclitaxel **protein-bound particles,** J9264
Pad
  correction, CTLSO, L1020–L1060
  gel pressure, E0185, E0196
  heat, *A9273,* E0210, E0215, E0217, E0238, E0249
  orthotic device interface, E1820
  sheepskin, E0188, E0189
  water circulating cold with pump, E0218
  water circulating heat with pump, E0217
  water circulating heat unit, E0249
Pail, **for use with commode chair,** E0167
Palate, **prosthetic implant,** L8618
Palifermin, J2425
Paliperidone **palmitate,** J2426
Palonosetron **HCl,** J2469
Pamidronate **disodium,** J2430
Pan, **for use with commode chair,** E0167
Panitumumab, J9303
Papanicolaou **(Pap) screening smear,** P3000, P3001, Q0091
Papaverine **HCl,** J2440
Paraffin, A4265
  bath unit, E0235
Parenteral **nutrition**
  administration kit, B4224
  pump, B9004, B9006
  solution, B4164–B5200
  supply kit, B4220, B4222
Paricalcitol, J2501
Parking **fee, nonemergency transport,** A0170
Paste, **conductive,** A4558
Pathology **and laboratory tests, miscellaneous,** P9010–P9615
Patient **support system,** E0636
Patient **transfer system,** E1035–E1036
Payment adjustment, hardship exemption, G8642, G8643
Pediculosis (lice) treatment, A9180
PEFR, **peak expiratory flow rate meter,** A4614
Pegademase **bovine,** J2504
Pegaptanib, J2503
Pegaspargase, J9266

Pegfilgrastim, J2505
Pegloticase, J2507 ◀
Pelvic
  belt/harness/boot, E0944
  traction, E0890, E0900, E0947
Pemetrexed, J9305
Penicillin
  G benzathine/G benzathine and penicillin G procaine, J0558, J0561
  G potassium, J2540
  G procaine, aqueous, J2510
Pentamidine **isethionate,** J2545, J7676
Pentastarch, **10% solution,** J2513
Pentazocine **HCl,** J3070
Pentobarbital **sodium,** J2515
Pentostatin, J9268
Percussor, E0480
Percutaneous **access system,** A4301
Perflexane **lipid microspheres,** Q9955
Perflutren **lipid microspheres,** Q9957
Peroneal **strap,** L0980
Peroxide, A4244
Perphenazine, J3310
Personal **care services,** T1019–T1021
Pessary, A4561, A4562
PET, G0219, G0235, G0252
Pharmacologic therapy, G8633
Phenobarbital **sodium,** J2560
Phentolamine **mesylate,** J2760
Phenylephrine **HCl,** J2370
Phenytoin **sodium,** J1165
Phisohex **solution,** A4246
Photofrin, *see* **Porfimer sodium**
Phototherapy **light,** E0202
Phytonadione, J3430
Pillow, **cervical,** E0943
Pinworm **examination,** Q0113
Placement
  transcatheter, stent, G0290, G0291, S2211
Plasma
  single donor, fresh frozen, P9017
  multiple donor, pooled, frozen, P9023
Plastazote, L3002, L3252, L3253, L3265, L5654–L5658
Platelet
  concentrate, each unit, P9019
  rich plasma, each unit, P9020
Platform **attachment**
  forearm crutch, E0153
  walker, E0154
Plerixafor, J2562
Plicamycin, J9270
Plumbing, **for home ESRD equipment,** A4870
Pneumatic
  appliance, E0655–E0673, L4350–L4379
  compressor, E0650–E0652
  splint, L4350–L4379
  ventricular assist device, Q0480–Q0505

◀ New   ← Revised   ✔ Reinstated   ~~deleted~~ Deleted

Pneumatic nebulizer
  administration set, small volume, filtered, A7006
  administration set, small volume, nonfiltered, A7003
  administration set, small volume, nonfiltered, non-
    disposable, A7005
  small volume, disposable, A7004
Pneumococcal
  vaccine, administration, G0009
Porfimer, J9600
Portable
  equipment transfer, R0070–R0076
  gaseous oxygen, K0741, K0742◄
  hemodialyzer system, E1635
  liquid oxygen system, E0433
  x-ray equipment, Q0092
Positioning seat, T5001
Positive airway pressure device, accessories,
  A7030–A7039, E0561–E0562
Positive expiratory pressure device, E0484
Post-coital examination, Q0115
Postural drainage board, E0606
Potassium
  chloride, J3480
  hydroxide (KOH) preparation, Q0112
Pouch
  fecal collection, A4330
  ostomy, A4375–A4378, A5051–A5054, A5061–A5065
  urinary, A4379–A4383, A5071–A5075
Pralatrexate, J9307
Practice, guidelines, oncology, G9056–G9062
Pralidoxime chloride, J2730
Prednisolone
  acetate, J2650
  oral, J7506, J7510
Prednisone, J7506
Preparation kits, dialysis, A4914
Preparatory prosthesis, L5510–L5595
  chemotherapy, J8999
  nonchemotherapy, J8499
Prescribing privilege, eligible, G8644
Pressure
  alarm, dialysis, E1540
  pad, A4640, E0180–E0199
Privigen, J1459
Procainamide HCl, J2690
Procedure
  HALO, L0810–L0861
  noncovered, G0293, G0294
  scoliosis, L1000–L1499
Prochlorperazine, J0780
Prolotherapy, M0076
Promazine HCl, J2950
Promethazine
  HCl, J2550
  and meperdine, J2180
Prophylaxis
  DVT, documentation, G8218
  thrombosis, deep, vein, documentation, G8218

Propranolol HCl, J1800
Prostate, cancer, screening, G0102, G0103
Prosthesis
  artificial larynx battery/accessory, L8505
  breast, L8000–L8035, L8600
  eye, L8610, L8611, V2623–V2629
  fitting, L5400–L5460, L6380–L6388
  foot/ankle one piece system, L5979
  hand, L6000–L6020, L6025
  implants, L8600–L8690
  larynx, L8500
  lower extremity, L5700–L5999, L8640–L8642
  mandible, L8617
  maxilla, L8616
  maxillofacial, provided by a non-physician,
    L8040–L8048
  miscellaneous service, L8499
  ocular, V2623–V2629
  repair of, L7520, L8049
  socks (shrinker, sheath, stump sock), L8400–L8485
  taxes, orthotic/prosthetic/other, L9999
  tracheo-esophageal, L8507–L8509
  upper extremity, L6000–L6999
  vacuum erection system, L7900
Prosthetic additions
  lower extremity, L5610–L5999
  upper extremity, L6600–L7405
Protamine sulfate, J2720
Protectant, skin, A6250
Protector, heel or elbow, E0191
Protein C Concentrate, J2724
Protirelin, J2725
Pulse generator, E2120
Pump
  alternating pressure pad, E0182
  ambulatory infusion, E0781
  ambulatory insulin, E0784
  blood, dialysis, E1620
  breast, E0602–E0604
  enteral infusion, B9000, B9002
  external infusion, E0779
  heparin infusion, E1520
  implantable infusion, E0782, E0783
  implantable infusion, refill kit, A4220
  infusion, supplies, A4230, A4232
  negative pressure wound therapy, E2402
  parenteral infusion, B9004, B9006
  suction, portable, E0600
  water circulating pad, E0236
  wound, negative, pressure, E2402
Purification system, E1610, E1615
Pyridoxine HCl, J3415

Q

Quad cane, E0105
Quinupristin/dalfopristin, J2770

◄ New   ← Revised   ✔ Reinstated   ~~deleted~~ Deleted

R

Rack/stand, **oxygen,** E1355
Radiesse, Q2026
Radioelements **for brachytherapy,** Q3001
Radiology **service,** R0070–R0076
Radiological, supplies, A4641, A4642
Radiopharmaceutical **diagnostic imaging**
   agent, A4641, A4642, A9500, A9532
Radiopharmaceutical, **therapeutic,** A9600, A9605
Radiosurgery, stereotactic, G0173, G0251, G0339,
   G0340
Rail
   bathtub, E0241, E0242, E0246
   bed, E0305, E0310
   toilet, E0243
Ranibizumab, J2778
Rasburicase, J2783
Reaching/grabbing **device,** A9281
Reagent **strip,** A4252
Reciprocating **peritoneal dialysis system,** E1630
Reclast, J3488
Reclining, wheelchair, E1014, E1050–E1070,
   E1100–E1110
Reconstruction, angiography, G0288
Red **blood cells,** P9021, P9022
Regadenoson, J2785
Regular **insulin,** J1820
Regulator, **oxygen,** E1353
Rehabilitation
   cardiac, S9472, S9473
   program, H2001
   psychosocial, H2017, H2018
   system, jaw, motion, E1700–E1702
   vestibular, S9476
Removal, cerumen, G0268
Renal, artery, angiography, G0275
Repair
   contract, ESRD, A4890
   maxillofacial prosthesis, L8049
   orthosis, L4000–L4130
   prosthetic, L7510
Replacement
   battery, A4630
   pad (alternating pressure), A4640
   tanks, dialysis, A4880
   tip for cane, crutches, walker, A4637
   underarm pad for crutches, A4635
Reporting, asthma measures group, G8645, G8646
RespiGam, *see* **Respiratory syncytial virus immune**
   globulin
Respiratory
   DME, A7000–A7527
   equipment, E0424–E0601
   function, therapeutic, procedure, G0237–G0239,
     S5180, S5181
   supplies, A4604–A4629

Restraint, **any type,** E0710
Reteplase, J2993
Rho(D) **immune globulin, human,** J2788, J2790,
   J2791, J2792
Rib **belt, thoracic,** A4572, L0220
Rilanocept, J2793
RimabotulinumtoxinB, J0587
Ringers **lactate infusion,** J7120
Ring, **ostomy,** A4404
Risk-adjusted functional status
   elbow, wrist or hand, G8667–G8670
   hip, G8651-G8654
   knee, G8647–G8650
   lower leg, foot or ankle, G8655–G8658
   lumbar spine, G8659–G8662
   neck, cranium, mandible, thoracic spine, ribs, or
     other, G8671–G8674
   shoulder, G8663–G8666
Risperidone, J2794
Rituximab, J9310
Robin-Aids, L6000, L6010, L6020, L6855, L6860
Rocking **bed,** E0462
Rollabout **chair,** E1031
Romidepsin, J9315
Romiplostim, J2796
Ropivacaine **HCl,** J2795
Rubidium **Rb-82,** A9555

S

Sacral **nerve stimulation test lead,** A4290
Safety **equipment,** E0700
   vest, wheelchair, E0980
Saline
   ~~hypertonic, J7130~~
   infusion, J7030–J7060
   solution, J7030–J7050, A4216–A4218
Saliva
   analysis, A0418
   artificial, A9155
Sargramostim **(GM-CSF),** J2820
Scoliosis, L1000–L1499
   additions, L1010–L1120, L1210–L1290
Screening
   cancer, cervical or vaginal, G0101
   colorectal, cancer, G0104–G0106, G0120–G0122,
     G0328, S3890
   cytopathology cervical or vaginal, G0123, G0124,
     G0141–G0148
   dysphagia, documentation, G8232, V5364
   enzyme immunoassay, G0432
   glaucoma, G0117, G0118
   infectious agent antibody detection, G0433, G0435
   language, V5363
   prostate, cancer, G0102, G0103
   speech,V5362
Sculptra, Q2027

◀ New   ← Revised   ✔ Reinstated   ~~deleted~~ Deleted

Sealant
 skin, A6250
Seat
 attachment, walker, E0156
 insert, wheelchair, E0992
 lift (patient), E0621, E0627–E0629
 upholstery, wheelchair, E0975
Secretin, J2850
Semen analysis, G0027
Semi-reclining, wheelchair, E1100, E1110
Sensitivity study, P7001
Sensory nerve conduction test, G0255
Sermorelin acetate, Q0515
Serum clotting time tube, A4771
Service
 hearing, V5000–V5999
 laboratory, P0000–P9999
 mental, health, training, G0177
 non-covered, A9270
 physician, for mobility device, G0372
 pulmonary, for LVRS, G0302–G0305
 speech-language, V5336–V5364
 vision, V2020–V2799
SEWHO, L3960–L3974
SEXA, G0130
Sheepskin pad, E0188, E0189
Shoes
 arch support, L3040–L3100
 for diabetics, A5500–A5508
 insert, L3000–L3030
 lift, L3300–L3334
 miscellaneous additions, L3500–L3595
 orthopedic, L3201–L3265
 positioning device, L3140–L3170
 transfer, L3600–L3649
 wedge, L3340–L3485
Shoulder
 disarticulation, prosthetic, L6300–L6320, L6550
 orthosis (SO), L3650–L3674
 spinal, cervical, L0100–L0200
Shoulder-elbow-wrist-hand orthosis (SEWHO),
 L3960–L3963
Shoulder sling, A4566
Shunt accessory for dialysis, A4740
 aqueous, L8612
Sigmoidoscopy, cancer screening, G0104, G0106
Sincalide, J2805
Sipuleucel-T, Q2043◀
Sirolimus, J7520
Sitz bath, E0160–E0162
Skin
 barrier, ostomy, A4362, A4363, A4369–A4373,
 A4385, A5120
 bond or cement, ostomy, A4364
 sealant, protectant, moisturizer, A6250
 substitute, Q4100–Q4140 ←
Sling, A4565
 patient lift, E0621, E0630, E0635

*Smear, **Papanicolaou, screening,** P3000, P3001,*
 Q0091
SNCT, G0255
*Social **worker, clinical, home, health,** G0155*
Social worker, nonemergency transport, A0160
Sock
 body sock, L0984
 prosthetic sock, L8420–L8435, L8470, L8480, L8485
 stump sock, L8470–L8485
Sodium
 chloride injection, J2912
 ferric gluconate complex in sucrose, J2916
 fluoride F-18, A9580
 hyaluronate
 Euflexxa, J7323
 Hyalgan, J7321
 Orthovisc, J7324
 Supartz, J7321
 Synvisc and Synvisc-One, J7325
 phosphate P32, A9563
 succinate, J1720
Solution
 calibrator, A4256
 dialysate, A4760
 elliotts b, J9175
 enteral formulae, B4149–B4156
 parenteral nutrition, B4164–B5200
*Solvent, **adhesive remover,** A4455*
Somatrem, J2940
Somatropin, J2941
Sorbent cartridge, ESRD, E1636
Special size, wheelchair, E1220–E1239
Specialty absorptive dressing, A6251–A6256
Spectinomycin HCl, J3320
Speech assessment, V5362–V5364
Speech generating device, E2500–E2599
Speech-Language, services, V5336–V5364
*Speech, **pathologist,** G0153*
Spinal orthosis
 cervical, L0100, L0200
 cervical-thoracic-lumbar-sacral (CTLSO), L0700,
 L0710
 DME, K0112–K0116
 halo, L0810–L0830
 multiple post collar, L0180–L0200
 scoliosis, L1000–L1499
 torso supports, L0960
Splint, A4570, L3100, L4350–L4379
 ankle, L4390–L4398
 dynamic, E1800, E1805, E1810, E1815, E1825,
 E1830, E1840
 footdrop, L4398
 supplies, miscellaneous, Q4051
*Standard, **wheelchair,** E1130, K0001*
Static progressive stretch, E1801, E1806, E1811,
 E1816, E1818, E1821
Status
 disease, oncology, G9063–G9139

◀ New   ← Revised   ✔ Reinstated   ~~deleted~~ **Deleted**

*Stent, **transcatheter, placement,** G0290, G0291, S2211*
Sterile cefuroxime sodium, J0697
Sterile water, A4216–A4217
*Stereotactic, **radiosurgery,** G0173, G0251, G0339, G0340*
Stimulators
  neuromuscular, E0744, E0745
  osteogenesis, electrical, E0747–E0749
  ultrasound, E0760
  salivary reflex, E0755
  stoma absorptive cover, A5083
  transcutaneous, electric, nerve, A4595, E0720–E0749
Stockings
  gradient, compression, A6530–A6549
  surgical, A4490–A4510
Stomach tube, B4083
*Stool, **guaiac,** G0394*
Streptokinase, J2995
Streptomycin, J3000
Streptozocin, J9320
Strip, blood glucose test, A4253, A4772
  urine reagent, A4250
Strontium-89 chloride, supply of, A9600
*Study, **bone density,** G0130*
Stump sock, L8470–L8485
Stylet, A4212
*Substance/Alcohol, **assessment,** G0396, G0397, H0001, H0003, H0049*
Succinylcholine chloride, J0330
Suction pump
  gastric, home model, E2000
  portable, E0600
  respiratory, home model, E0600
Sumatriptan succinate, J3030
Supartz, J7321
Supply/accessory/service, A9900
Supplies
  cast, A4580, A4590, Q4001–Q4051
  contraceptive, A4267–A4269
  dialysis, A4650–A4927
  DME, other, A4630–A4640
  enteral, therapy, B4000–B9999
  infusion, A4221, A4222, A4230–A4232, E0776–E0791
  ostomy, A4361–A4434, A5051–A5093, A5120–A5200
  parenteral, therapy, B4000–B9999
  radiological, A4641, A4642
  respiratory, A4604–A4629
  splint, Q4051
  surgical, miscellaneous, A4649
  urinary, external, A4356–A4358
Support
  arch, L3040–L3090
  cervical, L0100–L0200
  spinal, L0960
  stockings, L8100–L8239
Surgical
  arthroscopy, knee, G0289, S2112, S2113
  boot, L3208–L3211

Surgical (Continued)
  brush, dialysis, A4910
  dressing, A6196–A6406
  procedure, noncovered, G0293, G0294
  stocking, A4490–A4510
  supplies, A4649
  tray, A4550
Swabs, betadine or iodine, A4247
Syringe, A4213
  with needle, A4206–A4209
Synvisc and Synvisc-One, J7325
System
  external, ambulatory insulin, A9274
  rehabilitation, jaw, motion, E1700–E1702
  transport, E1035–E1039

T

Tables, bed, E0274, E0315
Tacrolimus
  oral, J7507
  parenteral, J7525
Tape, A4450–A4452
Taxi, non emergency transportation, A0100
*Team, **conference,** G0175, G9007, S0220, S0221*
Technetium TC 99M
  Arcitumomab, A9568
  Bicisate, A9557
  Depreotide, A9536
  Disofenin, A9510
  Exametazine, A9521
  Exametazine labeled autologous white blood cells, A9569
  Fanolesomab, A9566
  Glucepatate, A9550
  Labeled red blood cells, A9560
  Macroaggregated albumin, A9540
  Mebrofenin, A9537
  Mertiatide, A9562
  Oxidronate, A9561
  Pentetate, A9539, A9567
  Pertechnetate, A9512
  Pyrophosphate, A9538
  Sestamibi, A9500
  Succimer, A9551
  Sulfur colloid, A9541
  Teboroxime, A9501
  Tetrofosmin, A9502
TEEV, J0900
Telavancin, J3095
Telehealth, Q3014
Telehealth transmission, T1014
Televancin, J3095
Temozolomide
  injection, J9328
  oral, J8700
*Temporary **codes,** Q0000–Q9999, S0009–S9999*

◀ New   ← Revised   ✔ Reinstated   ~~deleted~~ Deleted

Temsirolimus, J9330
Tenecteplase, J3101
Teniposide, Q2017
TENS, A4595, E0720–E0749
Tent, oxygen, E0455
Terbutaline sulfate, J3105
    inhalation solution, concentrated, J7680
    inhalation solution, unit dose, J7681
Teriparatide, J3110
Terminal devices, L6700–L6895
Test
    occult, blood, G0394
    sensory, nerve, conduction, G0255
Testosterone
    aqueous, J3140
    cypionate and estradiol cypionate, J1060
    enanthate, J3120, J3130
    enanthate and estradiol valerate, J0900
    propionate, J3150
    suspension, J3140
Tetanus immune globulin, human, J1670
Tetracycline, J0120
Thallous Chloride TL 201, A9505
Theophylline, J2810
Therapeutic lightbox, A4634, E0203
Therapy
    ACE/ARB, G8468–G8475
    activity, G0176
    electromagnetic, G0295, G0329
    enteral, supplies, B4000–B9999
    medical, nutritional, G0270, G0271
    occupational, H5300, G0129, S9129
    occupational, health, G0152
    respiratory, function, procedure, G0237–G0239,
        S5180, S5181
    parenteral, supplies, B4000–B9999
    speech, home, G0153, S9128
    wound, negative, pressure, pump, E2402
Theraskin, Q4121
Thermometer, A4931–A4932
    dialysis, A4910
Thiamine HCl, J3411
Thiethylperazine maleate, J3280
Thiotepa, J9340
~~Thoracic-hip-knee-ankle (THKAO), L1500–L1520~~
Thoracic-lumbar-sacral orthosis (TLSO)
    scoliosis, L1200–L1290
    spinal, L0430–L0492
Thoracic orthosis, L0210
Thymol turbidity, blood, P2033
Thyrotropin Alfa, J3240
Tigecycline, J3243
Tinzaparin sodium, J1655
Tip (cane, crutch, walker) replacement, A4637
Tire, wheelchair, E0999
Tirofiban, J3246
Tissue marker, A4648
TLSO, L0430–L0492, L1200–L1290

Tobacco
    intervention, G9016
Tobramycin
    inhalation solution, unit dose, J7682, J7685
    sulfate, J3260
Tocilizumab, J2362
Toe device, E1831
Toilet accessories, E0167–E0179, E0243, E0244,
    E0625
Tolazoline HCl, J2670
Toll, non emergency transport, A0170
Topical hyperbaric oxygen chamber, A4575
Topotecan, J8705, J9351
Torsemide, J3265
Tositumomab, administration and supply, G3001
Tracheostoma heat moisture exchange system,
    A7501–A7509
Tracheostomy
    care kit, A4629
    filter, A4481
    speaking valve, L8501
    supplies, A4623, A4629, A7523–A7524
    tube, A7520–A7522
Tracheotomy mask or collar, A7525–A7526
Traction
    cervical, E0855, E0856
    extremity, E0870–E0880
    device, ambulatory, E0830
    equipment, E0840–E0948
    pelvic, E0890, E0900, E0947
Training
    diabetes, outpatient, G0108, G0109
    home health or hospice, G0164
    services, mental, health, G0177
Transcatheter, placement, stent, G0290, G0291, S2211
Transcutaneous electrical nerve stimulator
    (TENS), E0720–E0770
Transducer protector, dialysis, E1575
Transfer (shoe orthosis), L3600–L3640
Transfer system with seat, E1035
Transplant
    islet, G0341–G0343, S2102
Transparent film (for dressing), A6257–A6259
Transport
    chair, E1035–E1039
    system, E1035–E1039
    x-ray, R0070–R0076
Transportation
    ambulance, A0021–A0999, Q3019, Q3020
    corneal tissue, V2785
    EKG (portable), R0076
    handicapped, A0130
    non emergency, A0080–A0210, T2001–T2005
    service, including ambulance, A0021–A0999, T2006
    taxi, non emergency, A0100
    toll, non emergency, A0170
    volunteer, non emergency, A0080, A0090
    x-ray (portable), R0070, R0075

◄ New   ← Revised   ✔ Reinstated   ~~deleted~~ Deleted

Transtracheal **oxygen catheter,** A7018
Trapeze **bar,** E0910–E0912, E0940
Trauma, response, team, G0390
Tray
   insertion, A4310–A4316
   irrigation, A4320
   surgical (*see also* kits), A4550
   wheelchair, E0950
Treatment
   pediculosis (lice), A9180
   services, behavioral health, H0002–H2037
Treprostinil, J3285
Triamcinolone, J3301–J3303
   acetonide, J3300, J3301
   diacetate, J3302
   hexacetonide, J3303
   inhalation solution, concentrated, J7683
   inhalation solution, unit dose, J7684
Triflupromazine **HCl,** J3400
Trifocal, **glass or plastic,** V2300–V2399
Trimethobenzamide **HCl,** J3250
Trimetrexate **glucuoronate,** J3305
Trimming, nails, dystrophic, G0127
Triptorelin **pamoate,** J3315
Truss, L8300–L8330
Tube/Tubing
   anchoring device, A5200
   blood, A4750, A4755
   drainage extension, A4331
   gastrostomy, B4087, B4088
   irrigation, A4355
   larynectomy, A4622
   nasogastric, B4081, B4082
   oxygen, A4616
   serum clotting time, A4771
   stomach, B4083
   suction pump, each, A7002
   tire, K0091, K0093, K0095, K0097
   tracheostomy, A4622
   urinary drainage, K0280

U

Ultrasonic **nebulizer,** E0575
Ultrasound, G0389, S8055, S9024
Ultraviolet, cabinet/system, E0691–E0694
Ultraviolet **light therapy system,** A4633,
   E0691–E0694
Unclassified **drug,** J3490
Underpads, disposable, A4554
Unipuncture **control system, dialysis,** E1580
Upper **extremity addition, locking elbow,** L6693
Upper **extremity fracture orthosis,** L3980–L3999
Upper **limb prosthesis,** L6000–L7499
Urea, J3350
Ureterostomy **supplies,** A4454–A4590
Urethral **suppository, Alprostadil,** J0275

Urinal, E0325, E0326
Urinary
   catheter, A4338–A4346, A4351–A4353
   collection and retention (supplies), A4310–A4360
   incontinence, documentation, G8063, G8067
   supplies, external, A4335, A4356–A4358
   tract implant, collagen, L8603
   tract implant, synthetic, L8606
Urine
   sensitivity study, P7001
   tests, A4250
Urofollitropin, J3355
Urokinase, J3364, J3365
Ustekinumab, J3357
U-V **lens,** V2755

V

Vabra **aspirator,** A4480
Vaccination, **administration**
   hepatitis B, G0010
   influenza virus, G0008
   pneumococcal, G0009
Vaccine
   administration, influenza, G0008
   administration, pneumococcal, G0009
   hepatitis B, administration, G0010
Vaginal
   cancer, screening, G0101
   cytopathology, G0123, G0124, G0141–G0148
Vancomycin **HCl,** J3370
Vaporizer, E0605
Vascular
   catheter (appliances and supplies), A4300–A4306
   graft material, synthetic, L8670
Vasoxyl, J3390
Velaglucerase **alfa,** J3385
Venous **pressure clamp, dialysis,** A4918
Ventilator
   battery, A4611–A4613
   moisture exchanger, disposable, A4483
   negative pressure, E0460
   volume, stationary or portable, E0450,
      E0461–E0464
Ventricular **assist device,** Q0478–Q0506
Verteporfin, J3396
Vest, **safety, wheelchair,** E0980
Vinblastine **sulfate,** J9360
Vincristine **sulfate,** J9370
Vinorelbine **tartrate,** J9390
Vision **service,** V2020–V2799
Visit, emergency department, G0380–G0384
Vitamin **B-12 cyanocobalamin,** J3420
Vitamin **K,** J3430
Voice
   amplifier, L8510
   prosthesis, L8511–L8514

◄ New   ← Revised   ✔ Reinstated   ~~deleted~~ Deleted

Von **Willebrand Factor Complex, human,** J7183, J7187←
Voriconazole, J3465

W

Waiver, T2012–T2050
Walker, E0130–E0149
  accessories, A4636, A4637
  attachments, E0153–E0159
Walking splint, L4386
*Washer, **Gravlee jet,** A4470*
Water
  dextrose, J7042, J7060, J7070
  distilled (for nebulizer), A7018
  pressure pad/mattress, E0187, E0198
  purification system (ESRD), E1610, E1615
  softening system (ESRD), E1625
  sterile, A4714
WBC/CBC, G0306
Wedges, shoe, L3340–L3420
*Wellness **visit; annual,** G0438, G0439*
Wet mount, Q0111
Wheel attachment, rigid pickup walker, E0155
Wheelchair, E0950–E1298, K0001–K0108, *K0801–K0899*
  accessories, E0192, E0950–E1030, E1065–E1069, E2211–E2230, E2300–E2397
  amputee, E1170–E1200
  back, fully reclining, manual, E1226
  component or accessory, not otherwise specified, K0108
  cushions, E2601–E2625
  heavy duty, E1280–E1298, K0006, K0007, K0801–K0886
  lightweight, E1087–E1090, E1240–E1270, E2618
  narrowing device, E0969
  power add-on, E0983–E0984
  reclining, fully, E1014, E1050–E1070, E1100–E1110
  semi-reclining, E1100, E1110
  shock absorber, E1015–E1018
  specially sized, E1220, E1230
  standard, E1130, K0001
  stump support system, K0551
  tire, E0999
  transfer board or device, E0705
  tray, K0107
  van, non-emergency, A0130
  youth, E1091
WHFO with inflatable air chamber, L3807
WHO, wrist extension, L3914
Whirlpool equipment, E1300–E1310

Wig, A9282
Wipes, A4245, A4247
Wound
  cleanser, A6260
  closure, adhesive, G0168
  cover
    alginate dressing, A6196–A6198
    collagen dressing, A6020–A6024
    foam dressing, A6209–A6214
    hydrocolloid dressing, A6234–A6239
    hydrogel dressing, A6242–A6247
    non-contact wound warming cover, and accessory, E0231, E0232
    specialty absorptive dressing, A6251–A6256
  filler
    alginate dressing, A6199
    collagen based, A6010
    foam dressing, A6215
    hydrocolloid dressing, A6240, A6241
    hydrogel dressing, A6248
    not elsewhere classified, A6261, A6262
  matrix, Q4114
  pouch, A6154
  therapy, negative, pressure, pump, E2402
Wrist
  disarticulation prosthesis, L6050, L6055
  hand/finger orthosis (WHFO), E1805, E1825, L3800–L3954

X

Xenon Xe 133, A9558
Xylocaine HCl, J2000
X-ray
  equipment, portable, Q0092, R0070, R0075
  single, energy, absorptiometry (SEXA), G0130
  transport, R0070–R0076

Y

Yttrium Y-90 ibritumomab, A9543

Z

Ziconotide, J2278
Zidovudine, J3485
Ziprasidone mesylate, J3486
Zoledronic acid, J3487
Zometa, J3487

◀ New   ← Revised   ✔ Reinstated   ~~deleted~~ Deleted

2012
TABLE OF DRUGS

IA	Intra-arterial administration
IV	Intravenous administration
IM	Intramuscular administration
IT	Intrathecal
SC	Subcutaneous administration
INH	Administration by inhaled solution
VAR	Various routes of administration
OTH	Other routes of administration
ORAL	Administered orally

Intravenous administration includes all methods, such as gravity infusion, injections, and timed pushes. The "VAR" posting denotes various routes of administration and is used for drugs that are commonly administered into joints, cavities, tissues, or topical applications, in addition to other parenteral administrations. Listings posted with "OTH" indicate other administration methods, such as suppositories or catheter injections.

Blue typeface terms are added by publisher.

DRUG NAME	DOSAGE	METHOD OF ADMINISTRATION	HCPCS CODE
A			
Abatacept	10 mg		**J0129**
Abbokinase	5,000 IU vial	IV	J3364
	250,000 IU vial	IV	J3365
Abbokinase, Open Cath	5,000 IU vial	IV	J3364
Abciximab	10 mg	IV	**J0130**
Abelcet	10 mg	IV	J0287, J0288, J0289
Abilify	0.25 mg		J0400
Ablavar	1 ml		A9583
ABLC	50 mg	IV	J0285
AbobotulinumtoxintypeA	5 units		**J0586**
Acetaminophen	10 mg		**J0131** ◄
Abraxane	1 mg		J9264
Acetazolamide sodium	up to 500 mg	IM, IV	**J1120**
Acetylcysteine			◄
injection	100 mg		J0132
unit dose form	per gram	INH	**J7604, J7608**
Achromycin	up to 250 mg	IM, IV	J0120
Actemra	1 mg		J3262
ACTH	up to 40 units	IV, IM, SC	J0800
Acthar	up to 40 units	IV, IM, SC	J0800
Acthib			J3490
Acthrel	1 mcg		J0795
Actimmune	0.25 mg	SC	J1830
	3 million units	SC	J9216
Activase	1 mg	IV	J2997
Acyclovir	5 mg		**J0133**
			J8499
Adagen	25 IU		J2504
Adalimumab	20 mg		**J0135**

◄ New   ← Revised   ✔ Reinstated   ~~deleted~~ Deleted

DRUG NAME	DOSAGE	METHOD OF ADMINISTRATION	HCPCS CODE
Adenocard	6 mg	IV	J0150
	30 mg	IV	J0152
Adenoscan	30 mg	IV	J0152
Adenosine	6 mg	IV	J0150
	30 mg	IV	J0152
Adrenalin Chloride	up to 1 ml ampule	SC, IM	J0171
Adrenalin, epinephrine	0.1 mg	SC, IM	J0171
Adriamycin, PFS, RDF	10 mg	IV	J9000
Adrucil	500 mg	IV	J9190
Advate	per IU		J7192
Agalsidase beta	1 mg	IV	J0180
Aggrastat	0.25 mg	IM, IV	J3246
Aglucosidase alfa	10 mg	IV	J0220
A-hydroCort	up to 50 mg	IV, IM, SC	J1710
	up to 100 m		J1720
Akineton	per 5 mg	IM, IV	J0190
Alatrofloxacin mesylate, injection	100 mg	IV	J0200
Albuminar-5	50 ml		P9041
	250 ml		P9045
Albuminar-25	20 ml		P9046
	50 ml		P9047
Albumin-Zlb	50 ml, 5%		P9041
	250 ml, 5%		P9045
	50 ml, 25%		P9047
Albunex	250 ml		P9045
Alburx	50 ml		P9041
	250 ml		P9045
	20 ml		P9046
Albutein	20 ml		P9041
	250 ml		P9045
	20 ml		P9046
	50 ml		P9047
Albuterol	0.5 mg	INH	J7620
concentrated form	1 mg	INH	J7610, J7611
unit dose form	1 mg	INH	J7609, J7613
Aldesleukin	per single use vial	IM, IV	J9015
Aldomet	up to 250 mg	IV	J0210
Aldurazyme	0.1 mg		J1931
Alefacept	0.5 mg		J0215
Alemtuzumab	10 mg		J9010
Alferon N	250,000 IU	IM	J9215
Alglucerase	per 10 units	IV	J0205

◀ New　　← Revised　　✔ Reinstated　　~~deleted~~ Deleted

DRUG NAME	DOSAGE	METHOD OF ADMINISTRATION	HCPCS CODE	
Alglucosidase alfa	10 mg	IV	**J0220, J0221**	←
Alimta	10 mg		J9305	
Alkaban-AQ	1 mg	IV	J9360	
Alkeran	2 mg	ORAL	J8600	
	50 mg	IV	J9245	
Allopurinol Sodium			J9999	
Aloxi	25 mcg		J2469	
Alpha 1-proteinase inhibitor, human	10 mg	IV	**J0256, J0257**	←
Alphanate			**J7186**	
Alphanate	per IU		J7190, J7193, J7194	
Alprostadil				
injection	1.25 mcg	OTH injection	**J0270**	
urethral suppository	EA	OTH	**J0275**	
Alteplase recombinant	1 mg	IV	**J2997**	
Alupent	per 10 mg	INH	**J7667, J7668**	
noncompounded, unit dose	10 mg	INH	J7669	
AmBisome	10 mg	IV	J0289	
Amcort	per 5 mg	IM	J3302	
A-methaPred	up to 40 mg	IM, IV	J2920	
	up to 125 mg	IM, IV	J2930	
Amevive	0.5 mg		J0215	
Amgen	1 mcg	SC	J9212	
Amifostine	500 mg	IV	**J0207**	
Amikin	100 mg	IM, IV	J0278	
Amikacin sulfate	100 mg	IM, IV	**J0278**	
Aminocaproic Acid			J3490	
Aminolevalinic acid HCl	unit dose (354 mg)	OTH	**J7308**	
Aminolevulinate	1 gm	OTH	**J7309**	
Amiodarone HCl	30 mg	IV	**J0282**	
Amitriptyline HCl	up to 20 mg	IM	**J1320**	
Amobarbital	up to 125 mg	IM, IV	**J0300**	
Amphadase	up to 150 units		J3470	
Amphocin	50 mg	IV	J0285	
Amphotec	10 mg	IV	J0288	
Amphotericin B	50 mg	IV	**J0285**	
Amphotericin B, lipid complex	10 mg	IV	**J0287–J0289**	
Ampicillin				
sodium	up to 500 mg	IM, IV	**J0290**	
sodium/sulbactam sodium	per 1.5 gm	IM, IV	**J0295**	
Amygdalin			J3570	

◄ New   ← Revised   ✔ Reinstated   ~~deleted~~ Deleted

DRUG NAME	DOSAGE	METHOD OF ADMINISTRATION	HCPCS CODE
Amytal	up to 125 mg	IM, IV	J0300
Anabolin LA 100	up to 50 mg	IM	J2320
Anadulafungin	1 mg	IV	J0348
Ancef	500 mg	IV, IM	J0690
Andrest 90-4	up to 1 cc	IM	J0900
Andro-Cyp	up to 100 mg	IM	J1070
	1 cc, 200 mg	IM	J1080
Andro-Cyp 200	up to 100 mg	IM	J1070
	1 cc, 200 mg	IM	J1080
Andro L.A. 200	up to 100 mg	IM	J3120
	up to 200 mg	IM	J3130
Andro-Estro 90-4	up to 1 cc	IM	J0900
Andro/Fem	up to 1 ml	IM	J1060
Androgyn L.A	up to 1 cc	IM	J0900
Androlone-50	up to 50 mg		J2320
Androlone-D 100	up to 50 mg	IM	J2320
Andronaq-50	up to 50 mg	IM	J3140
Andronaq-LA	up to 100 mg	IM	J1070
	1 cc, 200 mg	IM	J1080
Andronate-200	up to 100 mg	IM	J1070
	1 cc, 200 mg	IM	J1080
Andronate-100	up to 100 mg	IM	J1070
	1 cc, 200 mg	IM	J1080
Andropository 100	up to 100 mg	IM	J3120
	up to 200 mg	IM	J3130
Andryl 200	up to 100 mg	IM	J3120
	up to 200 mg	IM	J3130
Anectine	up to 20 mg	IM, IV	J0330
Anergan 25	up to 50 mg	IM, IV	J2550
	12.5 mg	ORAL	Q0169
	25 mg	ORAL	Q0170
Anergan 50	up to 50 mg	IM, IV	J2550
	12.5 mg	ORAL	Q0169
	25 mg	ORAL	Q0170
Angiomax	1 mg		J0583
Anistreplase	30 units	IV	J0350
Antiflex	up to 60 mg		J2360
Anti-Inhibitor	per IU	IV	J7198
Antispas	up to 20 mg	IM	J0500
Antithrombin III (human)	per IU	IV	J7197
Antithrombin recombinant	50 IU		J7196
Antizol	15 mg		J1451

◀ New   ← Revised   ✔ Reinstated   ~~deleted~~ Deleted

DRUG NAME	DOSAGE	METHOD OF ADMINISTRATION	HCPCS CODE
Anzemet	10 mg	IV	J1260
	50 mg	ORAL	S0174
	100 mg	ORAL	Q0180
Apidra	per 50 units		J1817
	per 5 units		J1815
A.P.L.	per 1,000 USP units	IM	J0725
Apokyn	1 mg		J0364
Apomorphine Hydrochloride	1 mg		J0364
Apresoline	up to 20 mg	IV, IM	J0360
Aprotinin	10,000 kiu		J0365
AquaMEPHYTON	per 1 mg	IM, SC, IV	J3430
Aralast	10 mg	IV	J0256
Aralen	up to 250 mg	IM	J0390
Aramine	per 10 mg	IV, IM, SC	J0380
Aranesp			
ESRD use	1 mcg		J0882
Non-ESRD use	1 mcg		J0881
Arbutamine	1 mg	IV	J0395
Arcalyst	1 mg		J2793
Aredia	per 30 mg	IV	J2430
Arfonad, see Trimethaphan camsylate			
Arformoterol tartrate	15 mcg		J7605
Aridol	25% in 50 ml	IV	J2150
	5 mg	INH	J7665
Arimidex			J8999
Aripiprazole	0.25 mg		J0400
Aristocort Forte	per 5 mg	IM	J3302
Aristocort Intralesional	per 5 mg	IM	J3302
Aristopan	per 5 mg		J3303
Aristospan Intra-Articular	per 5 mg	VAR	J3303
Aristospan Intralesional	per 5 mg	VAR	J3303
Arixtra	per 0.5 m		J1652
Aromasin			J8999
Arranon	50 mg		J9261
Arrestin	up to 200 mg	IM	J3250
	250 mg	ORAL	Q0173
Arsenic trioxide	1 mg	IV	J9017
Arzerra	10 mg		J9302
Asparaginase	10,000 units	IV, IM	J9020
Astramorph PF	up to 10 mg	IM, IV, SC	J2270
	100 mg	IM, IV, SC	J2271
Atgam	250 mg	IV	J7504

◀ New   ← Revised   ✔ Reinstated   ~~deleted~~ Deleted

DRUG NAME	DOSAGE	METHOD OF ADMINISTRATION	HCPCS CODE
Ativan	2 mg	IM, IV	J2060
Atropine			
concentrated form	per mg	INH	J7635
unit dose form	per mg	INH	J7636
sulfate	0.01 mg, per mg	IV, IM, SC	J0461, J7636
Atrovent	per mg	INH	J7644, J7645
Atryn	50 IU		J7196
Aurothioglucose	up to 50 mg	IM	J2910
Autologous cultured chondrocytes implant			J7330
Autoplex T	per IU	IV	J7198, J7199
Avastin	10 mg		J9035
Avelox	100 mg		J2280
Avonex	11 mcg	IM	Q3025
	11 mcg	SC	Q3026
	33 mcg	IM	J1826
Azacitidine	1 mg		J9025
Azasan	50 mg		J7500
Azathioprine	50 mg	ORAL	J7500
Azathioprine			
parenteral	100 mg	IV	J7501
dihydrate	1 gm	ORAL	Q0144
injection	500 mg	IV	J0456
Azithromycin Bihydrate	500 mg		J0456
B			
Baci-RX			J3490
Baciim			J3490
Bacitracin			J3490
Baclofen	10 mg	IT	J0475
Baclofen for intrathecal trial	50 mcg	OTH	J0476
Bacteriostatic	10 ml		A4216
Bactocill	up to 250 mg	IM, IV	J2700
BAL in oil	per 100 mg	IM	J0470
Banflex	up to 60 mg	IV, IM	J2360
Basiliximab	20 mg	IV	J0480
Bayhep B			J3590
BayRho-D	50 mcg		J2788
BCG (Bacillus Calmette and Guérin), live	per vial	IV	J9031
Bebulin VH	per IU		J7194
Beclomethasone inhalation solution, unit dose form	per mg	INH	J7622, J7624
Belimumab	10 mg		J0490
Bena-D 10	up to 50 mg	IV, IM	J1200
Bena-D 50	up to 50 mg	IV, IM	J1200

◄ New   ← Revised   ✔ Reinstated   ~~deleted~~ Deleted

DRUG NAME	DOSAGE	METHOD OF ADMINISTRATION	HCPCS CODE
Benadryl	up to 50 mg	IV, IM	J1200
Benahist 10	up to 50 mg	IV, IM	J1200
Benahist 50	up to 50 mg	IV, IM	J1200
Ben-Allergin-50	up to 50 mg	IV, IM	J1200
	50 mg	ORAL	Q0163
Bendamustine HCl	1 mg		J9033
Benefix	per IU	IV	J7195
Benlysta	10 mg		J0490
Benoject-10	up to 50 mg	IV, IM	J1200
Benoject-50	up to 50 mg	IV, IM	J1200
Bentyl	up to 20 mg	IM	J0500
Benzacot	up to 200 mg		J3250
Benzocaine			J3490
Benztropine mesylate	per 1 mg	IM, IV	J0515
Berinert, see C-1 esterase inhibitor			
Berubigen	up to 1,000 mcg	IM, SC	J3420
Betalin 12	up to 1,000 mcg	IM, SC	J3420
Betameth	per 4 mg	IM, IV	J0702
Betamethasone acetate & betamethasone sodium phosphate	per 3 mg	IM	J0702
Betamethasone inhalation solution, unit dose form	per mg	INH	J7624
Betaseron	0.25 mg	SC	J1830
Bethanechol chloride	up to 5 mg	SC	J0520
Bevacizumab	10 mg		J9035
Bicillin C-R	100,000 units		J0558
Bicillin C-R 900/300	100,000 units	IM	J0558, J0561
Bicillin L-A	100,000 units	IM	J0561
BiCNU	100 mg	IV	J9050
Biperiden lactate	per 5 mg	IM, IV	J0190
Bitolterol mesylate			
concentrated form	per mg	INH	J7628
unit dose form	per mg	INH	J7629
Bivalirudin	1 mg		J0583
Blenoxane	15 units	IM, IV, SC	J9040
Bleomycin sulfate	15 units	IM, IV, SC	J9040
Boniva	1 mg		J1740
Bortezomib	0.1 mg		J9041
Botox	1 unit		J0585
Bravelle	75 IU		J3355
Brethine			
concentrated form	per 1 mg	INH	J7680
unit dose	per 1 mg	INH	J7681
	up to 1 mg	SC, IV	J3105

◄ New   ← Revised   ✔ Reinstated   ~~deleted~~ Deleted

DRUG NAME	DOSAGE	METHOD OF ADMINISTRATION	HCPCS CODE
Brevital Sodium			J3490
Bricanyl Subcutaneous	up to 1 mg	SC, IV	J3105
Brompheniramine maleate	per 10 mg	IM, SC, IV	**J0945**
Broncho Saline	10 ml		A4216
Bronkephrine, see Ethylnorepinephrine HCl			
Bronkosol			
concentrated form	per mg	INH	J7647, J7648
unit dose form	per mg	INH	J7649, J7650
Brovana			J7605, J7699
Budesonide inhalation solution			
concentrated form	0.25 mg	INH	**J7633, J7634**
unit dose form	0.5 mg	INH	**J7626, J7627**
Bumetanide			J3490
Buminate	50 ml		P9041
	250 ml		P9045
	20 ml		P9046
	50 ml		P9047
Bupivacaine			J3490
Buprenex	0.1 mg		J0592
Buprenorphine Hydrochloride	0.1 mg		**J0592, J3490**
Busulfan	1 mg		**J0594**
	2 mg	ORAL	**J8510**
Butorphanol tartrate	1 mg		**J0595**
C			
C1 Esterase Inhibitor	10 units		**J0597, J0598**
Cabazitaxel	1 mg		**J9043** ◄
Cabergoline	0.25 mg	ORAL	J8515
Cafcit	5 mg	IV	J0706
Caffeine citrate	5 mg	IV	**J0706**
Caine-1	10 mg	IV	J2001
Caine-2	10 mg	IV	J2001
Calcijex	0.1 mcg	IM	J0636
Calcimar	up to 400 units	SC, IM	J0630
Calcitonin-salmon	up to 400 units	SC, IM	**J0630**
Calcitriol	0.1 mcg	IM	J0636
Calcitriol in almond oil	0.1 mcg		J0636
Calcium Disodium Versenate	up to 1,000 mg	IV, SC, IM	J0600
Calcium gluconate	per 10 ml	IV	**J0610**
Calcium glycerophosphate and calcium lactate	per 10 ml	IM, SC	**J0620**
Calcium glycerophosphate and calcium lactate	10 ml	IM, SC	J0620
Calphosan	per 10 ml	IM, SC	J0620
Campath	10 mg		J9010

◄ New   ← Revised   ✔ Reinstated   ~~deleted~~ Deleted

DRUG NAME	DOSAGE	METHOD OF ADMINISTRATION	HCPCS CODE
Camptosar	20 mg	IV	J9206
Canakinumab	1 mg		J0638
Cancidas	5 mg		J0637
Capecitabine	150 mg	ORAL	J8520
	500 mg	ORAL	J8521
Capsaicin patch	per 10 sq cm	OTH	J7335
Carbocaine with Neo-Cobefrin	per 10 ml	VAR	J0670
Carbocaine	per 10 ml	VAR	J0670
Carboplatin	50 mg	IV	J9045
Carimune	500 mg		J1566
Carmustine	100 mg	IV	J9050
Carnitor	per 1 g	IV	J1955
Carticel			J7330
Caspofungin acetate	5 mg	IV	J0637
Cathflo Activase	1 mg		J2997
Caverject injection	1.25 mcg		J0270
Cayston, see Aztreonam			
Ceenu		ORAL	J8799
Cefadyl	up to 1 g	IV, IM	J0710
Cefazolin sodium	500 mg	IV, IM	J0690
Cefepime hydrochloride	500 mg	IV	J0692
Cefizox	per 500 mg	IM, IV	J0715
Cefotan			J3490
Cefotaxime sodium	per 1 g	IV, IM	J0698
Cefotetan			J3490
Cefoxitin sodium	1 g	IV, IM	J0694
Ceftaroline fosamil	1 mg		J0712
Ceftazidime	per 500 mg	IM, IV	J0713
Ceftizoxime sodium	per 500 mg	IV, IM	J0715
	per 250 mg	IV, IM	J0696
Cefuroxime sodium, sterile	per 750 mg	IM, IV	J0697
Celestone Soluspan	per 3 mg	IM	J0702
	per mg	ORAL	J7624
CellCept	250 mg	ORAL	J7517
Cel-U-Jec	per 4 mg	IM, IV	Q0511
Cenacort A-40	per 10 mg	IM	J3301
	per 5 mg		J3302
Cenacort Forte	per 5 mg	IM	J3302
Cephalothin sodium	up to 1 g	IM, IV	J1890
Cephapirin sodium	up to 1 g	IV, IM	J0710
Cerebyx	50 mg		Q2009
Ceredase	per 10 units	IV	J0205

◀ New   ← Revised   ✔ Reinstated   ~~deleted~~ Deleted

DRUG NAME	DOSAGE	METHOD OF ADMINISTRATION	HCPCS CODE
Cerezyme	10 units		J1786
Certolizumab pegol	1 mg		J0718
Cerubidine	10 mg	IV	J9150
Cetuximab	10 mg		J9055
Chealamide	per 150 mg	IV	J3520
Chloramphenicol sodium succinate	up to 1 g	IV	J0720
Chlordiazepoxide HCl	up to 100 mg	IM, IV	J1990
Chloromycetin Sodium Succinate	up to 1 g	IV	J0720
Chloroprocaine HCl	per 30 ml	VAR	J2400
	10 mg	ORAL	Q0171
	25 mg	ORAL	Q0172
	up to 50 mg	IM, IV	J3230
Chloroquine HCl	up to 250 mg	IM	J0390
Chlorothiazide sodium	per 500 mg	IV	J1205
Chlorpromazine HCl	up to 50 mg	IM, IV	J3230
Cholografin Meglumine	per ml		Q9961
Chorex-5	per 1,000 USP units	IM	J0725
Chorex-10	per 1,000 USP units	IM	J0725
Chorignon	per 1,000 USP units	IM	J0725
Chorionic gonadotropin	per 1,000 USP units	IM	J0725
Choron 10	per 1,000 USP units	IM	J0725
Cidofovir	375 mg	IV	J0740
Cimzia	1 mg		J0718
Cinryze	10 units		J0598
Cilastatin sodium, imipenem	per 250 mg	IV, IM	J0743
Cimetidine HCl			J3490
Cipro IV	200 mg	IV	J0706
Ciprofloxacin	200 mg	IV	J0706
			J3490
Cisplatin, powder or solution	per 10 mg	IV	J9060
Cladribine	per mg	IV	J9065
Claforan	per 1 gm	IM, IV	J0698
Cleocin Phosphate			J3490
Clincacort	per 5 mg		J3302
Clofarabine	1 mg		J9027
Clolar	1 mg		J9027
Clonidine Hydrochloride	1 mg	epidural	J0735
Cobal-1000	up to 1,000 mcg		J3420
Cobex	up to 1,000 mcg	IM, SC	J3420
Cobulin-M	up to 1,000 mcg		J3420
Codeine phosphate	per 30 mg	IM, IV, SC	J0745
Codimal-A	per 10 mg	IM, SC, IV	J0945

◄ New   ← Revised   ✔ Reinstated   ~~deleted~~ Deleted

DRUG NAME	DOSAGE	METHOD OF ADMINISTRATION	HCPCS CODE
Cogentin	per 1 mg	IM, IV	J0515
Colchicine	per 1 mg	IV	J0760
Colistimethate sodium	up to 150 mg	IM, IV	J0770, S0142
Collagenase, Clostridium Histolyticum	0.01 mg		J0775
Coly-Mycin M	up to 150 mg	IM, IV	J0770
Compa-Z	up to 10 mg	IM, IV	J0780
Compazine	up to 10 mg	IM, IV	J0780, J8498
	5 mg	ORAL	Q0164
	10 mg	ORAL	Q0165
Compro			J8498
Comptosar	20 mg		J9206
Conray	per ml		Q9961
Conray 30	per ml		Q9958
Conray 43	per ml		Q9960
Copaxone	20 mg		J1595
Cophene-B	per 10 mg	IM, SC, IV	J0945
Copper contraceptive, intrauterine		OTH	J7300
Cordarone	30 mg	IV	J0282
Corgonject-5	per 1,000 USP units	IM	J0725
Corticorelin ovine triflutate	1 mcg		J0795
Corticotropin	up to 40 units	IV, IM, SC	J0800
Cortisone Acetate			J3490
Cortrosyn	per 0.25 mg	IM, IV	J0835
Corvert	1 mg		J1742
Cosmegen	0.5 mg	IV	J9120
Cosyntropin	per 0.25 mg	IM, IV	J0833, J0834
Cotolone	up to 1 ml		J2650
	per 5 mg		J7510
Cotranzine	up to 10 mg	IM, IV	J0780
Crofab	up to 1 gram		J0840 ◄
Cromolyn sodium, unit dose form	per 10 mg	INH	J7631, J7632
Crotalidae Polyvalent Immune Fab	up to 1 gram		J0840 ◄
Crystal B-12	up to 1,000 mcg		J3420
Crysticillin 300 A.S.	up to 600,000 units	IM, IV	J2510
Crysticillin 600 A.S.	up to 600,000 units	IM, IV	J2510
Cubicin	1 mg		J0878
Cyano	up to 1,000 mcg		J3420
Cyanocobalamin	up to 1,000 mcg		J3420
Cyclophosphamide	100 mg	IV	J9070
oral	25 mg	ORAL	J8530
Cyclosporin A	250 mg		J7516

◄ New   ← Revised   ✔ Reinstated   ~~deleted~~ Deleted

DRUG NAME	DOSAGE	METHOD OF ADMINISTRATION	HCPCS CODE
Cyclosporine	25 mg	ORAL	J7515
	100 mg	ORAL	J7502
parenteral	250 mg	IV	J7516
Cymetra	1 cc		Q4112
Cyomin	up to 1,000 mcg		J3420
Cysto-Cornray LI	per ml		Q9958
Cystografin	per ml		Q9958
Cystografin-Dilute	per ml		Q9958
Cytarabine	100 mg	SC, IV	J9100
Cytarabine liposome	10 mg		J9098
CytoGam	per vial		J0850
Cytomegalovirus immune globulin intravenous (human)	per vial	IV	J0850
Cytosar-U	100 mg	SC, IV	J9100
Cytovene	500 mg	IV	J1570
Cytoxan	100 mg	IV	J9070
D			
D-5-W, infusion	1000 cc	IV	J7070
Dacarbazine	100 mg	IV	J9130
Daclizumab	25 mg	IV	J7513
Dactinomycin	0.5 mg	IV	J9120
Dalalone	1 mg	IM, IV, OTH	J1100
Dalalone L.A	1 mg	IM	J1094
Dalteparin sodium	per 2500 IU	SC	J1645
Daptomycin	1 mg		J0878
Darbepoetin Alfa	1 mcg		J0881, J0882
Daunorubicin citrate, liposomal formulation	10 mg	IV	J9151
Daunorubicin HCl	10 mg	IV	J9150
Daunoxome	10 mg	IV	J9151
DDAVP	1 mcg	IV, SC	J2597
Debioclip Kit	3.75 mg		J3310
Decadron Phosphate	1 mg	IM, IV, OTH	J1100
Decadron	1 mg	IM, IV, OTH	J1100
	0.25 mg		J8540
Decadron-LA	1 mg	IM	J1094
Deca-Durabolin	up to 50 mg	IM	J2320
Decaject	1 mg	IM, IV, OTH	J1100
Decaject-L.A.	1 mg	IM	J1094
Decitabine	1 mg		J0894
Decolone-50	up to 50 mg	IM	J2320
Decolone-100	up to 50 mg	IM	J2320
De-Comberol	up to 1 ml	IM	J1060
Decongest	per 10 mg		Q0163

◀ New   ← Revised   ✔ Reinstated   ~~deleted~~ Deleted

DRUG NAME	DOSAGE	METHOD OF ADMINISTRATION	HCPCS CODE
Deferoxamine mesylate	500 mg	IM, SC, IV	**J0895**
Definity	per ml		J3490, Q9957
Degarelix	1 mg		**J9155**
Dehist	per 10 mg	IM, SC, IV	J0945
Deladumone OB	up to 1 cc	IM	J0900
Deladumone	up to 1 cc	IM	J0900
Delatest	up to 100 mg	IM	J3120
	up to 200 mg	IM	J3130
Delatestadiol	up to 1 cc	IM	J0900
Delatestryl	up to 100 mg	IM	J3120
	up to 200 mg	IM	J3130
Delta-Cortef	5 mg	ORAL	J7510
Deltasone	5 mg		J7506
Delestrogen	up to 10 mg	IM	J1380
Demadex	10 mg/ml	IV	J3265
Demerol HCl	per 100 mg	IM, IV, SC	J2175
Denileukin diftitox	300 mcg		**J9160**
Denosumab	1 mg		**J0897**
DepAndro 100	up to 100 mg	IM	J1070
	1 cc, 200 mg	IM	J1080
	up to 100 mg		J3150
DepAndro 200	up to 100 mg	IM	J1070
	1 cc, 200 mg	IM	J1080
DepAndrogyn	up to 1 ml	IM	J1060
DepGynogen	up to 5 mg	IM	J1000
DepoCyt	10 mg		J9098
DepMedalone 40	20 mg	IM	J1020
	40 mg	IM	J1030
	80 mg	IM	J1040
DepMedalone 80	20 mg	IM	J1020
	40 mg	IM	J1030
	80 mg	IM	J1040
Depo-estradiol cypionate	up to 5 mg	IM	**J1000**
Depogen	up to 5 mg	IM	J1000
Depoject	20 mg	IM	J1020
	40 mg	IM	J1030
	80 mg	IM	J1040
Depo-Medrol	20 mg	IM	J1020
	40 mg	IM	J1030
	80 mg	IM	J1040

◄ New   ← Revised   ✔ Reinstated   -deleted- Deleted

DRUG NAME	DOSAGE	METHOD OF ADMINISTRATION	HCPCS CODE
Depopred-40	20 mg	IM	J1020
	40 mg	IM	J1030
	80 mg	IM	J1040
Depopred-80	20 mg	IM	J1020
	40 mg	IM	J1030
	80 mg	IM	J1040
Depo-Provera	50 mg	IM	J1051
	150 mg	IM	J1055
Depotest	up to 100 mg	IM	J1070
	1 cc, 200 mg	IM	J1080
Depo-Testadiol	up to 1 ml	IM	J1060
Depotestrogen	up to 1 ml	IM	J1060
Depo-Testosterone	1 cc, 200 mg	IM	J1080
	up to 100 mg	IM	J1070, J3120
Dermagraft	per square centimeter		Q4106
Desferal Mesylate	500 mg	IM, SC, IV	J0895
Desmopressin acetate	1 mcg	IV, SC	J2597
Dexacen LA-8	1 mg	IM	J1094
Dexacen-4	1 mg	IM, IV, OTH	J1100
Dexamethasone			
concentrated form	per mg	INH	J7637
intravitreal implant	0.1 mg	OTH	J7312
unit form	per mg	INH	J7638
oral	0.25 mg	ORAL	J8540
	1 mg		J1100
Dexamethasone acetate	1 mg	IM	J1094
Dexamethasone sodium phosphate	1 mg	IM, IV, OTH	J1100, J7638
Dexasone	1 mg	IM, IV, OTH	J1100
Dexasone L.A.	1 mg	IM	J1094
Dexferrum	50 mg		J1750
Dexone	0.25 mg	ORAL	J8540
	1 mg	IM, IV, OTH	J1100
Dexone LA	1 mg	IM	J1094
Dexpak	0.25 mg	ORAL	J8540
Dexrazoxane hydrochloride	250 mg	IV	J1190
Dextran 40	500 ml	IV	J7100
Dextran 70	500 ml		J7110
Dextran 75	500 ml	IV	J7110
Dextrose 5%/normal saline solution	500 ml = 1 unit	IV	J7042
Dextrose/water (5%)	500 ml = 1 unit	IV	J7060
D.H.E. 45	per 1 mg		J1110
Diamox	up to 500 mg	IM, IV	J1120

◀ New   ← Revised   ✔ Reinstated   ~~deleted~~ Deleted

DRUG NAME	DOSAGE	METHOD OF ADMINISTRATION	HCPCS CODE
Diazepam	up to 5 mg	IM, IV	J3360
Diazoxide	up to 300 mg	IV	J1730
Dibent	up to 20 mg	IM	J0500
Dicyclocot	up to 20 mg		J0500
Dicyclomine HCl	up to 20 mg	IM	J0500
Didronel	per 300 mg	IV	J1436
Diethylstilbestrol diphosphate	250 mg	IV	J9165
Diflucan	200 mg	IV	J1450
Digibind	per vial		J1162
DigiFab	per vial		J1162
Digoxin	up to 0.5 mg	IM, IV	J1160
Digoxin immune fab (ovine)	per vial		J1162
Dihydrex	up to 50 mg	IV, IM	J1200
	50 mg	ORAL	Q0163
Dihydroergotamine mesylate	per 1 mg	IM, IV	J1110
Dilantin	per 50 mg	IM, IV	J1165
Dilaudid	up to 4 mg	SC, IM, IV	J1170
	250 mg	OTH	S0092
Dilocaine	10 mg	IV	J2001
Dilomine	up to 20 mg	IM	J0500
Dilor	up to 500 mg	IM	J1180
Dimenhydrinate	up to 50 mg	IM, IV	J1240
Dimercaprol	per 100 mg	IM	J0470
Dimethyl sulfoxide	50%, 50 ml	OTH	J1212
Dinate	up to 50 mg	IM, IV	J1240
Dioval	up to 10 mg	IM	J1380
Dioval 40	up to 10 mg	IM	J1380
Dioval XX	up to 10 mg	IM	J1380
Diphenacen-50	up to 50 mg	IV, IM	J1200
	50 mg	ORAL	Q0163
Diphenhydramine HCl			
injection	up to 50 mg	IV, IM	J1200
oral	50 mg	ORAL	Q0163
Diprivan			J3490
Dipyridamole	per 10 mg	IV	J1245
Disotate	per 150 mg	IV	J3520
Di-Spaz	up to 20 mg	IM	J0500
Ditate-DS	up to 1 cc	IM	J0900
Diuril	per 500 mg	IV	J1205
Diuril Sodium	per 500 mg	IV	J1205
Dizac	up to 5 mg		J3360

◀ New　　← Revised　　✔ Reinstated　　~~deleted~~ Deleted

DRUG NAME	DOSAGE	METHOD OF ADMINISTRATION	HCPCS CODE
D-Med 80	20 mg	IM	J1020
	40 mg	IM	J1030
	80 mg	IM	J1040
DMSO, Dimethyl sulfoxide 50%	50 ml	OTH	J1212
Dobutamine HCl	per 250 mg	IV	J1250
Dobutrex	per 250 mg	IV	J1250
Docetaxel	20 mg	IV	J9170
Dolasetron mesylate			
injection	10 mg	IV	J1260
tablets	100 mg	ORAL	Q0180
Dolophine HCl	up to 10 mg	IM, SC	J1230
Dommanate	up to 50 mg	IM, IV	J1240
Donbax	10 mg		J1267
Dopamine	40 mg		J1265
Dopamine in D5W	40 mg		J1265
Dopamine HCl	40 mg		J1265
Doribax	10 mg		J1267
Doripenem	10 mg		J1267
Dornase alpha, unit dose form	per mg	INH	J7639
Doxercalciferol	1 mcg	IV	J1270
Doxil	10 mg	IV	J9001
Doxorubicin			
HCl	10 mg	IV	J9000
HCl, all lipid	10 mg	IV	J9001
Dramamine	up to 50 mg	IM, IV	J1240
Dramanate	up to 50 mg	IM, IV	J1240
Dramilin	up to 50 mg	IM, IV	J1240
Dramocen	up to 50 mg	IM, IV	J1240
Dramoject	up to 50 mg	IM, IV	J1240
Dronabinol	2.5 mg	ORAL	Q0167
	5 mg	ORAL	Q0168
Droperidol	up to 5 mg	IM, IV	J1790
Droxia		ORAL	J8799
Drug administered through a metered dose inhaler		INH	J3535
Droperidol and fentanyl citrate	up to 2 ml ampule	IM, IV	J1810
DTIC-Dome	100 mg	IV	J9130
Dua-Gen L.A.	up to 1 cc		J0900
DuoNeb	up to 2.5 mg		J7620
	up to 0.5 mg		J7620
Duoval P.A.	up to 1 cc	IM	J0900
Durabolin, see Nandrolone phenpropionate			
Duraclon	1 mg	epidural	J0735

◀ New   ← Revised   ✔ Reinstated   ~~deleted~~ Deleted

DRUG NAME	DOSAGE	METHOD OF ADMINISTRATION	HCPCS CODE
Dura-Estrin	up to 5 mg	IM	J1000
Duracillin A.S.	up to 600,000 units	IM, IV	J2510
Duragen-10	up to 10 mg	IM	J1380
Duragen-20	up to 10 mg	IM	J1380
Duragen-40	up to 10 mg	IM	J1380
Duralone-40	20 mg	IM	J1020
	40 mg	IM	J1030
	80 mg	IM	J1040
Duralone-80	20 mg	IM	J1020
	40 mg	IM	J1030
	80 mg	IM	J1040
Duralutin, see Hydroxyprogesterone Caproate			
Duramorph	10 mg	IM, IV, SC	J2271
	up to 10 mg	IM, IV, SC	J2270
	500 mg	OTH	S0093
Duratest-100	up to 100 mg	IM	J1070
	1 cc, 200 mg	IM	J1080
Duratest-200	up to 100 mg	IM	J1070
	1 cc, 200 mg	IM	J1080
Duratestrin	up to 1 ml	IM	J1060
Durathate-200	up to 100 mg	IM	J3120
	up to 200 mg	IM	J3130
Dymenate	up to 50 mg	IM, IV	J1240
Dyphylline	up to 500 mg	IM	J1180
Dysport	5 units		J0586
E			
Ecallantide	1 mg		J1290
Eculizumab	10 mg		J1300
Edetate calcium disodium	up to 1,000 mg	IV, SC, IM	J0600
Edetate disodium	per 150 mg	IV	J3520
Edex	per 1.25 millicurie		J0270
Edisylate	up to 10 mg		J0780
Elaprase	1 mg		J1743
Elavil	up to 20 mg	IM	J1320
Elitek	0.5 mg		J2783
Ellence	2 mg		J9178
Elliotts b solution	1 ml	OTH	J9175
Eloxatin	0.5 mg		J9263
Elspar	10,000 units	IV, IM	J9020
Emend	1 mg		J1453
Ememd	5 mg	ORAL	J8501
Emete-Con, see Benzquinamide			

◀ New   ← Revised   ✔ Reinstated   ~~deleted~~ Deleted

DRUG NAME	DOSAGE	METHOD OF ADMINISTRATION	HCPCS CODE
Eminase	30 units	IV	J0350
Enbrel	25 mg	IM, IV	J1438
Endrate ethylenediamine-tetra-acetic acid	per 150 mg	IV	J3520
Enfuvirtide	1 mg		J1324
Enovil	up to 20 mg	IM	J1320
Enoxaparin sodium	10 mg	SC	J1650
Eovist	1 ml		A9581
Epinephrine, adrenalin	0.1 mg	SC, IM	J0171
Epirubicin hydrochloride	2 mg		J9178, J7799
Epoetin alfa	1,000 units		Q4081
Epogen	1,000 units		J0885
			J0886
			Q4081
Epoprostenol	0.5 mg	IV	J1325
Eptifibatide, injection	5 mg	IM, IV	J1327
Eraxis	1 mg	IV	J0348
Erbitux	10 mg		J9055
Ergonovine maleate	up to 0.2 mg	IM, IV	J1330
Eribulin mesylate	0.1 mg		J9179
Ertapenem sodium	500 mg		J1335
Erthrocin	500 mg		J1364
Erythromycin lactobionate	500 mg	IV	J1364
Estra-D	up to 5 mg	IM	J1000
Estra-L 20	up to 10 mg	IM	J1380
	up to 40 mg	IM	J1370
Estra-L 40	up to 10 mg	IM	J1380
	up to 40 mg	IM	J1370
Estra-Testrin	up to 1 cc	IM	J0900
Estradiol Cypionate	up to 5 mg	IM	J1000, J1056, J1060
Estradiol			
L.A.	up to 10 mg	IM	J1380
	up to 40 mg	IM	J1370
L.A. 20	up to 10 mg	IM	J1380
	up to 40 mg	IM	J1370
L.A. 40	up to 10 mg	IM	J1380
	up to 40 mg	IM	J1370
Estradiol valerate	up to 10 mg	IM	J1380
Estragyn 5	per 1 mg		J1435
Estro-Cyp	up to 5 mg	IM	J1000
Estrogen, conjugated	per 25 mg	IV, IM	J1410
Estroject L.A.	up to 5 mg	IM	J1000

◀ New   ← Revised   ✔ Reinstated   deleted Deleted

DRUG NAME	DOSAGE	METHOD OF ADMINISTRATION	HCPCS CODE
Estrone	per 1 mg	IM	J1435
Estrone 5	per 1 mg	IM	J1435
Estrone Aqueous	per 1 mg	IM	J1435
Estronol	per 1 mg	IM	J1435
Estronol-L.A.	up to 5 mg	IM	J1000
Etanercept, injection	25 mg	IM, IV	J1438
Ethamolin	100 mg		J1430
Ethanolamine	100 mg		J1430, J3490
Ethyol	500 mg	IV	J0207
Etidronate disodium	per 300 mg	IV	J1436
Etonogestrel implant			J7307
Etopophos	10 mg	IV	J9181
Etoposide	10 mg	IV	J9181
oral	50 mg	ORAL	J8560
Euflexxa			J7323
Everolimus, oral	0.25 mg		J8561
Everone	up to 100 mg	IM	J3120
	up to 200 mg	IM	J3130
F			
Fabrazyme	1 mg	IV	J0180
Factor VIIa (coagulation factor, recombinant)	1 mcg	IV	J7189
Factor VIII (anti-hemophilic factor)			
human	per IU	IV	J7190
porcine	per IU	IV	J7191
recombinant	per IU	IV	J7185, J7192
Factor IX			
anti-hemophilic factor, purified, non-recombinant	per IU	IV	J7193
anti-hemophilic factor, recombinant	per IU	IV	J7195
complex	per IU	IV	J7194
Factors, other hemophilia clotting	per IU	IV	J7196
Factrel	per 100 mcg	SC, IV	J1620
Famotidine			J3490
Faraheme	1 mg		Q0138, Q0139
Faslodex	25 mg		J9395
Feiba VH Immuno	per IU	IV	J7196
Fentanyl citrate	0.1 mg	IM, IV	J3010
Ferrlecit	12.5 mg		J2916
Ferumoxytol	1 mg		Q0138, Q0139
Filgrastim (G-CSF)	300 mcg	SC, IV	J1440
	480 mcg	SC, IV	J1441
Firmagon	1 mg		J9155

◄ New   ← Revised   ✔ Reinstated   ~~deleted~~ Deleted

DRUG NAME	DOSAGE	METHOD OF ADMINISTRATION	HCPCS CODE
Flebogamma	500 mg	IV	J1572
	1 cc		J1460
Flexbumin	20 ml		P9046
	50 ml		P9047
Flexoject	up to 60 mg	IV, IM	J2360
Flexon	up to 60 mg	IV, IM	J2360
Flolan	0.5 mg	IV	J1325
Floxuridine	500 mg	IV	J9200
Fluconazole	200 mg	IV	J1450
Fludara	1 mg	ORAL	J8562
	50 mg	IV	J9185
Fludarabine phosphate	50 mg	IV	J9185
Flunisolide inhalation solution, unit dose form	per mg	INH	J7641
Fluocinolone			J7311
Fluorouracil	500 mg	IV	J9190
Flutamide			J8999
Folex	5 mg	IA, IM, IT, IV	J9250
	50 mg	IA, IM, IT, IV	J9260
Folex PFS	5 mg	IA, IM, IT, IV	J9250
	50 mg	IA, IM, IT, IV	J9260
Follutein	per 1,000 USP units	IM	J0725
Folotyn	1 mg		J9307
Fomepizole	15 mg		J1451
Fomivirsen sodium	1.65 mg	Intraocular	J1452
Fondaparinux sodium	0.5 mg		J1652
Formoterol	12 mcg	INH	J7640
Formoterol fumarate	20 mcg		J7606
	12 mcg		J7640
Fortaz	per 500 mg	IM, IV	J0713
Forteo	10 mcg		J3110
Fosaprepitant	1 mg		J1453
Foscarnet sodium	per 1,000 mg	IV	J1455
Foscavir	per 1,000 mg	IV	J1455
Fosphenytoin	50 mg		Q2009
Fragmin	per 2,500 IU		J1645
FUDR	500 mg	IV	J9200
Fulvestrant	25 mg		J9395
Fungizone intravenous	50 mg	IV	J0285
Furomide M.D.	up to 20 mg	IM, IV	J1940
Furosemide	up to 20 mg	IM, IV	J1940
Fuzeon	1 mg		J1324

◀ New   ← Revised   ✔ Reinstated   deleted Deleted

DRUG NAME	DOSAGE	METHOD OF ADMINISTRATION	HCPCS CODE
G			
Gablofen	10 mg		J0475
	50 mcg		J0476
Gadoxetate disodium	1 ml		**A9581**
Gallium nitrate	1 mg		**J1457**
Galsulfase	1 mg		**J1458**
Gamastan	1 cc	IM	J1460
	over 10 cc	IM	J1560
Gammagard Liquid	500 mg		**J1569**
Gammagard S/D			J1566
Gamma globulin	1 cc	IM	J1460
	over 10 cc	IM	J1560
Gammaplex	500 mg		**J1557** ◄
GammaGraft	per square centimeter		Q4111
Gammar	1 cc	IM	J1460
	over 10 cc	IM	J1560
Gammar-IV, see Immune globin intravenous (human)			
Gamulin RH			
immune globulin			J2791
immune globulin, human	1 dose package, 300 mcg	IM	J2790
immune globulin, human, solvent detergent	100 IU	IV	J2792
Gamunex	500 mg		**J1561**
Ganciclovir, implant	4.5 mg	OTH	**J7310**
Ganciclovir sodium	500 mg	IV	**J1570**
Ganirelix			J3490
Ganite	1 mg		J1457
Garamycin, gentamicin	up to 80 mg	IM, IV	**J1580**
Gastrografin	per ml		Q9963
Gastromark	per 100 ml		Q9954
Gatifloxacin	10 mg	IV	**J1590**
Gefitinib	250 mg		**J8565**
Gel-One	per dose		**J7326** ◄
Gemcitabine HCl	200 mg	IV	**J9201**
Gemsar	200 mg	IV	J9201
Gemtuzumab ozogamicin	5 mg	IV	**J9300**
Gengraf	100 mg		J7502
	25 mg	ORAL	J7515
	250 mg		J7516
Gentamicin Sulfate	up to 80 mg	IM, IV	J1580
Gentran	500 ml	IV	J7100
Gentran 75	500 ml	IV	J7110

◄ New ← Revised ✔ Reinstated deleted Deleted

DRUG NAME	DOSAGE	METHOD OF ADMINISTRATION	HCPCS CODE
Gentropin	1 mg		J2941
Geodon	10 mg		J3486
Geref Diagnostic	1 mcg		Q0515
Gesterol 50	per 50 mg		J2675
Glassia	10 mg		J0257
Glatiramer Acetate	20 mg		J1595
GlucaGen	per 1 mg		J1610
Glucagon HCl	per 1 mg	SC, IM, IV	J1610
Glukor	per 1,000 USP units	IM	J0725
Glycopyrrolate			
concentrated form	per 1 mg	INH	J7642
unit dose form	per 1 mg	INH	J7643
Gold sodium thiomalate	up to 50 mg	IM	J1600
Gonadorelin HCl	per 100 mcg	SC, IV	J1620
Gonal-F			J3490
Gonic	per 1,000 USP units	IM	J0725
Goserelin acetate implant	per 3.6 mg	SC	J9202
Graftjacket	per square centimeter		Q4107
Graftjacket express	1 cc		Q4113
Granisetron HCl			
injection	100 mcg	IV	J1626
oral	1 mg	ORAL	Q0166
Gynogen L.A. A10	up to 10 mg	IM	J1380
Gynogen L.A. A20	up to 10 mg	IM	J1380
Gynogen L.A. A40	up to 10 mg	IM	J1380
H			
Halaven, *see* Eribulin mesylate			
Haldol	up to 5 mg	IM, IV	J1630
Haloperidol	up to 5 mg	IM, IV	J1630
Haloperidol decanoate	per 50 mg	IM	J1631
Haloperidol Lactate	up to 5 mg		J1630
Hectoral	1 mcg	IV	J1270
Helixate FS	per IU		J7192
Hemin	1 mg		J1640
Hemofil M	per IU	IV	J7190
Hemophilia clotting factors (e.g., anti-inhibitors)	per IU	IV	J7198
NOC	per IU	IV	J7199
Hepagam B	0.5 ml	IM	J1571
	0.5 ml	IV	J1573
Hep Flush-10	per 10 units		J1642
Hep-Lock	10 units	IV	J1642
Hep-Lock Flush	per 10 units		J1642

◀ New   ← Revised   ✔ Reinstated   deleted Deleted

DRUG NAME	DOSAGE	METHOD OF ADMINISTRATION	HCPCS CODE
Hep-Lock U/P	10 units	IV	J1642
Heparin Combination	per 10 units		J1642
Heparin Lock Flush	per 10 units		J1642
Heparin (Procine) In D5W	per 1,000 units		J1644
Heparin (Procine) In Nacl	per 10 units		J1642
	per 1,000 units		J1644
Heparin (Procine) Lock Flush	per 10 units		J1642
Heparin sodium	1,000 units	IV, SC	J1644
Heparin Sodium (Bovine)	per 1,000 units		J1644
Heparin Sodium Flush	per 10 units		J1642
Heparin sodium (heparin lock flush)	10 units	IV	J1642
Heparin Sodium (Procine)	per 1,000 units		J1644
Herceptin	10 mg	IV	J9355
Hexabrix 320	per ml		Q9967
Hexadrol Phosphate	1 mg	IM, IV, OTH	J1100
Histaject	per 10 mg	IM, SC, IV	J0945
Histerone 50	up to 50 mg	IM	J3140
Histerone 100	up to 50 mg	IM	J3140
Histrelin			
acetate	10 mcg		J1675
implant	50 mg		J9225
Hizentra, see Immune globulin			
Humalog	per 5 units		J1815
	per 50 units		J1817
Human Albumin Grifols	50 ml		P9047
Human fibrinogen concentrate	100 mg		J1680
Humate-P	per IU		J7187
Humatrope	1 mg		J2941
Humira	20 mg		J0135
Humulin	per 5 units		J1815
	per 50 units		J1817
Hyalgan			J7321
Hyaluronic Acid			J3490
Hyaluronidase	up to 150 units	SC, IV	J3470
Hyaluronidase			
ovine	up to 999 units		J3471
ovine	per 1000 units		J3472
recombinant	1 usp		J3473
Hylutin			J3490
Hyate:C	per IU	IV	J7191
Hybolin Improved, see Nandrolone phenpropionate			
Hybolin Decanoate	up to 50 mg	IM	J2320

◄ New   ← Revised   ✔ Reinstated   ~~deleted~~ Deleted

DRUG NAME	DOSAGE	METHOD OF ADMINISTRATION	HCPCS CODE
Hycamtin	0.25 mg	ORAL	J8705
	4 mg	IV	J9351
Hydralazine HCl	up to 20 mg	IV, IM	**J0360**
Hydrate	up to 50 mg	IM, IV	J1240
Hydrea			J8999
Hydrocortisone acetate	up to 25 mg	IV, IM, SC	**J1700**
Hydrocortisone sodium phosphate	up to 50 mg	IV, IM, SC	**J1710**
Hydrocortisone succinate sodium	up to 100 mg	IV, IM, SC	**J1720**
Hydrocortone Acetate	up to 25 mg	IV, IM, SC	J1700
Hydrocortone Phosphate	up to 50 mg	IM, IV, SC	J1710
Hydromorphone HCl	up to 4 mg	SC, IM, IV	**J1170**
Hydroxyprogesterone Caproate	1 mg		**J1725** ◄
Hydroxocobalamin	up to 1,000 mcg		J3420
Hydroxyurea			J8999
Hydroxyzine HCl	up to 25 mg	IM	J3410
Hydroxyzine Pamoate	25 mg	ORAL	Q0177
	50 mg	ORAL	**Q0178**
Hylan G-F 20			J7322
Hyoscyamine sulfate	up to 0.25 mg	SC, IM, IV	**J1980**
Hypaque	per ml		Q9961, Q9963
Hypaque Sodium Oral	per ml		Q9958
Hyperhep B			J3590
Hyperrho S/D	300 mcg		J2790
	100 IU		J2792
Hyper-Sal	10 ml		A4216
Hyperstat IV	up to 300 mg	IV	J1730
Hyper-Tet	up to 250 units	IM	J1670
HypRho-D	300 mcg	IM	J2790
			J2791
	50 mcg		J2788
Hyrexin-50	up to 50 mg	IV, IM	J1200
Hyzine-50	up to 25 mg	IM	J3410
I			
Ibandronate sodium	1 mg		**J1740**
Ibutilide fumarate	1 mg	IV	**J1742**
Idamycin	5 mg	IV	J9211
Idarubicin HCl	5 mg	IV	**J9211**
Idursulfase	1 mg		J1743
Ifex	1 g	IV	J9208
Ifosfamide	1 g	IV	**J9208**
Ilaris	1 mg		J0638

◄ New   ← Revised   ✔ Reinstated   ~~deleted~~ Deleted

DRUG NAME	DOSAGE	METHOD OF ADMINISTRATION	HCPCS CODE
Iletin	per 5 units		J1815
	per 50 units		J1817
Iloprost	20 mcg		**Q4074**
Ilotycin, see Erythromycin gluceptate			
Imferon	50 mg		J1750, J1752
Imiglucerase	10 units	IV	**J1786**
Imitrex	6 mg	SC	J3030
Immune globulin			
Flebogamma	500 mg	IV	**J1572**
Gammagard Liquid	500 mg	IV	**J1569**
Gammaplex	500 mg		**J1557** ◀
Gamunex	500 mg	IV	**J1561**
HepaGam B	0.5 ml	IM	**J1571**
	0.5 ml	IV	**J1573**
Hizentra	100 mg		**J1559**
NOS	500 mg	IV	**J1566, J1599**
Octagam	500 mg	IV	**J1568**
Privigen	500 mg	IV	**J1459**
Rhophylac	100 IU	IM	**J2791**
Subcutaneous	100 mg		**J1562**
Immunosuppressive drug, not otherwise classified			**J7599**
Imuran	50 mg	ORAL	J7500
	100 mg		J7501
Inapsine	up to 5 mg	IM, IV	J1790
Incobotulinumtoxin type A	1 unit		**J0588** ◀
Increlex	1 mg		J2170
Inderal	up to 1 mg	IV	J1800
Infed	50 mg		J1750
Infergen	1 mcg	SC	J9212
Infliximab, injection	10 mg	IM, IV	**J1745**
Innohep	1,000 IU	SC	J1655
Innovar	up to 2 ml ampule	IM, IV	J1810
Insulin	5 units	SC	**J1815**
Insulin-Humalog	per 50 units		J1817
Insulin lispro	50 units	SC	**J1817**
Intal	per 10 mg	INH	J7631, J7632
Integrilin	5 mg	IM, IV	J1327
Intera-BMWD	per square centimeter		Q4104
Integra			
Bilayer Matrix Wound Dressing (BMWD)	per square centimeter		Q4104
Dermal Regeneration Template (DRT)	per square centimeter		Q4105
Flowable Wound Matrix	1 cc		Q4114
Matrix	per square centimeter		Q4108

◀ New   ← Revised   ✔ Reinstated   ~~deleted~~ Deleted

DRUG NAME	DOSAGE	METHOD OF ADMINISTRATION	HCPCS CODE
Interferon alphacon-1, recombinant	1 mcg	SC	J9212
Interferon alfa-2a, recombinant	3 million units	SC, IM	J9213
Interferon alfa-2b, recombinant	1 million units	SC, IM	J9214
Interferon alfa-n3 (human leukocyte derived)	250,000 IU	IM	J9215
Interferon beta-1a	30 mcg	IM	J1826
	11 mcg	IM	Q3025
	11 mcg	SC	Q3026
Interferon beta-1b	0.25 mg	SC	J1830
Interferon gamma-1b	3 million units	SC	J9216
Intrauterine copper contraceptive		OTH	J7300
Intron-A	1 million units		J9214
Invanz	500 mg		J1335
Invega Sustenna	1 mg		J2426
Ipilimumab	1 mg		J9228 ◄
Ipratropium bromide, unit dose form	per mg	INH	J7620, J7644, J7645, J3535
Iressa	250 mg	ORAL	J8565
Irinotecan	20 mg	IV	J9206
Iron dextran	50 mg	IV, IM	J1750
Iron sucrose	1 mg	IV	J1756
Irrigation solution for Tx of bladder calculi	per 50 ml	OTH	Q2004
Isocaine HCl	per 10 ml	VAR	J0670
Isoetharine HCl			
concentrated form	per mg	INH	J7647, J7648
unit dose form	per mg	INH	J7649, J7650
Isoproterenol HCl			
concentrated form	per mg	INH	J7657, J7658
unit dose form	per mg	INH	J7659, J7660
Isovue-200	per ml		Q9966
Isovue-250	per ml		Q9966
Isovue-300	per ml		Q9967
Isovue-370	per ml		Q9967
Istodax	1 mg		J9315
Isuprel			
concentrated form	per mg	INH	J7657, J7658
unit dose form	per mg	INH	J7659, J7660
Itraconazole	50 mg	IV	J1835
Ixabepilone	1 mg		J9207
Ixempra	1 mg		J9207
J			
Jenamicin	up to 80 mg	IM, IV	J1580
Jevtana	1 mg		J9043 ◄

◄ New   ← Revised   ✔ Reinstated   ~~deleted~~ Deleted

2012 TABLE OF DRUGS I–J

DRUG NAME	DOSAGE	METHOD OF ADMINISTRATION	HCPCS CODE
K			
Kabikinase	per 250,000 IU	IV	J2995
Kalbitor	1 mg		J1290
Kaleinate	per 10 ml	IV	J0610
Kanamycin sulfate	up to 75 mg	IM, IV	**J1850**
	up to 500 mg	IM, IV	**J1840**
Kantrex	up to 75 mg	IM, IV	J1850
	up to 500 mg	IM, IV	J1840
Kay-Pred 25	up to 1 ml		J2650
Keflin	up to 1 g	IM, IV	J1890
Kefurox	per 750 mg		J0697
Kefzol	500 mg	IV, IM	J0690
Kenaject-40	per 10 mg	IM	J3301
	1 mg		J3300
Kenalog-10	per 10 mg	IM	J3301
	1 mg		J3300
Kenalog-40	per 10 mg	IM	J3301
	1 mg		J3300
Kepivance	50 mcg		J2425
Keppra	10 mg		J1953
Kestrone 5	per 1 mg	IM	J1435
Ketorolac tromethamine	per 15 mg	IM, IV	**J1885**
Key-Pred 25	up to 1 ml	IM	J2650
Key-Pred 50	up to 1 ml	IM	J2650
Key-Pred-SP, see Prednisolone sodium phosphate			
K-Flex	up to 60 mg	IV, IM	J2360
Kineret			J3490
Kinlytic	250,000 IU		J3365
Klebcil	up to 75 mg	IM, IV	J1850
	up to 500 mg	IM, IV	J1840
Koate-HP (anti-hemophilic factor)			
human	per IU	IV	J7190
porcine	per IU	IV	J7191
recombinant	per IU	IV	J7192
Kogenate			
human	per IU	IV	**J7190**
porcine	per IU	IV	**J7191**
recombinant	per IU	IV	**J7192**
FS	per IU		J7192
Konakion	per 1 mg	IM, SC, IV	J3430
Konyne-80	per IU	IV	J7194, J7195
Krystexxa	1 mg		J2507

◄ New   ← Revised   ✔ Reinstated   ~~deleted~~ Deleted

DRUG NAME	DOSAGE	METHOD OF ADMINISTRATION	HCPCS CODE
Kytril	1 mg	ORAL	Q0166
	1 mg	IV	S0091
	100 mcg	IV	J1626
L			
Lactated Ringers	up to 1,000 cc		J7120
L.A.E. 20	up to 10 mg	IM	J1380
Laetrile, Amygdalin, vitamin B-17			J3570
Lanoxin	up to 0.5 mg	IM, IV	J1160
Lanreotide	1 mg		J1930
Lantus	per 5 units		J1815
	per 50 units		J1817
Largon, see Propiomazine HCl			
Laronidase	0.1 mg		J1931
Lasix	up to 20 mg	IM, IV	J1940
L-Caine	10 mg	IV	J2001
L-Carnitine	per 1 gm		J1955
Lepirudin	50 mg		J1945
Leucovorin calcium	per 50 mg	IM, IV	J0640
Leukeran			J8999
Leukine	50 mcg	IV	J2820
Leuprolide acetate (for depot suspension)	per 3.75 mg	IM	J1950
	7.5 mg	IM	J9217
Leuprolide acetate	per 1 mg	IM	J9218
Leuprolide acetate implant	65 mg		J9219
Leustatin	per mg	IV	J9065
Levalbuterol HCl			
concentrated form	0.5 mg	INH	J7607, J7612
unit dose form	0.5 mg	INH	J7614, J7615
Levaquin I.U.	250 mg	IV	J1956
Levetiracetam	10 mg		J1953
Levocarnitine	per 1 gm	IV	J1955
Levo-Dromoran	up to 2 mg	SC, IV	J1960
Levofloxacin	250 mg	IV	J1956
Levoleucovorin calcium	0.5 mg		J0641
Levonorgestrel implant			J7306
Levonorgestrel-releasing intrauterine contraceptive system	52 mg	OTH	J7302
Levorphanol tartrate	up to 2 mg	SC, IV	J1960
Levsin	up to 0.25 mg	SC, IM, IV	J1980
Levulan Kerastick	unit dose (354 mg)	OTH	J7308
Lexiscan	0.1 mg		J2785
Librium	up to 100 mg	IM, IV	J1990
Lidocaine HCl	10 mg	IV	J2001

◄ **New**   ← **Revised**   ✔ **Reinstated**   ~~deleted~~ **Deleted**

DRUG NAME	DOSAGE	METHOD OF ADMINISTRATION	HCPCS CODE
Lidoject-1	10 mg	IV	J2001
Lidoject-2	10 mg	IV	J2001
Lincocin	up to 300 mg	IV	J2010
Lincomycin HCl	up to 300 mg	IV	J2010
Linezolid	200 mg	IV	J2020
Liquaemin Sodium	1,000 units	IV, SC	J1644
Liquid Pred	5 mg		J7506
Lioresal	10 mg	IT	J0475
			J0476
Lispro	per 5 units		J1815
LMD (10%)	500 ml	IV	J7100
Lovenox	10 mg	SC	J1650
Lorazepam	2 mg	IM, IV	J2060
Lucentis	0.1 mg		J2778
Lufyllin	up to 500 mg	IM	J1180
Luminal	up to 120 mg		J2560
Luminal Sodium	up to 120 mg	IM, IV	J2560
Lumizyme	10 mg		J0220, J0221 ◄
Lunelle	5 mg/25 mg	IM	J1056
Lupon Depot	7.5 mg		J9217
Lupon Depot-Ped	7.5 mg		J9216
Lupron	per 1 mg	IM	J9218
	per 3.75 mg	IM	J1950
	7.5 mg	IM	J9217
Lymphocyte immune globulin			
anti-thymocyte globulin, equine	250 mg	IV	J7504
anti-thymocyte globulin, rabbit	25 mg	IV	J7511
Lyophilized			J1566
M			
Macugen	0.3 mg		J2503
Magnesium sulfate	500 mg		J3475
Magnevist	per ml		A9579
Makena	1 mg		J1725 ◄
Malulane			J8999
Mannitol	25% in 50 ml	IV	J2150
	5 mg	INH	J7665 ◄
Marcaine			J3490
Marinol	2.5 mg	ORAL	Q0167
	5 mg	ORAL	Q0168
Marmine	up to 50 mg	IM, IV	J1240
Maxipime	500 mg	IV	J0692
MD-76R	per ml		Q9963

◄ New   ← Revised   ✔ Reinstated   ~~deleted~~ Deleted

DRUG NAME	DOSAGE	METHOD OF ADMINISTRATION	HCPCS CODE
MD Gastroview	per ml		Q9963
Mecasermin	1 mg		J2170
Mechlorethamine HCl (nitrogen mustard), HN2	10 mg	IV	J9230
Medralone 40	20 mg	IM	J1020
	40 mg	IM	J1030
	80 mg	IM	J1040
Medralone 80	20 mg	IM	J1020
	40 mg	IM	J1030
	80 mg	IM	J1040
Medrol	per 4 mg	ORAL	J7509
Medroxyprogesterone acetate	50 mg	IM	J1051
	150 mg	IM	J1055
Medroxyprogesterone acetate/estradiol cypionate	5 mg/25 mg	IM	J1056
Mefoxin	1 g	IV, IM	J0694
Megace			J8999
Megestrol Acetate			J8999
Melphalan HCl	50 mg	IV	J9245
Melphalan, oral	2 mg	ORAL	J8600
Menoject LA	up to 1 ml	IM	J1060
Mepergan Injection	up to 50 mg	IM, IV	J2180
Meperidine HCl	per 100 mg	IM, IV, SC	J2175
Meperidine and promethazine HCl	up to 50 mg	IM, IV	J2180
Mepivacaine HCl	per 10 ml	VAR	J0670
Mercaptopurine			J8999
Meropenem	100 mg		J2185
Merrem	100 mg		J2185
Mesna	200 mg	IV	J9209
Mesnex	200 mg	IV	J9209
Metaprel			
concentrated form	per 10 mg	INH	J7667, J7668
unit dose form	per 10 mg	INH	J7669, J7670
Metaproterenol sulfate			
concentrated form	per 10 mg	INH	J7667, J7668
unit dose form	per 10 mg	INH	J7669, J7670
Metaraminol bitartrate	per 10 mg	IV, IM, SC	J0380
Metastron	per millicurie		A9600
Methacholine chloride	1 mg		J7674
Methadone HCl	up to 10 mg	IM, SC	J1230
Methergine, see Methylergonovine maleate			
Methocarbamol	up to 10 ml	IV, IM	J2800
Methotrexate, oral	2.5 mg	ORAL	J8610

◄ New   ← Revised   ✔ Reinstated   ~~deleted~~ Deleted

DRUG NAME	DOSAGE	METHOD OF ADMINISTRATION	HCPCS CODE
Methotrexate sodium	5 mg	IV, IM, IT, IA	**J9250**
	50 mg	IV, IM, IT, IA	**J9260**
Methotrexate LPF	5 mg	IV, IM, IT, IA	J9250
	50 mg	IV, IM, IT, IA	J9260
Methyldopate HCl	up to 250 mg	IV	**J0210**
Methylpred	20 mg		J1020
Methylpred DP	per 4 mg		J7509
Methylprednisolone	40 mg		J1030
Methylprednisolone, oral	per 4 mg	ORAL	**J7509**
Methylprednisolone acetate	20 mg	IM	**J1020**
	40 mg	IM	**J1030**
	80 mg	IM	**J1040**
Methylprednisolone sodium succinate	up to 40 mg	IM, IV	**J2920**
	up to 125 mg	IM, IV	**J2930**
Metoclopramide HCl	up to 10 mg	IV	**J2765**
Metrodin	75 IU		J3355
Metronidazole			J3490
Metvixia, see Aminolevulinate			
Miacalcin	up to 400 units	SC, IM	J0630
Micafungin sodium	1 mg		**J2248**
MicRhoGAM	50 mcg		J2788
Midazolam HCl	per 1 mg	IM, IV	**J2250**
Millipred		ORAL	J8499
Milrinone lactate	5 mg	IV	**J2260**
Minocine	1 mg		J2265
Minocycline Hydrochloride	1 mg		**J2265**
Mirena	52 mg	OTH	J7302
Mithracin	2,500 mcg	IV	J9270
Mitomycin	5 mg	IV	**J9280**
Mitoxantrone HCl	per 5 mg	IV	**J9293**
Monocid, see Cefonicic sodium			
Monoclate-P			
human	per IU	IV	J7190
porcine	per IU	IV	J7191
recombinant	per IU	IV	J7192
Monoclonal antibodies, parenteral	5 mg	IV	**J7505**
Monoject Prefill Advanced	10 ml		A4216
Mononine	per IU	IV	J7193
Morphine sulfate	up to 10 mg	IM, IV, SC	**J2270**
	100 mg	IM, IV, SC	**J2271**
preservative-free	per 10 mg	SC, IM, IV	**J2275**
Moxifloxacin	100 mg		**J2280**

◀ New   ← Revised   ✔ Reinstated   ~~deleted~~ Deleted

DRUG NAME	DOSAGE	METHOD OF ADMINISTRATION	HCPCS CODE
Mozobil	1 mg		J2562
M-Prednisol-40	20 mg	IM	J1020
	40 mg	IM	J1030
	80 mg	IM	J1040
M-Prednisol-80	20 mg	IM	J1020
	40 mg	IM	J1030
	80 mg	IM	J1040
Mucomyst			
unit dose form	per gram	INH	J7604, J7608
Mucosol			
injection	100 mg		J0132
unit dose	per gram	INH	J7604, J7608
Muromonab-CD3	5 mg	IV	J7505
Muse		OTH	J0275
	1.25 mcg	OTH	J0270
Mustargen	10 mg	IV	J9230
Mutamycin	5 mg	IV	J9280
Mycamine	1 mg		J2248
Mycophenolic acid	180 mg		J7518
Mycophenolate Mofetil	250 mg	ORAL	J7517
Myfortic	180 mg		J7518
Myleran	1 mg		J0594
	2 mg	ORAL	J8510
Mylotarg	5 mg	IV	J9300
Myobloc	per 100 units	IM	J0587
Myochrysine	up to 50 mg	IM	J1600
Myolin	up to 60 mg	IV, IM	J2360
Myozyme	10 mg		J0220
N			
Nabi-HB			J3590
Nabilone	1 mg	ORAL	J8650
N-acetyl-L-cysteine	per gram		J7604
Nafcillin			J3490
Naglazyme	1 mg		J1458
Nalbuphine HCl	per 10 mg	IM, IV, SC	J2300
Naloxone HCl	per 1 mg	IM, IV, SC	J2310, J3490
Naltrexone			J3490
Naltrexone, depot form	1 mg		J2315
Nandrobolic L.A.	up to 50 mg	IM	J2320
Nandrolone decanoate	up to 50 mg	IM	J2320
Narcan	1 mg	IM, IV, SC	J2310
Naropin	1 mg		J2795

◄ New   ← Revised   ✔ Reinstated   ~~deleted~~ Deleted

DRUG NAME	DOSAGE	METHOD OF ADMINISTRATION	HCPCS CODE
Nasahist B	per 10 mg	IM, SC, IV	J0945
Nasal vaccine inhalation		INH	J3530
Natalizumab	1 mg		J2323
Natrecor	0.1 mg		J2325
Navane, see Thiothixene			
Navelbine	per 10 mg	IV	J9390
ND Stat	per 10 mg	IM, SC, IV	J0945
Nebcin	up to 80 mg	IM, IV	J3260
	per 300 mg		J7682
NebuPent	per 300 mg	INH	J2545, J7676
	300 mg	IM, IV	S0080
inhalation solution			J7699
Nelarabine	50 mg	IV	J9261
Nembutal Sodium Solution	per 50 mg	IM, IV, OTH	J2515
Neocyten	up to 60 mg	IV, IM	J2360
Neo-Durabolic	up to 50 mg	IM	J2320
Neoral	100 mg		J7502
	25 mg		J7515
Neoquess	up to 20 mg	IM	J0500
Neosar	100 mg	IV	J9070
Neostigmine methylsulfate	up to 0.5 mg	IM, IV, SC	J2710
Neo-Synephrine	up to 1 ml	SC, IM, IV	J2370
Nervidox-6 S	up to 1,000 mcg		J3420
Nervocaine 1%	10 mg	IV	J2001
Nervocaine 2%	10 mg	IV	J2001
Nesacaine	per 30 ml	VAR	J2400
Nesacaine-MPF	per 30 ml	VAR	J2400
Nesiritide	0.1 mg		J2325
Neulasta	6 mg		J2505
Neumega	5 mg	SC	J2355
Neupogen	300 mcg	SC, IV	J1440
	480 mcg	SC, IV	J1441
Neuroforte-R	up to 1,000 mcg		J3420
Neutrexin	per 25 mg	IV	J3305
Nipent	per 10 mg	IV	J9268
Nolvadex			J8999
Nordiflex	1 mg		J2941
Norditropin	1 mg		J2941
Nordryl	up to 50 mg	IV, IM	J1200
	50 mg	ORAL	Q0163
Norflex	up to 60 mg	IV, IM	J2360

◀ New   ← Revised   ✔ Reinstated   ~~deleted~~ Deleted

DRUG NAME	DOSAGE	METHOD OF ADMINISTRATION	HCPCS CODE
Norzine			
injection	up to 10 mg	IM	J3280
oral	10 mg	ORAL	Q0174
Not otherwise classified drugs			**J3490**
other than inhalation solution administered thru DME			**J7799**
inhalation solution administered thru DME			**J7699**
anti-neoplastic			**J9999**
chemotherapeutic		ORAL	**J8999**
immunosuppressive			**J7599**
nonchemotherapeutic		ORAL	**J8499**
Novantrone	per 5 mg	IV	J9293
Novarel	per 1,000 USP Units		J0725
Novolin	per 5 units		J1815
	per 50 units		J1817
Novolog	per 5 units		J1815
	per 50 units		J1817
Novo Seven	1 mcg	IV	J7189
NPH	5 units	SC	J1815
Nplate	100 units		J0587
	10 mcg		J2796
Nubain	per 10 mg	IM, IV, SC	J2300
Nulicaine	10 mg	IV	J2001
Numorphan	up to 1 mg	IV, SC, IM	J2410
Numorphan H.P.	up to 1 mg	IV, SC, IM	J2410
Nutropin	1 mg		J2941
O			
Oasis Burn Matrix	per square centimeter		Q4103
Oasis Wound Matrix	per square centimeter		Q4102
Octagam	500 mg		**J1568**
Octreotide Acetate, injection	1 mg	IM	J2353
	25 mcg	IV, SQ	J2354
Oculinum	per unit	IM	J0585
Ofatumumab	10 mg		**J9302**
Ofirmev	10 mg		J0131
O-Flex	up to 60 mg	IV, IM	J2360
Oforta	10 mg		J8562
Olanzapine	1 mg		J2358
Omalizumab	5 mg		J2357
Omnipaque	per ml		Q9965, Q9967
Omnipen-N	up to 500 mg	IM, IV	J0290
	per 1.5 gm	IM, IV	J0295
Omniscan	per ml		A9579

◄ New   ← Revised   ✔ Reinstated   ~~deleted~~ Deleted

DRUG NAME	DOSAGE	METHOD OF ADMINISTRATION	HCPCS CODE
Omnitrope	1 mg		J2941
OnabotulinumtoxinA	1 unit		**J0585**
Oncaspar	per single dose vial	IM, IV	J9266
Oncovin	1 mg	IV	J9370
Ondansetron HCl	1 mg	IV	**J2405**
	1 mg	ORAL	**Q0162**
Ontak	300 mcg		J9160
Onxol	30 mg		J9265
Opana	up to 1 mg		J2410
Oprelvekin	5 mg	SC	**J2355**
Optimark	per ml		A9579
Optiray 300	per ml		Q9967
Optiray 320	per ml		Q9967
Optiray 350	per ml		Q9967
Optison	per ml		Q9956
Oraminic II	per 10 mg	IM, SC, IV	J0945
Orfro	up to 60 mg		J2360
Ormazine	10 mg	ORAL	Q0171
	25 mg	ORAL	Q0172
	up to 50 mg	IM, IV	J3230
Orphenadrine citrate	up to 60 mg	IV, IM	**J2360**
Orphenate	up to 60 mg	IV, IM	J2360
Orencia	10 mg		J0129
Orthoclone OKT3	5 mg		J7505
Orthovisc			**J7324**
Or-Tyl	up to 20 mg	IM	**J0500**
Osmitrol			J7799
Ovidrel			J3490
Oxacillin sodium	up to 250 mg	IM, IV	**J2700**
Oxaliplatin	0.5 mg		**J9263**
Oxilan 300	per ml		Q9967
Oxilan 350	per ml		Q9967
Oxymorphone HCl	up to 1 mg	IV, SC, IM	**J2410**
Oxytetracycline HCl	up to 50 mg	IM	**J2460**
Oxytocin	up to 10 units	IV, IM	**J2590**
Ozurdex	0.1 mg		J7312
P			
Paclitaxel	30 mg	IV	**J9265**
Paclitaxel protein-bound particles	1 mg		**J9264**
Palifermin	50 mcg		**J2425**
Paliperidone Palmitate	1 mg		**J2426**
Palonosetron HCl	25 mcg		**J2469**

◀ New   ← Revised   ✔ Reinstated   deleted Deleted

DRUG NAME	DOSAGE	METHOD OF ADMINISTRATION	HCPCS CODE
Pamidronate disodium	per 30 mg	IV	J2430
Panglobulin NF	500 mg		J1566
Panhematin	1 mg		J1640
Panitumumab	10 mg		J9303
Papaverine HCl	up to 60 mg	IV, IM	J2440
Paragard T 380 A		OTH	J7300
Paraplatin	50 mg	IV	J9045
Paricalcitol, injection	1 mcg	IV, IM	J2501
Pegademase bovine	25 IU		J2504
Pegaptinib	0.3 mg		J2503
Pegaspargase	per single dose vial	IM, IV	J9266
Pegasys			J3490
Pegfilgrastim	6 mg		J2505
Peg-Intron			J3490
Pegloticase	1 mg		J2507
Pemetrexed	10 mg		J9305
Penicillin G benzathine	up to 100,000 units	IM	J0561
Penicillin G benzathine and penicillin G procaine	100,000 units	IM	J0558
Penicillin G potassium	up to 600,000 units	IM, IV	J2540
Penicillin G procaine, aqueous	up to 600,000 units	IM, IV	J2510
Penicillin G Sodium			J3490
Pentam	per 300 mg		J7676
Pentamidine isethionate	per 300 mg	INH	J2545, J7676
Pentastarch, 10%	100 ml		J2513
Pentazocine HCl	30 mg	IM, SC, IV	J3070
Pentobarbital sodium	per 50 mg	IM, IV, OTH	J2515
Pentostatin	per 10 mg	IV	J9268
Peforomist	20 mcg		J7606
Permapen	up to 600,000	IM	J0561
Perphenazine			
injection	up to 5 mg	IM, IV	J3310
tablets	4 mg	ORAL	Q0175
	8 mg	ORAL	Q0176
Persantine IV	per 10 mg	IV	J1245
Pfizerpen	up to 600,000 units	IM, IV	J2540
Pfizerpen A.S.	up to 600,000 units	IM, IV	J2510
Phenadoz			J8498
Phenazine 25	up to 50 mg	IM, IV	J2550
	12.5 mg	ORAL	Q0169
	25 mg	ORAL	Q0170

◄ New   ← Revised   ✔ Reinstated   ~~deleted~~ Deleted

DRUG NAME	DOSAGE	METHOD OF ADMINISTRATION	HCPCS CODE
Phenazine 50	up to 50 mg	IM, IV	J2550
	12.5 mg	ORAL	Q0169
	25 mg	ORAL	Q0170
Phenergan	12.5 mg	ORAL	Q0169
	25 mg	ORAL	Q0170
	up to 50 mg	IM, IV	J2550, J8498
Phenobarbital sodium	up to 120 mg	IM, IV	J2560
Phentolamine mesylate	up to 5 mg	IM, IV	J2760
Phenylephrine HCl	up to 1 ml	SC, IM, IV	J2370
Phenylephrine HCl, other			J7799
Phenytoin sodium	per 50 mg	IM, IV	J1165
Photofrin	75 mg	IV	J9600
Phytonadione (Vitamin K)	per 1 mg	IM, SC, IV	J3430
Piperacillin/Tazobactam Sodium, injection	1.125 g	IV	J2543, J3490
Pitocin	up to 10 units	IV, IM	J2590
Plantinol AQ	10 mg	IV	J9060
Plas+SD	each unit	IV	P9023
Plasma			
cryoprecipitate reduced	each unit		P9044
pooled multiple donor, frozen	each unit	IV	P9023
Plasbumin	20 ml		P9046
Plasbumin-5	50 ml		P9041
	250 ml		P9045
Plasbumin-25	20 ml		P9046
	50 ml		P9047
Plasmanate	50 ml		P9043, P9047
Plerixafor	1 mg		J2562
Plicamycin	2,500 mcg	IV	J9270
Polocaine	per 10 ml	VAR	J0670
Poly Bio-Set	per IU		J7192
Polycillin-N	up to 500 mg	IM, IV	J0290
	per 1.5 gm	IM, IV	J0295
Porfimer Sodium	75 mg	IV	J9600
Potassium chloride	per 2 mEq	IV	J3480
Pralatrexate	1 mg		J9307
Pralidoxime chloride	up to 1 g	IV, IM, SC	J2730
Predalone-50	up to 1 ml	IM	J2650
Predcor-25	up to 1 ml	IM	J2650
Predcor-50	up to 1 ml	IM	J2650
Predicort-50	up to 1 ml	IM	J2650
Prelone	5 mg		J7510
Prednicot	5 mg		J7506, J7510

◀ New   ← Revised   ✔ Reinstated   ~~deleted~~ Deleted

DRUG NAME	DOSAGE	METHOD OF ADMINISTRATION	HCPCS CODE
Prednisone	per 5 mg	ORAL	**J7506**
Prednisolone, oral	5 mg	ORAL	**J7510**
Prednisolone acetate	up to 1 ml	IM	**J2650**
Predoject-50	up to 1 ml	IM	J2650
Pregnyl	per 1,000 USP units	IM	J0725
Premarin Intravenous	per 25 mg	IV, IM	J1410
Prescription, chemotherapeutic, not otherwise specified		ORAL	**J8999**
Prescription, nonchemotherapeutic, not otherwise specified		ORAL	**J8499**
Prialt	1 mcg		J2278
Primacor	5 mg	IV	J2260
Primatrix	per square centimeter		Q4110
Primaxin	per 250 mg	IV, IM	J0743
Priscoline HCl	up to 25 mg	IV	J2670
Privigen	500 mg		**J1459**
Pro-Depo, see Hydroxyprogesterone Caproate			
Procainamide HCl	up to 1 g	IM, IV	**J2690**
Prochlorperazine	up to 10 mg	IM, IV	**J0780**
			J8498
Prochlorperazine maleate	5 mg	ORAL	**Q0164**
	10 mg	ORAL	**Q0165**
			S0183
Procrit			J0885
			J0886
			Q4081
Prodrox			J3490
Profasi HP	per 1,000 USP units	IM	J0725
Profilnine Heat-Treated			
non-recombinant	per IU	IV	J7193
recombinant	per IU	IV	J7195
complex	per IU	IV	J7194
Profilnine-SD	per IU		J7193, J7194, J7195
Progestaject	per 50 mg		J2675
Progesterone	per 50 mg		**J2675**
Prograf			
oral	per 1 mg	ORAL	J7507
parenteral	5 mg		J7525
Prokine	50 mcg	IV	J2820
Prolastin	10 mg	IV	J0256
Prolastin-C	10 mg		J0256
Proleukin	per single use vial	IM, IV	J9015

◄ New   ← Revised   ✔ Reinstated   ̶d̶e̶l̶e̶t̶e̶d̶ Deleted

DRUG NAME	DOSAGE	METHOD OF ADMINISTRATION	HCPCS CODE
Prolixin Decanoate, see Fluphenazine decanoate			
	25 mg	IM, SC	J2680
Promazine HCl	up to 25 mg	IM	J2950
Promethazine			J8498
Promethazine HCl			
injection	up to 50 mg	IM, IV	J2550
oral	12.5 mg	ORAL	Q0169
oral	25 mg	ORAL	Q0170
Promethegan			J8498
Pronestyl	up to 1 g	IM, IV	J2690
Proplex T			
non-recombinant	per IU	IV	J7193
recombinant	per IU	IV	J7195
complex	per IU	IV	J7194
Proplex SX-T			
non-recombinant	per IU	IV	J7193
recombinant	per IU	IV	J7195
complex	per IU	IV	J7194
Propofol			J3490
Propranolol HCl	up to 1 mg	IV	J1800
Prorex-25			
	up to 50 mg	IM, IV	J2550
	12.5 mg	ORAL	Q0169
	25 mg	ORAL	Q0170
Prorex-50			
	up to 50 mg	IM, IV	J2550
	12.5 mg	ORAL	Q0169
	25 mg	ORAL	Q0170
Prostaphlin	up to 1 g	IM, IV	J2690
Prostigmin	up to 0.5 mg	IM, IV, SC	J2710
Protamine sulfate	per 10 mg	IV	J2720
Protein C Concentrate	10 IU		J2724
Protirelin	per 250 mcg	IV	J2725
Prothazine	up to 50 mg	IM, IV	J2550
	12.5 mg	ORAL	Q0169
	25 mg	ORAL	Q0170
Protonix			J3490
Protopam Chloride	up to 1 g	IV, IM, SC	J2730
Proventil			
concentrated form	1 mg	INH	J7610, J7611
unit dose form	1 mg	INH	J7609, J7613
Provocholine	per 1 mg		J7674

◀ **New**   ← **Revised**   ✔ **Reinstated**   ~~deleted~~ **Deleted**

DRUG NAME	DOSAGE	METHOD OF ADMINISTRATION	HCPCS CODE
Prozine-50	up to 25 mg	IM	J2950
Pulmicort	0.25 mg	INH	J7633
	up to 0.5 mg		J7626
Pulmicort Respules	0.5 mg	INH	J7627, J7626
	per 0.25 mg		J7633
	up to 0.5 mg		J7626
noncompounded, concentrated	0.25 mg	INH	J7626
Pulmozyme	per mg		J7639
Purinethol	50 mg		J8999
Pyridoxine HCl	100 mg		J3415
Q			
Quelicin	up to 20 mg	IV, IM	J0330
Quinupristin/dalfopristin	500 mg (150/350)	IV	J2770
Qutenza	per 10 square cm		J7335
R			
Ranibizumab	0.1 mg		J2778
Ranitidine HCl, injection	25 mg	IV, IM	J2780
Rapamune	1 mg	ORAL	J7520
Rasburicase	0.5 mg		J2783
Rebetron Kit	1 million units		J9214
Rebif	11 mcg		Q3026
Reclast	1 mg		J3488
Recombinate (anti-hemophilic factor)			
human	per IU	IV	J7190
porcine	per IU	IV	J7191
recombinant	per IU	IV	J7192
Recombivax			J3490
Redisol	up to 1,000 mcg	IM, SC	J3420
Regadenoson	0.1 mg		J2785
Refacto	per IU		J7192
Refludan	50 mg		J1945
Regitine	up to 5 mg	IM, IV	J2760
Reglan	up to 10 mg	IV	J2765
Regular	5 units	SC	J1815
Relefact TRH	per 250 mcg	IV	J2725
Relion	per 5 units		J1815
	per 50 units		J1817
Remicade	10 mg	IM, IV	J1745
Remodulin	1 mg		J3285
Reno-30	per ml		Q9958
Reno-60	per ml		Q9961
Reno-Dip	per ml		Q9958

◀ New   ← Revised   ✔ Reinstated   ~~deleted~~ Deleted

DRUG NAME	DOSAGE	METHOD OF ADMINISTRATION	HCPCS CODE
Renocal-76	per ml		Q9963
Renografin-60	per ml		Q9961
Reno-M60	per ml		Q9961
ReoPro	10 mg	IV	J0130
Rep-Pred 40	20 mg	IM	J1020
	40 mg	IM	J1030
	80 mg	IM	J1040
Rep-Pred 80	20 mg	IM	J1020
	40 mg	IM	J1030
	80 mg	IM	J1040
Resectisol			J7799
Restall	up to 25 mg		J3410
Retavase	18.1 mg	IV	J2993
Reteplase	18.1 mg	IV	J2993
Retisert			J7311
Retrovir	10 mg	IV	J3485
Rheomacrodex	500 ml	IV	J7100
Rhesonativ	1 dose package/ 300 mcg	IM	J2790
	50 mg		J2788
Rheumatrex Dose Pack	2.5 mg	ORAL	J8610
Rho(D)			
immune globulin			J2791
immune globulin, human	1 dose package/ 300 mcg	IM	J2790
	50 mg		J2788
immune globulin, human, solvent detergent	100	IU, IV	J2792
RhoGAM	1 dose package, 300 mcg	IM	J2790
	50 mg		J2788
Rhophylac	100 IU		J2791
Riastap	100 mg		J1680
Rifadin			J3490
Rifampin			J3490
Rilonacept	1 mg		J2793
RimabotulinumtoxinB	100 units		J0587
Rimso-50	50 ml		J1212
Ringers lactate infusion	up to 1,000 cc	IV	J7120
Risperdal Costa	0.5 mg		J2794
Risperidone	0.5 mg		J2794
Rituxan	100 mg	IV	J9310
Rituximab	100 mg	IV	J9310

◄ New   ← Revised   ✔ Reinstated   ~~deleted~~ Deleted

DRUG NAME	DOSAGE	METHOD OF ADMINISTRATION	HCPCS CODE
Robaxin	up to 10 ml	IV, IM	J2800
Robinul	per mg		J7643
Rocephin	per 250 mg	IV, IM	J0696
Rodex	100 mg		J3415
Roferon-A	3 million units	SC, IM	J9213
Romidepsin	1 mg		J9315
Romiplostim	10 mcg		J2796
Ropivacaine Hydrochloride	1 mg		J2795
Rubex	10 mg	IV	J9000
Rubramin PC	up to 1,000 mcg	IM, SC	J3420
S			
Saizen	1 mg		J2941
Saline solution	10 ml		A4216
5% dextrose	500 ml	IV	J7042
infusion	250 cc	IV	J7050
	1,000 cc	IV	J7030
sterile	500 ml = 1 unit	IV, OTH	J7040
Sandimmune	25 mg	ORAL	J7515
	100 mg	ORAL	J7502
	250 mg	OTH	J7516
Sandoglobulin, see Immune globin intravenous (human)			
Sandostatin, Lar Depot	25 mcg		J2354
	1 mg	IM	J2353
Sargramostim (GM-CSF)	50 mcg	IV	J2820
Selestoject	per 4 mg	IM, IV	J0702
Sensorcaine MPF			J3490
Sermorelin acetate	1 mcg		Q0515
Serostim	1 mg		J2941
Simulect	20 mg		J0480
Sincalide	5 mcg		J2805
Sinografin	per ml		Q9963
Sinusol-B	per 10 mg	IM, SC, IV	J0945
Sirolimus	1 mg	ORAL	J7520
Smz-TMP			J3490
Sodium Chloride	1,000 cc		J7030
	10 ml		A4216
	500 ml = 1 unit		J7040
	500 ml		A4217
	250 cc		J7050
inhalation solution			J7699
Sodium Chloride Bacteriostatic	10 ml		A4216
Sodium Chloride Concentrate			J7799

◄ New   ← Revised   ✔ Reinstated   ~~deleted~~ Deleted

DRUG NAME	DOSAGE	METHOD OF ADMINISTRATION	HCPCS CODE
Sodium ferricgluconate in sucrose	12.5 mg		**J2916**
Sodium Hyaluronate			J3490
Euflexxa			**J7323**
Hyalgan			**J7321**
Orthovisc			**J7324**
Supartz			**J7321**
Solganal	up to 50 mg	IM	J2910
Soliris	10 mg		J1300
Solu-Cortef	up to 50 mg	IV, IM, SC	J1710
	100 mg		J1720
Solu-Medrol	up to 40 mg	IM, IV	J2920
	up to 125 mg	IM, IV	J2930
Solurex	1 mg	IM, IV, OTH	J1100
Solurex LA	1 mg	IM	J1094
Somatrem	1 mg		**J2940**
Somatropin	1 mg		**J2941**
Somatulin Depot	1 mg		J1930
Sparine	up to 25 mg	IM	J2950
Spasmoject	up to 20 mg	IM	J0500
Spectinomycin HCl	up to 2 g	IM	**J3320**
Sporanox	50 mg	IV	J1835
Stadol	1 mg		J0595
Staphcillin, see Methicillin sodium			
Stelara, see Ustekinumab			
Sterapred	5 mg		J7506
Stilphostrol	250 mg	IV	J9165
Streptase	250,000 IU	IV	J2995
Streptokinase	per 250,000	IU, IV	**J2995**
Streptomycin Sulfate	up to 1 g	IM	J3000
Streptomycin	up to 1 g	IM	**J3000**
Streptozocin	1 gm	IV	**J9320**
Strontium-89 chloride	per millicurie		**A9600**
Sublimaze	0.1 mg	IM, IV	J3010
Succinylcholine chloride	up to 20 mg	IV, IM	**J0330**
Sufenta			J3490
Sufentanil Citrate			J3490
Sumarel Dosepro	6 mg		J3030
Sumatriptan succinate	6 mg	SC	**J3030**
Supartz			J7321
SurgiMend Inguinal Fenestrated Oval			C9358
SurgiMend Inguinal Rectangle			C9358
SurgiMend Strip			C9358

◄ New   ← Revised   ✔ Reinstated   ~~deleted~~ Deleted

DRUG NAME	DOSAGE	METHOD OF ADMINISTRATION	HCPCS CODE
SurgiMend Thick			C9358
SurgiMend Thin			C9358
Surostrin	up to 20 mg	IV, IM	J0330
Sus-Phrine	up to 1 ml ampule	SC, IM	J0171
Synagis	per 50 mg		C9003
Synercid	500 mg (150/350)	IV	J2770
Synkavite	per 1 mg	IM, SC, IV	J3430
Syntocinon	up to 10 units	IV, IM	J2590
Synvisc and Synvisc-One	1 mg		J7322, J7325
Syrex	10 ml		A4216
Sytobex	1,000 mcg	IM, SC	J3420
T			
Tacrolimus			
oral	per 1 mg	ORAL	J7507
parenteral	5 mg		J7525
Talwin	30 mg	IM, SC, IV	J3070
Tamiflu	per 75 mg		G9035
Tamoxifen Citrate			J8999
Taractan, see Chlorprothixene			
Taxol	30 mg	IV	J9265
Taxotere	20 mg	IV	J9171
Tazicef	per 500 mg		J0713
Tazidime, see Ceftazidime Technetium TC Sestambi	per dose		A9500
			J0713
TEEV	up to 1 cc	IM	J0900
Teflaro	1 mg		J0712
Telavancin	10 mg		J3095
Temodar	5 mg	ORAL	J8700, J9328
Temozolomide	1 mg		J8700
	5 mg	ORAL	J9328
Temsirolimus	1 mg		J9330
Tenecteplase	1 mg		J3101
Teniposide	50 mg		Q2017
Tequin	10 mg	IV	J1590
Terbutaline sulfate	up to 1 mg	SC, IV	J3105
concentrated form	per 1 mg	INH	J7680
unit dose form	per 1 mg	INH	J7681
Teriparatide	10 mcg		J3110
Terramycin IM	up to 50 mg	IM	J2460
Testa-C	up to 100 mg	IM	J1070
	1 cc, 200 mg	IM	J1080
Testadiate	up to 1 cc	IM	J0900

◄ New   ← Revised   ✔ Reinstated   ~~deleted~~ Deleted

DRUG NAME	DOSAGE	METHOD OF ADMINISTRATION	HCPCS CODE
Testadiate-Depo	up to 100 mg	IM	J1070
	1 cc, 200 mg	IM	J1080
Testaject-LA	up to 100 mg	IM	J1070
	1 cc, 200 mg	IM	J1080
Testaqua	up to 50 mg	IM	J3140
Test-Estro Cypionates	up to 1 ml	IM	J1060
Test-Estro-C	up to 1 ml	IM	J1060
Testex	up to 100 mg	IM	J3150
Testo AQ	up to 50 mg		J3140
Testoject-50	up to 50 mg	IM	J3140
Testoject-LA	up to 100 mg	IM	J1070
	1 cc, 200 mg	IM	J1080
Testone			
LA 200	up to 100 mg	IM	J3120
	up to 200 mg	IM	J3130
LA 100	up to 100 mg	IM	J3120
	up to 200 mg	IM	J3130
Testosterone	up to 50 mg		J3140
Testosterone Aqueous	up to 50 mg	IM	J3140
Testosterone enanthate and estradiol valerate	up to 1 cc	IM	J0900
Testosterone enanthate	up to 100 mg	IM	J3120
	up to 200 mg	IM	J3130
Testosterone cypionate	up to 100 mg	IM	J1070
	1 cc, 200 mg	IM	J1080
Testosterone cypionate and estradiol cypionate	up to 1 ml	IM	J1060
Testosterone propionate	up to 100 mg	IM	J3150
Testosterone suspension	up to 50 mg	IM	J3140
Testradiol 90/4	up to 1 cc	IM	J0900
Testrin PA	up to 100 mg	IM	J3120
	up to 200 mg	IM	J3130
Testro AQ	up to 50 mg		J3140
Tetanus immune globulin, human	up to 250 units	IM	J1670
Tetracycline	up to 250 mg	IM, IV	J0120
Tev-Tropin	1 mg		J2941
Thallous Chloride TI–201	per MCI		A9505
Theelin Aqueous	per 1 mg	IM	J1435
Theophylline	per 40 mg	IV	J2810
TheraCys	per vial	IV	J9031
Thiamine HCl	100 mg		J3411
Thiethylenecthiophosphoramide/T	15 mg		J9340

◄ New   ← Revised   ✔ Reinstated   ~~deleted~~ Deleted

DRUG NAME	DOSAGE	METHOD OF ADMINISTRATION	HCPCS CODE
Thiethylperazine maleate			
injection	up to 10 mg	IM	J3280
oral	10 mg	ORAL	Q0174
Thiotepa	15 mg	IV	J9340
Thorazine	10 mg	ORAL	Q0171
	25 mg	ORAL	Q0172
	up to 50 mg		J3230, J8498
Thrombate III	per IU		J7197
Thymoglobulin, see Immune globin, anti-thymocyte			
	25 mg		J7511
Thypinone	per 250 mcg	IV	J2725
Thyrogen	0.9 mg	IM, SC	J3240
Thyrotropin Alfa, injection	0.9 mg	IM, SC	J3240
Tice BCG	per vial	IV	J9031
injection	up to 200 mg	IM	J3250
Ticon			
injection	up to 200 mg	IM	J3250
oral	250 mg	ORAL	Q0173
Tigan			
injection	up to 200 mg	IM	J3250
oral	250 mg	ORAL	Q0173
Tigecycline	1 mg		J3243
Tiject-20	up to 200 mg	IM	J3250
	250 mg	ORAL	Q0173
Timentin			J3490
Tinzaparin	1,000 IU	SC	J1655
Tirofiban Hydrochloride, injection	0.25 mg	IM, IV	J3246
TNKase	1 mg		J3101
Tobi	300 mg	INH	J7682, J7685
Tobramycin, inhalation solution	300 mg	INH	J7682, J7685
Tobramycin sulfate	up to 80 mg	IM, IV	J3260, J7685
Tocilizumab	1 mg		J3262
Tofranil, see Imipramine HCl			
Tolazoline HCl	up to 25 mg	IV	J2670
Topotecan	0.25 mg	ORAL	J8705
	40.1 mg	IV	J9351
Toradol	per 15 mg	IM, IV	J1885
Torecan	10 mg	ORAL	Q0174
	up to 10 mg	IM	J3280
Torisel	1 mg		J9330

◄ New   ← Revised   ✔ Reinstated   ~~deleted~~ Deleted

DRUG NAME	DOSAGE	METHOD OF ADMINISTRATION	HCPCS CODE
Tornalate			
concentrated form	per mg	INH	J7628
unit dose	per mg	INH	J7629
Torsemide	10 mg/ml	IV	**J3265**
Torsiel	1 mg		J3390
Totacillin-N	up to 500 mg	IM, IV	J0290
	per 1.5 gm	IM, IV	J0295
Trastuzumab	10 mg	IV	**J9355**
Trasylol	10,000 KIU		J0365
Treanda	1 mg		J9033
Trelstar Depot	3.75 mg		J3315
Trelstar LA	3.75 mg		J3315
Treprostinil	1 mg		**J3285**
Trexall	2.5 mg	ORAL	J8610
Triethylenethosphoramide	15 mg		J9340
Tri-Kort	1 mg		J3300
	per 10 mg	IM	J3301
Triam-A	1 mg		J3300
	per 10 mg	IM	J3301
Triamcinolone			
concentrated form	per 1 mg	INH	**J7683**
unit dose	per 1 mg	INH	**J7684**
Triamcinolone acetonide	1 mg		**J3300**
	per 10 mg	IM	**J3301**
Triamcinolone diacetate	per 5 mg	IM	**J3302**
Triamcinolone hexacetonide	per 5 mg	VAR	**J3303**
Triamcot	per 5 mg		J3302
Triesence	1 mg		J3300
	per 10 mg	IM	J3301
Triflupromazine HCl	up to 20 mg	IM, IV	**J3400**
Trilafon	4 mg	ORAL	Q0175
	8 mg	ORAL	Q0176
	up to 5 mg	IM, IV	J3310
Trilog	1 mg		J3300
	per 10 mg	IM	J3301
Trilone	per 5 mg		J3302
Trimethobenzamide HCl			
injection	up to 200 mg	IM	**J3250**
oral	250 mg	ORAL	**Q0173**
Trimetrexate glucuronate	per 25 mg	IV	**J3305**
Triptorelin Pamoate	3.75 mg		**J3315**
Trisenox	1 mg	IV	J9017

◄ New   ← Revised   ✔ Reinstated   ~~deleted~~ Deleted

DRUG NAME	DOSAGE	METHOD OF ADMINISTRATION	HCPCS CODE
Trobicin	up to 2 g	IM	J3320
Trovan	100 mg	IV	J0200
Truxadryl	50 mg		J1200
Twinrix			J3490
Tysabri	1 mg		J2323
Tyvaso	1.74 mg		J7686
			J7699
U			
Ultra Filtered Plus	50 mcg		J2788
Ultravist 150	per ml		Q9965
Ultravist 240	per ml		Q9966
Ultravist 300	per ml		Q9966
Ultravist 370	per ml		Q9967
Ultrazine-10	up to 10 mg	IM, IV	J0780
Unasyn	per 1.5 gm	IM, IV	J0295
Unclassified drugs (see also Not elsewhere classified)			**J3490**
Unspecified oral antiemetic			**Q0181**
Urea	up to 40 g	IV	**J3350**
Ureaphil	up to 40 g	IV	J3350
Urecholine	up to 5 mg	SC	J0520
Urofollitropin	75 IU		**J3355**
Urokinase	5,000 IU vial	IV	**J3364**
	250,000 IU vial	IV	**J3365**
Ustekinumab	1 mg		**J3357**
V			
V-Gan 25	up to 50 mg	IM, IV	J2550
	12.5 mg	ORAL	Q0169
	25 mg	ORAL	Q0170
V-Gan 50	up to 50 mg	IM, IV	J2550
	12.5 mg	ORAL	Q0169
	25 mg	ORAL	Q0170
Valcyte			J3490
Valergen 10	10 mg	IM	J1380
Valergen 20	10 mg	IM	J1380
Valergen 40	up to 10 mg	IM	J1380
Valertest No. 1	up to 1 cc	IM	J0900
			J1060
Valertest No. 2	up to 1 cc	IM	J0900
Valium	up to 5 mg	IM, IV	J3360
Valrubicin, intravesical	200 mg	OTH	**J9357**
Valstar	200 mg	OTH	J9357
Vancocin	500 mg	IV, IM	J3370

◄ New   ← Revised   ✔ Reinstated   deleted Deleted

DRUG NAME	DOSAGE	METHOD OF ADMINISTRATION	HCPCS CODE
Vancoled	500 mg	IV, IM	J3370
Vancomycin HCl	500 mg	IV, IM	J3370
Vantas	50 mg		J9226
Vasceze	per 10 mg		J1642
Vasceze Sodium Chloride	10 ml		A4216
Vasoxyl, see Methoxamine HCl			
Vectibix	10 mg		J9303
Velaglucerase alfa	100 units		J3385
Velban	1 mg	IV	J9360
Velcade	0.1 mg		J9041
Velosulin BR (RDNA)	per 50 units		J1817
Velsar	1 mg	IV	J9360
Venofer	1 mg	IV	J1756
Ventavis	20 mcg		Q4080
Ventolin	0.5 mg	INH	J7620
concentrated form	1 mg	INH	J7610, J7611
unit dose form	1 mg	INH	J7609, J7613
VePesid			
	10 mg	IV	J9181
	50 mg	ORAL	J8560
Veritas Collagen Matrix			J3490
Versed	per 1 mg	IM, IV	J2250
Verteporfin	0.1 mg	IV	J3396
Vesprin	up to 20 mg	IM, IV	J3400
VFEND IV	10 mg		J3465
VGan	up to 50 mg		J2550
Viadur	65 mg		J9219
Vibativ	10 mg		J3095
Vidaza	1 mg		J9025
Vinblastine sulfate	1 mg	IV	J9360
Vincasar PFS	1 mg	IV	J9370
Vincristine sulfate	1 mg	IV	J9370
Vinorelbine tartrate	per 10 mg	IV	J9390
Vispaque 320	per ml		Q9967
Vistacot	up to 25 mg		J3410
Vistaject-25	up to 25 mg	IM	J3410
Vistaril	up to 25 mg	IM	J3410
	25 mg	ORAL	Q0177
	50 mg	ORAL	Q0178
Vistide	375 mg	IV	J0740
Visudyne	0.1 mg	IV	J3396
Vita #12	up to 1,000 mcg		J3420

◄ New   ← Revised   ✔ Reinstated   ~~deleted~~ Deleted

DRUG NAME	DOSAGE	METHOD OF ADMINISTRATION	HCPCS CODE	
Vitamin B6	100 mg		J2415	
Vitamin K, phytonadione, menadione, menadiol sodium diphosphate	per 1 mg	IM, SC, IV	**J3430**	
Vitamin B-12 cyanocobalamin	up to 1,000 mcg	IM, SC	**J3420**	
Vitrase	up to 150 units		J3470	
	per 1 USP unit		J3471	
	per 1,000 USP units		J3472	
Vivaglobulin	100 mg		J1562	
Vivitrol	1 mg		J2315	
Von Willebrand Factor Complex, human	per IU VWF:RCo	IV	**J7187**	
	per 100 IU VWF:RCo	IV	**J7183**	←
Voriconazole	10 mg		**J3465**	
Vpriv	100 units		J3385	
Vumon	50 mg		Q2017	
W				
Water for injection bacteriostatic	10 ml		A4216	
Water for irrigation	500 ml		A4217	
Wehamine	up to 50 mg	IM, IV	J1240	
Wehdryl	up to 50 mg	IM, IV	J1200	
	50 mg	ORAL	Q0163	
Wellcovorin	per 50 mg	IM, IV	J0640	
Wilate	per IU	IV	J7187	
Win Rho SD	100 IU	IV	J2792	
Wyamine Sulfate, see Mephentermine sulfate				
Wycillin	up to 600,000 units	IM, IV	J2510	
Wydase	up to 150 units	SC, IV	J3470	
X				
Xeloda	150 mg	ORAL	J8520	
	500 mg	ORAL	J8521	
Xeomin	1 unit		J0588	◄
Xgeva	1 mg		J0897	◄
Xiaflex	0.01 mg		J0775	
Xolair	5 mg		J2357	
Xopenex	0.5 mg	INH	J7620	
concentrated form	1 mg	INH	J7610, J7611, J7612	
unit dose form	1 mg	INH	J7609, J7613, J7614	
Xylocaine HCl	10 mg	IV	J2001	
Xyntha	per IU IV		J7185, J7192	
Y				
Yervoy	1 mg		J9228	◄

◄ New   ← Revised   ✔ Reinstated   ~~deleted~~ Deleted

DRUG NAME	DOSAGE	METHOD OF ADMINISTRATION	HCPCS CODE
Z			
Zanosar	1 g	IV	J9320
Zantac	25 mg	IV, IM	J2780
Zemaira	10 mg	IV	J0256
Zemplar	1 mcg	IM, IV	J2501
Zenapax	25 mg	IV	J7513
Zetran	up to 5 mg	IM, IV	J3360
Ziconotide	1 mcg		**J2278**
Zidovudine	10 mg	IV	**J3485**
Zinacef	per 750 mg	IM, IV	J0697
Ziprasidone Mesylate	10 mg		**J3486**
Zithromax	1 g	ORAL	Q0144
I.V.	500 mg	IV	J0456
Zithromax Tri-Pak	1 g		Q0144
Zithromax Z-Pak	1 g		Q0144
Zmax	1 g		Q0144
Zofran	1 mg	IV	J2405
	1 mg	ORAL	Q0162
Zoladex	per 3.6 mg	SC	J9202
Zoledronic Acid	1 mg		**J3487**
Zolicef	500 mg	IV, IM	J0690
Zometa	1 mg		**J3487**
Zortress, oral	0.25 mg		J8561
Zorbtive	1 mg		J2941
Zosyn	1.125 g	IV	J2543
Zovirax	5 mg		J8499
Zyprexa Relprevv	1 mg		J2358
Zyvox	200 mg	IV	J2020

◄ New   ← Revised   ✔ Reinstated   ~~deleted~~ Deleted

HCPCS 2012: LEVEL II NATIONAL CODES

2012 HCPCS quarterly updates available
on the companion website at:
http://www.codingupdates.com

DISCLAIMER

Every effort has been made to make this text complete and accurate,
but no guarantee, warranty, or representation is made for its accu-
racy or completeness. This text is based on the Centers for Medicare
and Medicaid Services Healthcare Common Procedure Coding System (HCPCS).

INTRODUCTION

2012 HCPCS quarterly updates available on the companion website at: http:/evolve.elsevier.com/Buck/HCPCS/.

The Centers for Medicare and Medicaid Services (CMS) (formerly Health Care Financing Administration [HCFA]) Healthcare Common Procedure Coding System (HCPCS) is a collection of codes and descriptors that represent procedures, supplies, products, and services that may be provided to Medicare beneficiaries and to individuals enrolled in private health insurance programs. The codes are divided as follows:

Level I: Codes and descriptors copyrighted by the American Medical Association's (AMA's) Current Procedural Terminology, ed. 4 (CPT-4). These are 5 position numeric codes representing physician and nonphysician services.

Level II: Includes codes and descriptors copyrighted by the American Dental Association's current dental terminology, seventh edition (CDT-7/8). These are 5 position alpha-numeric codes comprising the D series. All other Level II codes and descriptors are approved and maintained jointly by the alpha-numeric editorial panel (consisting of CMS, the Health Insurance Association of America, and the Blue Cross and Blue Shield Association). These are 5 position alpha-numeric codes representing primarily items and nonphysician services that are not represented in the Level I codes.

Level III: The CMS eliminated Level III local codes. See Program Memorandum AB-02-113.

Headings are provided as a means of grouping similar or closely related items. The placement of a code under a heading does not indicate additional means of classification, nor does it relate to any health insurance coverage categories.

HCPCS also contains modifiers, which are two-position codes and descriptors used to indicate that a service or procedure that has been performed has been altered by some specific circumstance but not changed in its definition or code. Modifiers are grouped by the levels. Level I modifiers and descriptors are copyrighted by the AMA. Level II modifiers are HCPCS modifiers. Modifiers in the D series are copyrighted by the ADA.

HCPCS is designed to promote uniform reporting and statistical data collection of medical procedures, supplies, products, and services.

HCPCS Disclaimer

Inclusion or exclusion of a procedure, supply, product, or service does not imply any health insurance coverage or reimbursement policy.

HCPCS makes as much use as possible of generic descriptions, but the inclusion of brand names to describe devices or drugs is intended only for indexing purposes; it is not meant to convey endorsement of any particular product or drug.

Updating HCPCS

The primary updates are made annually. Quarterly updates are also issued by CMS.

Legend

CMS Updates:
- ▶ New
- → Revised
- ✔ Reinstated
- ✖ Deleted
- ☺ Special coverage instructions
- ◆ Not covered or valid by Medicare
- ✳ Carrier discretion

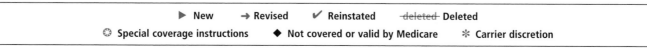

▶ New   → Revised   ✔ Reinstated   ~~deleted~~ Deleted
☺ Special coverage instructions   ◆ Not covered or valid by Medicare   ✳ Carrier discretion

INTRODUCTION

LEVEL II NATIONAL MODIFIERS

Do not report HCPCS modifiers with PQRI CPT Category II codes, rather use Category II modifiers (i.e., 1P, 2P, 3P, or 8P) or the claim may be returned or denied.

* **A1**   Dressing for one wound
* **A2**   Dressing for two wounds
* **A3**   Dressing for three wounds
* **A4**   Dressing for four wounds
* **A5**   Dressing for five wounds
* **A6**   Dressing for six wounds
* **A7**   Dressing for seven wounds
* **A8**   Dressing for eight wounds
* **A9**   Dressing for nine or more wounds
* **AA**   Anesthesia services performed personally by anesthesiologist
  IOM: 100-04, 12, 90.4
* **AD**   Medical supervision by a physician: more than four concurrent anesthesia procedures
  IOM: 100-04, 12, 90.4
* **AE**   Registered dietician
* **AF**   Specialty physician
* **AG**   Primary physician
* **AH**   Clinical psychologist
  IOM: 100-04, 12, 170
* **AI**   Principal physician of record
* **AJ**   Clinical social worker
  IOM: 100-04, 12, 170
  IOM: 100-04, 12, 150
* **AK**   Nonparticipating physician
* **AM**   Physician, team member service
  Not assigned for Medicare
* **AP**   Determination of refractive state was not performed in the course of diagnostic ophthalmological examination
* **AQ**   Physician providing a service in an unlisted health professional shortage area (HPSA)
* **AR**   Physician provider services in a physician scarcity area
* **AS**   Physician assistant, nurse practitioner, or clinical nurse specialist services for assistant at surgery

* **AT**   Acute treatment (this modifier should be used when reporting service 98940, 98941, 98942)
* **AU**   Item furnished in conjunction with a urological, ostomy, or tracheostomy supply
* **AV**   Item furnished in conjunction with a prosthetic device, prosthetic or orthotic
* **AW**   Item furnished in conjunction with a surgical dressing
* **AX**   Item furnished in conjunction with dialysis services
▶ * **AY**   Item or service furnished to an ESRD patient that is not for the treatment of ESRD
▶ ◆ **AZ**   Physician providing a service in a dental health professional shortage area for the purpose of an electronic health record incentive payment
* **BA**   Item furnished in conjunction with parenteral enteral nutrition (PEN) services
* **BL**   Special acquisition of blood and blood products
* **BO**   Orally administered nutrition, not by feeding tube
* **BP**   The beneficiary has been informed of the purchase and rental options and has elected to purchase the item
* **BR**   The beneficiary has been informed of the purchase and rental options and has elected to rent the item
* **BU**   The beneficiary has been informed of the purchase and rental options and after 30 days has not informed the supplier of his/her decision
* **CA**   Procedure payable only in the inpatient setting when performed emergently on an outpatient who expires prior to admission
* **CB**   Service ordered by a renal dialysis facility (RDF) physician as part of the ESRD beneficiary's dialysis benefit, is not part of the composite rate, and is separately reimbursable
* **CC**   Procedure code change (Use CC when the procedure code submitted was changed either for administrative reasons or because an incorrect code was filed)
* **CD**   AMCC test has been ordered by an ESRD facility or MCP physician that is part of the composite rate and is not separately billable

▶ New   → Revised   ✔ Reinstated   ~~deleted~~ Deleted
◎ Special coverage instructions   ◆ Not covered or valid by Medicare   * Carrier discretion

⊙ **CE** AMCC test has been ordered by an ESRD facility or MCP physician that is a composite rate test but is beyond the normal frequency covered under the rate and is separately reimbursable based on medical necessity

⊙ **CF** AMCC test has been ordered by an ESRD facility or MCP physician that is not part of the composite rate and is separately billable

✳ **CG** Policy criteria applied

✳ **CR** Catastrophe/Disaster related

▶ ✳ **CS** Item or service related, in whole or in part, to an illness, injury, or condition that was caused by or exacerbated by the effects, direct or indirect, of the 2010 oil spill in the Gulf of Mexico, including but not limited to subsequent clean-up activities

▶ ✳ **DA** Oral health assessment by a licensed health professional other than a dentist

✳ **E1** Upper left, eyelid

✳ **E2** Lower left, eyelid

✳ **E3** Upper right, eyelid

✳ **E4** Lower right, eyelid

⊙ **EA** Erythropoetic stimulating agent (ESA) administered to treat anemia due to anti-cancer chemotherapy

CMS requires claims for non-ESRD ESAs (J0881 and J0885) to include one of three modifiers: EA, EB, EC.

⊙ **EB** Erythropoetic stimulating agent (ESA) administered to treat anemia due to anti-cancer radiotherapy

CMS requires claims for non-ESRD ESAs (J0881 and J0885) to include one of three modifiers: EA, EB, EC.

⊙ **EC** Erythropoetic stimulating agent (ESA) administered to treat anemia not due to anti-cancer radiotherapy or anti-cancer chemotherapy

CMS requires claims for non-ESRD ESAs (J0881 and J0885) to include one of three modifiers: EA, EB, EC.

⊙ **ED** Hematocrit level has exceeded 39% (or hemoglobin level has exceeded 13.0 g/dl) for 3 or more consecutive billing cycles immediately prior to and including the current cycle

⊙ **EE** Hematocrit level has not exceeded 39% (or hemoglobin level has not exceeded 13.0 g/dl) for 3 or more consecutive billing cycles immediately prior to and including the current cycle

⊙ **EJ** Subsequent claims for a defined course of therapy, e.g., EPO, sodium hyaluronate, infliximab

⊙ **EM** Emergency reserve supply (for ESRD benefit only)

✳ **EP** Service provided as part of Medicaid early periodic screening diagnosis and treatment (EPSDT) program

✳ **ET** Emergency services

✳ **EY** No physician or other licensed health care provider order for this item or service

Items billed before a signed and dated order has been received by the supplier must be submitted with an -EY modifier added to each related HCPCS code.

✳ **F1** Left hand, second digit

✳ **F2** Left hand, third digit

✳ **F3** Left hand, fourth digit

✳ **F4** Left hand, fifth digit

✳ **F5** Right hand, thumb

✳ **F6** Right hand, second digit

✳ **F7** Right hand, third digit

✳ **F8** Right hand, fourth digit

✳ **F9** Right hand, fifth digit

✳ **FA** Left hand, thumb

◆ **FB** Item provided without cost to provider, supplier or practitioner, or full credit received for replaced device (examples, but not limited to, covered under warranty, replaced due to defect, free samples)

⊙ **FC** Partial credit received for replaced device

✳ **FP** Service provided as part of family planning program

✳ **G1** Most recent URR reading of less than 60

✳ **G2** Most recent URR reading of 60 to 64.9

✳ **G3** Most recent URR reading of 65 to 69.9

✳ **G4** Most recent URR reading of 70 to 74.9

✳ **G5** Most recent URR reading of 75 or greater

✳ **G6** ESRD patient for whom less than six dialysis sessions have been provided in a month

⊙ **G7** Pregnancy resulted from rape or incest or pregnancy certified by physician as life threatening

IOM: 100-02, 15, 20.1; 100-03, 3, 170.3

▶ New   → Revised   ✔ Reinstated   ~~deleted~~ Deleted   ⊙ Special coverage instructions   ◆ Not covered or valid by Medicare   ✳ Carrier discretion

CE – G7 LEVEL II NATIONAL MODIFIERS

✳ **G8**   Monitored anesthesia care (MAC) for deep complex, complicated, or markedly invasive surgical procedure

✳ **G9**   Monitored anesthesia care for patient who has history of severe cardiopulmonary condition

→ ✳ **GA**   Waiver of liability statement issued as required by payer policy, individual case

An item/service is expected to be denied as not reasonable and necessary and an ABN is on file. Modifier -GA can be used on either a specific or a miscellaneous HCPCS code. Modifiers -GA and -GY should never be reported together on the same line for the same HCPCS code.

✳ **GB**   Claim being resubmitted for payment because it is no longer covered under a global payment demonstration

◎ **GC**   This service has been performed in part by a resident under the direction of a teaching physician.

IOM: 100-04, 12, 90.4, 100

✳ **GD**   Units of service exceeds medically unlikely edit value and represents reasonable and necessary services

◎ **GE**   This service has been performed by a resident without the presence of a teaching physician under the primary care exception

✳ **GF**   Non-physician (e.g., nurse practitioner (NP), certified registered nurse anesthetist (CRNA), certified registered nurse (CRN), clinical nurse specialist (CNS), physician assistant (PA)) services in a critical access hospital

✳ **GG**   Performance and payment of a screening mammogram and diagnostic mammogram on the same patient, same day

✳ **GH**   Diagnostic mammogram converted from screening mammogram on same day

✳ **GJ**   "Opt out" physician or practitioner emergency or urgent service

✳ **GK**   Reasonable and necessary item/service associated with a GA or GZ modifier

An upgrade is defined as an item that goes beyond what is medically necessary under Medicare's coverage requirements. An item can be considered an upgrade even if the physician has signed an order for it. When suppliers know that an item will not be paid in full because it does not meet the coverage criteria stated in the LCD, the supplier can still obtain partial payment at the time of initial determination if the claim is billed using one of the upgrade modifiers (GK or GL). (https://www.cms.gov/manuals/downloads/clm104c01.pdf)

✳ **GL**   Medically unnecessary upgrade provided instead of non-upgraded item, no charge, no Advance Beneficiary Notice (ABN)

✳ **GM**   Multiple patients on one ambulance trip

✳ **GN**   Services delivered under an outpatient speech language pathology plan of care

✳ **GO**   Services delivered under an outpatient occupational therapy plan of care

✳ **GP**   Services delivered under an outpatient physical therapy plan of care

✳ **GQ**   Via asynchronous telecommunications system

✳ **GR**   This service was performed in whole or in part by a resident in a department of Veterans Affairs medical center or clinic, supervised in accordance with VA policy

◎ **GS**   Dosage of EPO or darbepoetin alfa has been reduced and maintained in response to hematocrit or hemoglobin level

◎ **GT**   Via interactive audio and video telecommunication systems

▶ ✳ **GU**   Waiver of liability statement issued as required by payer policy, routine notice

◎ **GV**   Attending physician not employed or paid under arrangement by the patient's hospice provider

◎ **GW**   Service not related to the hospice patient's terminal condition

▶ ✳ **GX**   Notice of liability issued, voluntary under payer policy

GX modifier must be submitted with non-covered charges only. This modifier differentiates from the required uses in conjunction with ABN. (https://www.cms.gov/manuals/downloads/clm104c01.pdf)

▶ New   → Revised   ✔ Reinstated   ~~deleted~~ Deleted

◎ Special coverage instructions   ◆ Not covered or valid by Medicare   ✳ Carrier discretion

◆ **GY**   Item or service statutorily excluded, does not meet the definition of any Medicare benefit or, for non-Medicare insurers, is not a contract benefit

Examples of "statutorily excluded" include: Infusion drug not administered using a durable infusion pump, a wheelchair that is for use for mobility outside the home or hearing aids. GA and GY should never be coded together on the same line for the same HCPCS code. (https://www.cms.gov/manuals/downloads/clm104c01.pdf)

◆ **GZ**   Item or service expected to be denied as not reasonable or necessary

Used when an ABN is not on file and can be used on either a specific or a miscellaneous HCPCS code. It would never be correct to place any combination of GY, GZ or GA modifiers on the same claim line and will result in rejected or denied claim for invalid coding. (https://www.cms.gov/manuals/downloads/clm104c01.pdf)

◆ **H9**   Court-ordered
◆ **HA**   Child/adolescent program
◆ **HB**   Adult program, nongeriatric
◆ **HC**   Adult program, geriatric
◆ **HD**   Pregnant/parenting women's program
◆ **HE**   Mental health program
◆ **HF**   Substance abuse program
◆ **HG**   Opioid addiction treatment program
◆ **HH**   Integrated mental health/substance abuse program
◆ **HI**   Integrated mental health and mental retardation/developmental disabilities program
◆ **HJ**   Employee assistance program
◆ **HK**   Specialized mental health programs for high-risk populations
◆ **HL**   Intern
◆ **HM**   Less than bachelor degree level
◆ **HN**   Bachelors degree level
◆ **HO**   Masters degree level
◆ **HP**   Doctoral level
◆ **HQ**   Group setting
◆ **HR**   Family/couple with client present
◆ **HS**   Family/couple without client present
◆ **HT**   Multi-disciplinary team
◆ **HU**   Funded by child welfare agency
◆ **HV**   Funded by state addictions agency

◆ **HW**   Funded by state mental health agency
◆ **HX**   Funded by county/local agency
◆ **HY**   Funded by juvenile justice agency
◆ **HZ**   Funded by criminal justice agency
∗ **J1**   Competitive acquisition program no-pay submission for a prescription number
∗ **J2**   Competitive acquisition program, restocking of emergency drugs after emergency administration
∗ **J3**   Competitive acquisition program (CAP), drug not available through CAP as written, reimbursed under average sales price methodology
∗ **J4**   DMEPOS item subject to DMEPOS competitive bidding program that is furnished by a hospital upon discharge
∗ **JA**   Administered intravenously

This modifier is informational only (not a payment modifier) and may be submitted with all injection codes. According to Medicare, reporting this modifier is voluntary. (CMS Pub. 100-04, chapter 8, section 60.2.3.1 and Pub. 100-04, chapter 17, section 80.11)

∗ **JB**   Administered subcutaneously
∗ **JC**   Skin substitute used as a graft
∗ **JD**   Skin substitute not used as a graft
∗ **JW**   Drug amount discarded/not administered to any patient

Use JW to identify unused drugs or biologicals from single use vial/package that are appropriately discarded. Bill on separate line for payment of discarded drug/biological.

∗ **K0**   Lower extremity prosthesis functional Level 0 - does not have the ability or potential to ambulate or transfer safely with or without assistance and a prosthesis does not enhance their quality of life or mobility.

∗ **K1**   Lower extremity prosthesis functional Level 1 - has the ability or potential to use a prosthesis for transfers or ambulation on level surfaces at fixed cadence. Typical of the limited and unlimited household ambulator.

∗ **K2**   Lower extremity prosthesis functional Level 2 - has the ability or potential for ambulation with the ability to traverse low level environmental barriers such as curbs, stairs or uneven surfaces. Typical of the limited community ambulator.

GY – K2   LEVEL II NATIONAL MODIFIERS

▶ New   → Revised   ✔ Reinstated   ~~deleted~~ Deleted
⊗ Special coverage instructions   ◆ Not covered or valid by Medicare   ∗ Carrier discretion

* **K3** Lower extremity prosthesis functional Level 3 - has the ability or potential for ambulation with variable cadence. Typical of the community ambulator who has the ability to traverse most environmental barriers and may have vocational, therapeutic, or exercise activity that demands prosthetic utilization beyond simple locomotion.

* **K4** Lower extremity prosthesis functional Level 4 - has the ability or potential for prosthetic ambulation that exceeds the basic ambulation skills, exhibiting high impact, stress, or energy levels, typical of the prosthetic demands of the child, active adult, or athlete.

* **KA** Add on option/accessory for wheelchair

* **KB** Beneficiary requested upgrade for ABN, more than 4 modifiers identified on claim

* **KC** Replacement of special power wheelchair interface

* **KD** Drug or biological infused through DME

* **KE** Bid under round one of the DMEPOS competitive bidding program for use with non-competitive bid base equipment

* **KF** Item designated by FDA as Class III device

* **KG** DMEPOS item subject to DMEPOS competitive bidding program number 1

* **KH** DMEPOS item, initial claim, purchase or first month rental

* **KI** DMEPOS item, second or third month rental

* **KJ** DMEPOS item, parenteral enteral nutrition (PEN) pump or capped rental, months four to fifteen

* **KK** DMEPOS item subject to DMEPOS competitive bidding program number 2

* **KL** DMEPOS item delivered via mail

* **KM** Replacement of facial prosthesis including new impression/moulage

* **KN** Replacement of facial prosthesis using previous master model

* **KO** Single drug unit dose formulation

* **KP** First drug of a multiple drug unit dose formulation

* **KQ** Second or subsequent drug of a multiple drug unit dose formulation

* **KR** Rental item, billing for partial month

☉ **KS** Glucose monitor supply for diabetic beneficiary not treated with insulin

* **KT** Beneficiary resides in a competitive bidding area and travels outside that competitive bidding area and receives a competitive bid item

* **KU** DMEPOS item subject to DMEPOS competitive bidding program number 3

* **KV** DMEPOS item subject to DMEPOS competitive bidding program that is furnished as part of a professional service

* **KW** DMEPOS item subject to DMEPOS competitive bidding program number 4

* **KX** Requirements specified in the medical policy have been met

* **KY** DMEPOS item subject to DMEPOS competitive bidding program number 5

* **KZ** New coverage not implemented by managed care

* **LC** Left circumflex coronary artery

* **LD** Left anterior descending coronary artery

* **LL** Lease/rental (use the LL modifier when DME equipment rental is to be applied against the purchase price)

* **LR** Laboratory round trip

☉ **LS** FDA-monitored intraocular lens implant

* **LT** Left side (used to identify procedures performed on the left side of the body)

* **M2** Medicare secondary payer (MSP)

* **MS** Six month maintenance and servicing fee for reasonable and necessary parts and labor which are not covered under any manufacturer or supplier warranty

▶ * **NB** Nebulizer system, any type, FDA-cleared for use with specific drug

* **NR** New when rented (use the NR modifier when DME which was new at the time of rental is subsequently purchased)

* **NU** New equipment

* **P1** A normal healthy patient

* **P2** A patient with mild systemic disease

* **P3** A patient with severe systemic disease

* **P4** A patient with severe systemic disease that is a constant threat to life

* **P5** A moribund patient who is not expected to survive without the operation

* **P6** A declared brain-dead patient whose organs are being removed for donor purposes

---

▶ New → Revised ✔ Reinstated ~~deleted~~ Deleted

☉ Special coverage instructions ◆ Not covered or valid by Medicare * Carrier discretion

◆ **PA**   Surgical or other invasive procedure on wrong body part

◆ **PB**   Surgical or other invasive procedure on wrong patient

◆ **PC**   Wrong surgery or other invasive procedure on patient

▶ ✳ **PD**   Diagnostic or related non diagnostic item or service provided in a wholly owned or operated entity to a patient who is admitted as an inpatient within 3 days

✳ **PI**   Positron emission tomography (PET) or PET/computed tomography (CT) to inform the initial treatment strategy of tumors that are biopsy proven or strongly suspected of being cancerous based on other diagnostic testing

✳ **PL**   Progressive addition lenses

✳ **PS**   Positron emission tomography (PET) or PET/computed tomography (CT) to inform the subsequent treatment strategy of cancerous tumors when the beneficiary's treating physician determines that the PET study is needed to inform subsequent anti-tumor strategy

▶ ✳ **PT**   Colorectal cancer screening test; converted to diagnostic text or other procedure

Assign this modifier with the appropriate CPT procedure code for colonoscopy, flexible sigmoidoscopy, or barium enema when the service is initiated as a colorectal cancer screening service but then becomes a diagnostic service. (MLN Matters article MM7012 (PDF, 75 KB)

⊘ **Q0**   Investigational clinical service provided in a clinical research study that is in an approved clinical research study

⊘ **Q1**   Routine clinical service provided in a clinical research study that is in an approved clinical research study

✳ **Q2**   HCFA/ORD demonstration project procedure/service

✳ **Live kidney donor surgery and related services**

✳ **Q4**   Service for ordering/referring physician qualifies as a service exemption

⊘ **Q5**   Service furnished by a substitute physician under a reciprocal billing arrangement

IOM: 100-04, 1, 30.2.10

⊘ **Q6**   Service furnished by a locum tenens physician

IOM: 100-04, 1, 30.2.11

✳ **Q7**   One Class A finding

✳ **Q8**   Two Class B findings

✳ **Q9**   One Class B and two Class C findings

✳ **QC**   Single channel monitoring

✳ **QD**   Recording and storage in solid state memory by a digital recorder

✳ **QE**   Prescribed amount of oxygen is less than 1 liter per minute (LPM)

✳ **QF**   Prescribed amount of oxygen exceeds 4 liters per minute (LPM) and portable oxygen is prescribed

✳ **QG**   Prescribed amount of oxygen is greater than 4 liters per minute (LPM)

✳ **QH**   Oxygen conserving device is being used with an oxygen delivery system

⊘ **QJ**   Services/items provided to a prisoner or patient in state or local custody, however, the state or local government, as applicable, meets the requirements in 42 CFR 411.4 (B)

⊘ **QK**   Medical direction of two, three, or four concurrent anesthesia procedures involving qualified individuals

IOM: 100-04, 12, 50K, 90

✳ **QL**   Patient pronounced dead after ambulance called

✳ **QM**   Ambulance service provided under arrangement by a provider of services

✳ **QN**   Ambulance service furnished directly by a provider of services

⊘ **QP**   Documentation is on file showing that the laboratory test(s) was ordered individually or ordered as a CPT-recognized panel other than automated profile codes 80002-80019, G0058, G0059, and G0060.

⊘ **QS**   Monitored anesthesia care service

IOM: 100-04, 12, 30.6, 501

✳ **QT**   Recording and storage on tape by an analog tape recorder

✳ **QW**   CLIA-waived test

✳ **QX**   CRNA service: with medical direction by a physician

⊘ **QY**   Medical direction of one certified registered nurse anesthetist (CRNA) by an anesthesiologist

IOM: 100-04, 12, 50K, 90

✳ **QZ**   CRNA service: without medical direction by a physician

---

▶ New   → Revised   ✔ Reinstated   ~~deleted~~ Deleted

⊘ Special coverage instructions   ◆ Not covered or valid by Medicare   ✳ Carrier discretion

PA – QZ   LEVEL II NATIONAL MODIFIERS

→ * **RA**   Replacement of a DME, orthotic or prosthetic item

Contractors will deny claims for replacement parts when furnished in conjunction with the repair of a capped rental item and billed with modifier -RB, including claims for parts submitted using code E1399, that are billed during the capped rental period (i.e., the last day of the 13th month of continuous use or before). Repair includes all maintenance, servicing, and repair of capped rental DME because it is included in the allowed rental payment amounts. (Pub 100-20 One-Time Notification Centers for Medicare & Medicaid Services, Transmittal: 901, May 13, 2011)

→ * **RB**   Replacement of a part of a DME, orthotic or prosthetic item furnished as part of a repair

* **RC**   Right coronary artery

* **RD**   Drug provided to beneficiary, but not administered "incident-to"

* **RE**   Furnished in full compliance with FDA-mandated risk evaluation and mitigation strategy (REMS)

* **RR**   Rental (use the 'RR' modifier when DME is to be rented)

* **RT**   Right side (used to identify procedures performed on the right side of the body)

♦ **SA**   Nurse practitioner rendering service in collaboration with a physician

♦ **SB**   Nurse midwife

→ * **SC**   Medically necessary service or supply

♦ **SD**   Services provided by registered nurse with specialized, highly technical home infusion training

♦ **SE**   State and/or federally funded programs/services

* **SF**   Second opinion ordered by a professional review organization (PRO) per Section 9401, P.L. 99-272 (100% reimbursement - no Medicare deductible or coinsurance)

* **SG**   Ambulatory surgical center (ASC) facility service

♦ **SH**   Second concurrently administered infusion therapy

♦ **SJ**   Third or more concurrently administered infusion therapy

♦ **SK**   Member of high risk population (use only with codes for immunization)

♦ **SL**   State supplied vaccine

♦ **SM**   Second surgical opinion

♦ **SN**   Third surgical opinion

♦ **SQ**   Item ordered by home health

♦ **SS**   Home infusion services provided in the infusion suite of the IV therapy provider

♦ **ST**   Related to trauma or injury

♦ **SU**   Procedure performed in physician's office (to denote use of facility and equipment)

♦ **SV**   Pharmaceuticals delivered to patient's home but not utilized

* **SW**   Services provided by a certified diabetic educator

♦ **SY**   Persons who are in close contact with member of high-risk population (use only with codes for immunization)

* **T1**   Left foot, second digit

* **T2**   Left foot, third digit

* **T3**   Left foot, fourth digit

* **T4**   Left foot, fifth digit

* **T5**   Right foot, great toe

* **T6**   Right foot, second digit

* **T7**   Right foot, third digit

* **T8**   Right foot, fourth digit

* **T9**   Right foot, fifth digit

* **TA**   Left foot, great toe

* **TC**   Technical component; under certain circumstances, a charge may be made for the technical component alone; under those circumstances the technical component charge is identified by adding modifier TC to the usual procedure number; technical component charges are institutional charges and not billed separately by physicians; however, portable x-ray suppliers only bill for technical component and should utilize modifier TC; the charge data from portable x-ray suppliers will then be used to build customary and prevailing profiles.

♦ **TD**   RN

♦ **TE**   LPN/LVN

♦ **TF**   Intermediate level of care

♦ **TG**   Complex/high tech level of care

♦ **TH**   Obstetrical treatment/services, prenatal or postpartum

♦ **TJ**   Program group, child and/or adolescent

♦ **TK**   Extra patient or passenger, non-ambulance

▶ New   → Revised   ✔ Reinstated   ~~deleted~~ Deleted

☺ Special coverage instructions   ♦ Not covered or valid by Medicare   * Carrier discretion

◆ **TL** Early intervention/individualized family service plan (IFSP)

◆ **TM** Individualized education program (IEP)

◆ **TN** Rural/outside providers' customary service area

◆ **TP** Medical transport, unloaded vehicle

◆ **TQ** Basic life support transport by a volunteer ambulance provider

◆ **TR** School-based individual education program (IEP) services provided outside the public school district responsible for the student

✳ **TS** Follow-up service

◆ **TT** Individualized service provided to more than one patient in same setting

◆ **TU** Special payment rate, overtime

◆ **TV** Special payment rates, holidays/weekends

◆ **TW** Back-up equipment

◆ **U1** Medicaid Level of Care 1, as defined by each State

◆ **U2** Medicaid Level of Care 2, as defined by each State

◆ **U3** Medicaid Level of Care 3, as defined by each State

◆ **U4** Medicaid Level of Care 4, as defined by each State

◆ **U5** Medicaid Level of Care 5, as defined by each State

◆ **U6** Medicaid Level of Care 6, as defined by each State

◆ **U7** Medicaid Level of Care 7, as defined by each State

◆ **U8** Medicaid Level of Care 8, as defined by each State

◆ **U9** Medicaid Level of Care 9, as defined by each State

◆ **UA** Medicaid Level of Care 10, as defined by each State

◆ **UB** Medicaid Level of Care 11, as defined by each State

◆ **UC** Medicaid Level of Care 12, as defined by each State

◆ **UD** Medicaid Level of Care 13, as defined by each State

✳ **UE** Used durable medical equipment

◆ **UF** Services provided in the morning

◆ **UG** Services provided in the afternoon

◆ **UH** Services provided in the evening

◆ **UJ** Services provided at night

◆ **UK** Services provided on behalf of the client to someone other than the client (collateral relationship)

✳ **UN** Two patients served

✳ **UP** Three patients served

✳ **UQ** Four patients served

✳ **UR** Five patients served

✳ **US** Six or more patients served

→ ✳ **V5** Vascular catheter (alone or with any other vascular access)

→ ✳ **V6** Arteriovenous graft (or other vascular access not including a vascular catheter)

→ ✳ **V7** Arteriovenous fistula only (in use with two needles)

✳ **V8** Infection present

✳ **V9** No infection present

✳ **VP** Aphakic patient

TL – VP   LEVEL II NATIONAL MODIFIERS

▶ New   → Revised   ✔ Reinstated   ~~deleted~~ Deleted

◯ Special coverage instructions   ◆ Not covered or valid by Medicare   ✳ Carrier discretion

Ambulance Modifiers

Modifiers that are used on claims for ambulance services are created by combining two alpha characters. Each alpha character, with the exception of X, represents an origin (source) code or a destination code. The pair of alpha codes creates one modifier. The first position alpha-code = origin; the second position alpha-code = destination. On form CMS-1491, used to report ambulance services, Item 12 should contain the origin code and Item 13 should contain the destination code. Origin and destination codes and their descriptions are as follows:

D	Diagnostic or therapeutic site other than P or H when these are used as origin codes
E	Residential, domiciliary, custodial facility (other than an 1819 facility)
G	Hospital-based dialysis facility (hospital or hospital related)
H	Hospital
I	Site of transfer (e.g., airport or helicopter pad) between modes of ambulance transport
J	Non–hospital-based dialysis facility
N	Skilled nursing facility (SNF) (1819 facility)
P	Physician's office (includes HMO non-hospital facility, clinic, etc.)
R	Residence
S	Scene of accident or acute event
X	Destination code only. Intermediate stop at physician's office en route to the hospital (includes non-hospital facility, clinic, etc.)

TRANSPORT SERVICES INCLUDING AMBULANCE (A0000-A0999)

A0021-A099: Bill local carrier

◆ **A0021** Ambulance service, outside state per mile, transport (Medicaid only)
Cross Reference A0030

◆ **A0080** Non-emergency transportation, per mile - vehicle provided by volunteer (individual or organization), with no vested interest

◆ **A0090** Non-emergency transportation, per mile - vehicle provided by individual (family member, self, neighbor) with vested interest

◆ **A0100** Non-emergency transportation; taxi

◆ **A0110** Non-emergency transportation and bus, intra or inter state carrier

◆ **A0120** Non-emergency transportation: mini-bus, mountain area transports, or other transportation systems

◆ **A0130** Non-emergency transportation: wheel chair van

◆ **A0140** Non-emergency transportation and air travel (private or commercial), intra or inter state

◆ **A0160** Non-emergency transportation: per mile - caseworker or social worker

◆ **A0170** Transportation: ancillary: parking fees, tolls, other

◆ **A0180** Non-emergency transportation: ancillary: lodging - recipient

◆ **A0190** Non-emergency transportation: ancillary: meals - recipient

◆ **A0200** Non-emergency transportation: ancillary: lodging - escort

◆ **A0210** Non-emergency transportation: ancillary: meals - escort

◆ **A0225** Ambulance service, neonatal transport, base rate, emergency transport, one way

◆ **A0380** BLS mileage (per mile)
Cross Reference A0425

∗ **A0382** BLS routine disposable supplies

∗ **A0384** BLS specialized service disposable supplies; defibrillation (used by ALS ambulances and BLS ambulances in jurisdictions where defibrillation is permitted in BLS ambulances)

◆ **A0390** ALS mileage (per mile)
Cross Reference A0425

∗ **A0392** ALS specialized service disposable supplies; defibrillation (to be used only in jurisdictions where defibrillation cannot be performed in BLS ambulances)

∗ **A0394** ALS specialized service disposable supplies; IV drug therapy

∗ **A0396** ALS specialized service disposable supplies; esophageal intubation

∗ **A0398** ALS routine disposable supplies

* **A0420**   Ambulance waiting time (ALS or BLS), one half (½) hour increments

	Waiting Time Table		
UNITS	**TIME**	**UNITS**	**TIME**
1	½ to 1 hr.	6	3 to 3½ hrs.
2	1 to 1½ hrs.	7	3½ to 4 hrs.
3	1½ to 2 hrs.	8	4 to 4½ hrs.
4	2 to 2½ hrs.	9	4½ to 5 hrs.
5	2½ to 3 hrs.	10	5 to 5½ hrs.

* **A0422**   Ambulance (ALS or BLS) oxygen and oxygen supplies, life sustaining situation

* **A0424**   Extra ambulance attendant, ground (ALS or BLS) or air (fixed or rotary winged); (requires medical review)

* **A0425**   Ground mileage, per statute mile

* **A0426**   Ambulance service, advanced life support, non-emergency transport, Level 1 (ALS1)

* **A0427**   Ambulance service, advanced life support, emergency transport, Level 1 (ALS1-Emergency)

* **A0428**   Ambulance service, basic life support, non-emergency transport (BLS)

* **A0429**   Ambulance service, basic life support, emergency transport (BLS-Emergency)

* **A0430**   Ambulance service, conventional air services, transport, one way (fixed wing)

* **A0431**   Ambulance service, conventional air services, transport, one way (rotary wing)

* **A0432**   Paramedic intercept (PI), rural area, transport furnished by a volunteer ambulance company, which is prohibited by state law from billing third party payers

* **A0433**   Advanced life support, Level 2 (ALS2)

* **A0434**   Specialty care transport (SCT)

* **A0435**   Fixed wing air mileage, per statute mile

* **A0436**   Rotary wing air mileage, per statute mile

◆ **A0888**   Noncovered ambulance mileage, per mile (e.g., for miles traveled beyond closest appropriate facility)
MCM 2125

◆ **A0998**   Ambulance response and treatment, no transport
IOM: 100-02, 10, 20

☼ **A0999**   Unlisted ambulance service
IOM: 100-02, 10, 20

MEDICAL AND SURGICAL SUPPLIES (A4000-A9999)

* **A4206**   Syringe with needle, sterile 1cc or less, each
If "incident to" a physician's service, do not bill; otherwise, bill DME/MAC.

* **A4207**   Syringe with needle, sterile 2cc, each
If "incident to" a physician's service, do not bill; otherwise, bill DME/MAC.

* **A4208**   Syringe with needle, sterile 3cc, each
If "incident to" a physician's service, do not bill; otherwise, bill DME/MAC.

* **A4209**   Syringe with needle, sterile 5cc or greater, each
If "incident to" a physician's service, do not bill; otherwise, bill DME/MAC.

◆ **A4210**   Needle-free injection device, each
IOM: 100-03, 4, 280.1
Bill DME/MAC

☼ **A4211**   Supplies for self-administered injections
Bill local carrier
If "incident to" a physican service, do not bill; otherwise, bill DME/MAC.
IOM: 100-02, 15, 50

* **A4212**   Non-coring needle or stylet with or without catheter

* **A4213**   Syringe, sterile, 20 cc or greater, each
If "incident to" a physican service, do not bill; otherwise, bill DME/MAC.

* **A4215**   Needle, sterile, any size, each
If "incident to" a physican service, do not bill; otherwise, bill DME/MAC.

☼ **A4216**   Sterile water, saline and/or dextrose diluent/flush, 10 ml
If "incident to" a physican service, do not bill; otherwise, bill DME/MAC.
Other: Broncho Saline, Hyper-Sal, Monoject Prefill advanced, Sodium Chloride, Sodium Chloride Bacteriostatic, Syrex, Vasceze Sodium Chloride, Water for Injection Bacteriostatic
IOM: 100-02, 15, 50

▶ **New**	→ **Revised**	✔ **Reinstated**	~~deleted~~ **Deleted**
☼ **Special coverage instructions**		◆ **Not covered or valid by Medicare**	* **Carrier discretion**

✿ **A4217** Sterile water/saline, 500 ml

If "incident to" a physican service, do not bill; otherwise, bill DME/MAC.

Other: Sodium Chloride

IOM: 100-02, 15, 50

✿ **A4218** Sterile saline or water, metered dose dispenser, 10 ml

If "incident to" a physican service, do not bill; otherwise, bill DME/MAC.

✿ **A4220** Refill kit for implantable infusion pump

Bill local carrier

Do not report with 95990 or 95991 since Medicare payment for these codes includes the refill kit.

IOM: 100-03, 4, 280.1

✳ **A4221** Supplies for maintenance of drug infusion catheter, per week (list drug separately)

If "incident to" a physican service, do not bill; otherwise, bill DME/MAC. Includes dressings for catheter site and flush solutions not directly related to drug infusion

✳ **A4222** Infusion supplies for external drug infusion pump, per cassette or bag (list drug separately)

If "incident to" physician service, do not bill; otherwise bill DME/MAC Includes cassette or bag, diluting solutions, tubing and/or administration supplies, port cap changes, compounding charges, and preparation charges.

✳ **A4223** Infusion supplies not used with external infusion pump, per cassette or bag (list drugs separately)

If "incident to" physician service, do not bill; otherwise bill DME/MAC

IOM: 100-03, 4, 280.1

✿ **A4230** Infusion set for external insulin pump, non-needle cannula type

If "incident to" physician service, do not bill; otherwise bill DME/MAC Requires prior authorization and copy of invoice.

IOM: 100-03, 4, 280.1

✿ **A4231** Infusion set for external insulin pump, needle type

If "incident to" physician service, do not bill; otherwise bill DME/MAC Requires prior authorization and copy of invoice.

IOM: 100-03, 4, 280.1

◆ **A4232** Syringe with needle for external insulin pump, sterile, 3cc

If "incident to" physician service, do not bill; otherwise bill DME/MAC Reports insulin reservoir for use with external insulin infusion pump (E0784); may be glass or plastic; includes needle for drawing up insulin. Does not include insulin for use in reservoir.

IOM: 100-03, 4, 280.1

✳ **A4233** Replacement battery, alkaline (other than J cell), for use with medically necessary home blood glucose monitor owned by patient, each

If "incident to" physician service, do not bill; otherwise bill DME/MAC

✳ **A4234** Replacement battery, alkaline, J cell, for use with medically necessary home blood glucose monitor owned by patient, each

If "incident to" a physician's service, do not bill; otherwise, bill DME/MAC.

✳ **A4235** Replacement battery, lithium, for use with medically necessary home blood glucose monitor owned by patient, each

If "incident to" a physician's service, do not bill; otherwise, bill DME/MAC.

✳ **A4236** Replacement battery, silver oxide, for use with medically necessary home blood glucose monitor owned by patient, each

If "incident to" a physician's service, do not bill; otherwise, bill DME/MAC.

✳ **A4244** Alcohol or peroxide, per pint

If "incident to" a physician's service, do not bill; otherwise, bill DME/MAC.

✳ **A4245** Alcohol wipes, per box

If "incident to" a physician's service, do not bill; otherwise, bill DME/MAC.

✳ **A4246** Betadine or pHisoHex solution, per pint

If "incident to" a physician's service, do not bill; otherwise, bill DME/MAC.

✳ **A4247** Betadine or iodine swabs/wipes, per box

If "incident to" a physician's service, do not bill; otherwise, bill DME/MAC.

✳ **A4248** Chlorhexidine containing antiseptic, 1 ml

If "incident to" a physician's service, do not bill; otherwise, bill DME/MAC.

▶ New   → Revised   ✔ Reinstated   ~~deleted~~ Deleted
✿ Special coverage instructions   ◆ Not covered or valid by Medicare   ✳ Carrier discretion

◆ **A4250** Urine test or reagent strips or tablets (100 tablets or strips)

If "incident to" a physician's service, do not bill; otherwise, bill DME/MAC.

IOM: 100-02, 15, 110

◆ **A4252** Blood ketone test or reagent strip, each

Bill DME/MAC

Medicare Statute 1861(n)

⊘ **A4253** Blood glucose test or reagent strips for home blood glucose monitor, per 50 strips

Bill DME/MAC

Test strips (1 unit = 50 strips); non-insulin treated (every 3 months) 100 test strips (1×/day testing), 100 lancets (1×/day testing); modifier KS

IOM: 100-03, 1, 40.2

⊘ **A4255** Platforms for home blood glucose monitor, 50 per box

Bill DME/MAC

IOM: 100-03, 1, 40.2

⊘ **A4256** Normal, low and high calibrator solution/chips

Bill DME/MAC

IOM: 100-03, 1, 40.2

✳ **A4257** Replacement lens shield cartridge for use with laser skin piercing device, each

Bill DME/MAC

⊘ **A4258** Spring-powered device for lancet, each

Bill DME/MAC

IOM: 100-03, 1, 40.2

⊘ **A4259** Lancets, per box of 100

Bill DME/MAC

IOM: 100-03, 1, 40.2

◆ **A4261** Cervical cap for contraceptive use

Bill local carrier

Medicare Statute 1862A1

⊘ **A4262** Temporary, absorbable lacrimal duct implant, each

Bill local carrier

⊘ **A4263** Permanent, long term, non-dissolvable lacrimal duct implant, each

Bill local carrier

Bundled if performed in physician office.

IOM: 100-04, 12, 30.4

◆ **A4264** Permanent implantable contraceptive intratubal occlusion device(s) and delivery system

Reports the Essure device.

⊘ **A4265** Paraffin, per pound

If "incident to" a physician's service, do not bill; otherwise, bill DME/MAC.

IOM: 100-03, 4, 280.1

◆ **A4266** Diaphragm for contraceptive use

Bill local carrier

◆ **A4267** Contraceptive supply, condom, male, each

Bill local carrier

◆ **A4268** Contraceptive supply, condom, female, each

Bill local carrier

◆ **A4269** Contraceptive supply, spermicide (e.g., foam, gel), each

Bill local carrier

✳ **A4270** Disposable endoscope sheath, each

Bill local carrier

✳ **A4280** Adhesive skin support attachment for use with external breast prosthesis, each

Bill DME/MAC

✳ **A4281** Tubing for breast pump, replacement

Bill DME/MAC

✳ **A4282** Adapter for breast pump, replacement

Bill DME/MAC

✳ **A4283** Cap for breast pump bottle, replacement

Bill DME/MAC

✳ **A4284** Breast shield and splash protector for use with breast pump, replacement

Bill DME/MAC

✳ **A4285** Polycarbonate bottle for use with breast pump, replacement

Bill DME/MAC

✳ **A4286** Locking ring for breast pump, replacement

Bill DME/MAC

✳ **A4290** Sacral nerve stimulation test lead, each

Bill local carrier

▶ New → Revised ✔ Reinstated deleted Deleted
⊘ Special coverage instructions ◆ Not covered or valid by Medicare ✳ Carrier discretion

Vascular Catheters

⊗ **A4300** Implantable access catheter, (e.g., venous, arterial, epidural subarachnoid, or peritoneal, etc.) external access

Bill local carrier

Bundled if performed in physician office.

IOM: 100-02, 15, 120

✻ **A4301** Implantable access total; catheter, port/reservoir (e.g., venous, arterial, epidural, subarachnoid, peritoneal, etc.)

Bill local carrier

✻ **A4305** Disposable drug delivery system, flow rate of 50 ml or greater per hour

If "incident to" a physician's service, do not bill; otherwise, bill DME/MAC.

✻ **A4306** Disposable drug delivery system, flow rate of less than 50 ml per hour

If "incident to" a physician's service, do not bill; otherwise, bill DME/MAC.

Incontinence Appliances and Care Supplies

A4310-A4355: If provided in the physician's office for a temporary condition, the item is incident to the physician's service and billed to the local carrier. If provided in the physician's office or other place of service for a permanent condition, the item is a prosthetic device and billed to the DME/MAC.

⊗ **A4310** Insertion tray without drainage bag and without catheter (accessories only)

IOM: 100-02, 15, 120

⊗ **A4311** Insertion tray without drainage bag with indwelling catheter, Foley type, two-way latex with coating (Teflon, silicone, silicone elastomer, or hydrophilic, etc.)

IOM: 100-02, 15, 120

⊗ **A4312** Insertion tray without drainage bag with indwelling catheter, Foley type, two-way, all silicone

IOM: 100-02, 15, 120

⊗ **A4313** Insertion tray without drainage bag with indwelling catheter, Foley type, three-way, for continuous irrigation

IOM: 100-02, 15, 120

⊗ **A4314** Insertion tray with drainage bag with indwelling catheter, Foley type, two-way latex with coating (Teflon, silicone, silicone elastomer or hydrophilic, etc.)

IOM: 100-02, 15, 120

⊗ **A4315** Insertion tray with drainage bag with indwelling catheter, Foley type, two-way, all silicone

IOM: 100-02, 15, 120

⊗ **A4316** Insertion tray with drainage bag with indwelling catheter, Foley type, three-way, for continuous irrigation

IOM: 100-02, 15, 120

⊗ **A4320** Irrigation tray with bulb or piston syringe, any purpose

IOM: 100-02, 15, 120

⊗ **A4321** Therapeutic agent for urinary catheter irrigation

⊗ **A4322** Irrigation syringe, bulb, or piston, each

IOM: 100-02, 15, 120

⊗ **A4326** Male external catheter with integral collection chamber, any type, each

IOM: 100-02, 15, 120

⊗ **A4327** Female external urinary collection device; meatal cup, each

IOM: 100-02, 15, 120

⊗ **A4328** Female external urinary collection device; pouch, each

IOM: 100-02, 15, 120

⊗ **A4330** Perianal fecal collection pouch with adhesive, each

IOM: 100-02, 15, 120

⊗ **A4331** Extension drainage tubing, any type, any length, with connector/adaptor, for use with urinary leg bag or urostomy pouch, each

IOM: 100-02, 15, 120

⊗ **A4332** Lubricant, individual sterile packet, each

IOM: 100-02, 15, 120

⊗ **A4333** Urinary catheter anchoring device, adhesive skin attachment, each

IOM: 100-02, 15, 120

⊗ **A4334** Urinary catheter anchoring device, leg strap, each

IOM: 100-02, 15, 120

▶ New   → Revised   ✔ Reinstated   ~~deleted~~ Deleted

⊗ **Special coverage instructions**   ◆ **Not covered or valid by Medicare**   ✻ **Carrier discretion**

⊕ **A4335** Incontinence supply; miscellaneous

IOM: 100-02, 15, 120

⊕ **A4336** Incontinence supply, urethral insert, any type, each

⊕ **A4338** Indwelling catheter; Foley type, two-way latex with coating (Teflon, silicone, silicone elastomer, or hydrophilic, etc.), each

IOM: 100-02, 15, 120

⊕ **A4340** Indwelling catheter; specialty type (e.g., coude, mushroom, wing, etc.), each

IOM: 100-02, 15, 120

⊕ **A4344** Indwelling catheter, Foley type, two-way, all silicone, each

IOM: 100-02, 15, 120

⊕ **A4346** Indwelling catheter; Foley type, three way for continuous irrigation, each

IOM: 100-02, 15, 120

⊕ **A4349** Male external catheter, with or without adhesive, disposable, each

IOM: 100-02, 15, 120

⊕ **A4351** Intermittent urinary catheter; straight tip, with or without coating (Teflon, silicone, silicone elastomer, or hydrophilic, etc.), each

IOM: 100-02, 15, 120

⊕ **A4352** Intermittent urinary catheter; coude (curved) tip, with or without coating (Teflon, silicone, silicone elastomeric, or hydrophilic, etc.), each

IOM: 100-02, 15, 120

⊕ **A4353** Intermittent urinary catheter, with insertion supplies

IOM: 100-02, 15, 120

⊕ **A4354** Insertion tray with drainage bag but without catheter

IOM: 100-02, 15, 120

⊕ **A4355** Irrigation tubing set for continuous bladder irrigation through a three-way indwelling Foley catheter, each

IOM: 100-02, 15, 120

External Urinary Supplies

⊕ **A4356** External urethral clamp or compression device (not to be used for catheter clamp), each

If provided in the physician's office for a temporary condition, the item is incident to the physician's service and billed to the local carrier. If provided in the physician's office or other place of service for a permanent condition, the item is a prosthetic device and billed to the DME/MAC.

IOM: 100-02, 15, 120

⊕ **A4357** Bedside drainage bag, day or night, with or without anti-reflux device, with or without tube, each

If provided in the physician's office for a temporary condition, the item is incident to the physician's service and billed to the local carrier. If provided in the physician's office or other place of service for a permanent condition, the item is a prosthetic device and billed to the DME/MAC.

IOM: 100-02, 15, 120

⊕ **A4358** Urinary drainage bag, leg or abdomen, vinyl, with or without tube, with straps, each

If provided in the physician's office for a temporary condition, the item is incident to the physician's service and billed to the local carrier. If provided in the physician's office or other place of service for a permanent condition, the item is a prosthetic device and billed to the DME/MAC.

IOM: 100-02, 15, 120

⊕ **A4360** Disposable external urethral clamp or compression device, with pad and/or pouch, each

If provided in the physician's office for a temporary condition, the item is incident to the physician's service and billed to the local carrier. If provided in the physician's office or other place of service for a permanent condition, the item is a prosthetic device and billed to the DME/MAC.

Added to the consolidated billing supply code list January 1, 2010.

▶ New	→ Revised	✔ Reinstated	~~deleted~~ Deleted

⊕ Special coverage instructions   ◆ Not covered or valid by Medicare   ✳ Carrier discretion

Ostomy Supplies

A4361-A4434: If provided in the physician's office for a temporary condition, the item is incident to the physician's service and billed to the local carrier. If provided in the physician's office or other place of service for a permanent condition, the item is a prosthetic device and billed to the DME/MAC.

⊛ **A4361** Ostomy faceplate, each

IOM: 100-02, 15, 120

⊛ **A4362** Skin barrier; solid, 4 × 4 or equivalent; each

IOM: 100-02, 15, 120

⊛ **A4363** Ostomy clamp, any type, replacement only, each

⊛ **A4364** Adhesive, liquid or equal, any type, per oz

Fee schedule category: Ostomy, tracheostomy, and urologicals items.

IOM: 100-02, 15, 120

✳ **A4366** Ostomy vent, any type, each

⊛ **A4367** Ostomy belt, each

IOM: 100-02, 15, 120

✳ **A4368** Ostomy filter, any type, each

⊛ **A4369** Ostomy skin barrier, liquid (spray, brush, etc), per oz

IOM: 100-02, 15, 120

⊛ **A4371** Ostomy skin barrier, powder, per oz

IOM: 100-02, 15, 120

⊛ **A4372** Ostomy skin barrier, solid 4 × 4 or equivalent, standard wear, with built-in convexity, each

IOM: 100-02, 15, 120

⊛ **A4373** Ostomy skin barrier, with flange (solid, flexible, or accordian), with built-in convexity, any size, each

IOM: 100-02, 15, 120

⊛ **A4375** Ostomy pouch, drainable, with faceplate attached, plastic, each

IOM: 100-02, 15, 120

⊛ **A4376** Ostomy pouch, drainable, with faceplate attached, rubber, each

IOM: 100-02, 15, 120

⊛ **A4377** Ostomy pouch, drainable, for use on faceplate, plastic, each

IOM: 100-02, 15, 120

⊛ **A4378** Ostomy pouch, drainable, for use on faceplate, rubber, each

IOM: 100-02, 15, 120

⊛ **A4379** Ostomy pouch, urinary, with faceplate attached, plastic, each

IOM: 100-02, 15, 120

⊛ **A4380** Ostomy pouch, urinary, with faceplate attached, rubber, each

IOM: 100-02, 15, 120

⊛ **A4381** Ostomy pouch, urinary, for use on faceplate, plastic, each

IOM: 100-02, 15, 120

⊛ **A4382** Ostomy pouch, urinary, for use on faceplate, heavy plastic, each

IOM: 100-02, 15, 120

⊛ **A4383** Ostomy pouch, urinary, for use on faceplate, rubber, each

IOM: 100-02, 15, 120

⊛ **A4384** Ostomy faceplate equivalent, silicone ring, each

IOM: 100-02, 15, 120

⊛ **A4385** Ostomy skin barrier, solid 4 × 4 or equivalent, extended wear, without built-in convexity, each

IOM: 100-02, 15, 120

⊛ **A4387** Ostomy pouch closed, with barrier attached, with built-in convexity (1 piece), each

IOM: 100-02, 15, 120

⊛ **A4388** Ostomy pouch, drainable, with extended wear barrier attached (1 piece), each

IOM: 100-02, 15, 120

⊛ **A4389** Ostomy pouch, drainable, with barrier attached, with built-in convexity (1 piece), each

IOM: 100-02, 15, 120

⊛ **A4390** Ostomy pouch, drainable, with extended wear barrier attached, with built-in convexity (1 piece), each

IOM: 100-02, 15, 120

⊛ **A4391** Ostomy pouch, urinary, with extended wear barrier attached (1 piece), each

IOM: 100-02, 15, 120

⊛ **A4392** Ostomy pouch, urinary, with standard wear barrier attached, with built-in convexity (1 piece), each

IOM: 100-02, 15, 120

⊛ **A4393** Ostomy pouch, urinary, with extended wear barrier attached, with built-in convexity (1 piece), each

IOM: 100-02, 15, 120

⚙ **A4394** Ostomy deodorant, with or without lubricant, for use in ostomy pouch, per fluid ounce

IOM: 100-02, 15, 20

⚙ **A4395** Ostomy deodorant for use in ostomy pouch, solid, per tablet

IOM: 100-02, 15, 20

⚙ **A4396** Ostomy belt with peristomal hernia support

IOM: 100-02, 15, 120

⚙ **A4397** Irrigation supply; sleeve, each

IOM: 100-02, 15, 120

⚙ **A4398** Ostomy irrigation supply; bag, each

IOM: 100-02, 15, 120

→ ⚙ **A4399** Ostomy irrigation supply; cone/catheter, with or without brush

IOM: 100-02, 15, 120

⚙ **A4400** Ostomy irrigation set

IOM: 100-02, 15, 120

⚙ **A4402** Lubricant, per ounce

IOM: 100-02, 15, 120

⚙ **A4404** Ostomy ring, each

IOM: 100-02, 15, 120

⚙ **A4405** Ostomy skin barrier, non-pectin based, paste, per ounce

IOM: 100-02, 15, 120

⚙ **A4406** Ostomy skin barrier, pectin-based, paste, per ounce

IOM: 100-02, 15, 120

⚙ **A4407** Ostomy skin barrier, with flange (solid, flexible, or accordion), extended wear, with built-in convexity, 4 × 4 inches or smaller, each

IOM: 100-02, 15, 120

⚙ **A4408** Ostomy skin barrier, with flange (solid, flexible, or accordion), extended wear, with built-in convexity, larger than 4 × 4 inches, each

IOM: 100-02, 15, 120

⚙ **A4409** Ostomy skin barrier, with flange (solid, flexible, or accordion), extended wear, without built-in convexity, 4 × 4 inches or smaller, each

IOM: 100-02, 15, 120

⚙ **A4410** Ostomy skin barrier, with flange (solid, flexible, or accordion), extended wear, without built-in convexity, larger than 4 × 4 inches, each

IOM: 100-02, 15, 120

⚙ **A4411** Ostomy skin barrier, solid 4 × 4 or equivalent, extended wear, with built-in convexity, each

⚙ **A4412** Ostomy pouch, drainable, high output, for use on a barrier with flange (2 piece system), without filter, each

IOM: 100-02, 15, 120

⚙ **A4413** Ostomy pouch, drainable, high output, for use on a barrier with flange (2 piece system), with filter, each

IOM: 100-02, 15, 120

⚙ **A4414** Ostomy skin barrier, with flange (solid, flexible, or accordion), without built-in convexity, 4 × 4 inches or smaller, each

IOM: 100-02, 15, 120

⚙ **A4415** Ostomy skin barrier, with flange (solid, flexible, or accordion), without built-in convexity, larger than 4 × 4 inches, each

IOM: 100-02, 15, 120

⚹ **A4416** Ostomy pouch, closed, with barrier attached, with filter (1 piece), each

⚹ **A4417** Ostomy pouch, closed, with barrier attached, with built-in convexity, with filter (1 piece), each

⚹ **A4418** Ostomy pouch, closed; without barrier attached, with filter (1 piece), each

⚹ **A4419** Ostomy pouch, closed; for use on barrier with non-locking flange, with filter (2 piece), each

⚹ **A4420** Ostomy pouch, closed; for use on barrier with locking flange (2 piece), each

⚹ **A4421** Ostomy supply; miscellaneous

⚙ **A4422** Ostomy absorbent material (sheet/pad/crystal packet) for use in ostomy pouch to thicken liquid stomal output, each

IOM: 100-02, 15, 120

⚹ **A4423** Ostomy pouch, closed; for use on barrier with locking flange, with filter (2 piece), each

⚹ **A4424** Ostomy pouch, drainable, with barrier attached, with filter (1 piece), each

⚹ **A4425** Ostomy pouch, drainable; for use on barrier with non-locking flange, with filter (2 piece system), each

⚹ **A4426** Ostomy pouch, drainable; for use on barrier with locking flange (2 piece system), each

⚹ **A4427** Ostomy pouch, drainable; for use on barrier with locking flange, with filter (2 piece system), each

---

▶ New → Revised ✔ Reinstated ~~deleted~~ Deleted

⚙ Special coverage instructions ◆ Not covered or valid by Medicare ⚹ Carrier discretion

✳ **A4428** Ostomy pouch, urinary, with extended wear barrier attached, with faucet-type tap with valve (1 piece), each

✳ **A4429** Ostomy pouch, urinary, with barrier attached, with built-in convexity, with faucet-type tap with valve (1 piece), each

✳ **A4430** Ostomy pouch, urinary, with extended wear barrier attached, with built-in convexity, with faucet-type tap with valve (1 piece), each

✳ **A4431** Ostomy pouch, urinary; with barrier attached, with faucet-type tap with valve (1 piece), each

✳ **A4432** Ostomy pouch, urinary; for use on barrier with non-locking flange, with faucet-type tap with valve (2 piece), each

✳ **A4433** Ostomy pouch, urinary; for use on barrier with locking flange (2 piece), each

✳ **A4434** Ostomy pouch, urinary; for use on barrier with locking flange, with faucet-type tap with valve (2 piece), each

Miscellaneous Supplies

⊘ **A4450** Tape, non-waterproof, per 18 square inches

If "incident to" physician service, do not bill separately; otherwise bill DME/MAC. If used with surgical dressings, billed with AW modifier (in addition to appropriate A1-A9 modifier).

IOM: 100-02, 15, 120

⊘ **A4452** Tape, waterproof, per 18 square inches

If "incident to" physician service, do not bill separately; otherwise, bill DME/MAC. If used with surgical dressings, billed with AW modifier (in addition to appropriate A1-A9 modifier).

IOM: 100-02, 15, 120

⊘ **A4455** Adhesive remover or solvent (for tape, cement or other adhesive), per ounce

If "incident to" a physician service, do not bill; otherwise, bill DME/MAC.

IOM: 100-02, 15, 120

⊘ **A4456** Adhesive remover, wipes, any type, each

Added to the consolidated billing supply code list January 1, 2010. May be reimbursed for male or female clients to home health DME providers and DME medical suppliers in the home setting.

✳ **A4458** Enema bag with tubing, reusable

Bill DME/MAC

✳ **A4461** Surgical dressing holder, non-reusable, each

If "incident to" a physician's service, do not bill; otherwise, bill DME/MAC.

✳ **A4463** Surgical dressing holder, reusable, each

If "incident to" a physician's service, do not bill; otherwise, bill DME/MAC.

✳ **A4465** Non-elastic binder for extremity

Bill DME/MAC

◆ **A4466** Garment, belt, sleeve or other covering, elastic or similar stretchable material, any type, each

⊘ **A4470** Gravlee jet washer

Bill local carrier

IOM: 100-02, 16, 90; 100-03, 4, 230.5

⊘ **A4480** VABRA aspirator

Bill local carrier

IOM: 100-02, 16, 90; 100-03, 4, 230.6

⊘ **A4481** Tracheostoma filter, any type, any size, each

If "incident to" a physician's service, do not bill; otherwise, bill DME/MAC.

IOM: 100-02, 15, 120

⊘ **A4483** Moisture exchanger, disposable, for use with invasive mechanical ventilation

Bill DME/MAC

IOM: 100-02, 15, 120

◆ **A4490** Surgical stockings above knee length, each

Bill DME/MAC

IOM: 100-02, 15, 100; 100-02, 15, 110; 100-03, 4, 280.1

◆ **A4495** Surgical stockings thigh length, each

Bill DME/MAC

IOM: 100-02, 15, 100; 100-02, 15, 110; 100-03, 4, 280.1

◆ **A4500** Surgical stockings below knee length, each

Bill DME/MAC

IOM: 100-02, 15, 100; 100-02, 15, 110; 100-03, 4, 280.1

◆ **A4510** Surgical stockings full length, each

Bill DME/MAC

IOM: 100-02, 15, 100; 100-02, 15, 110; 100-03, 4, 280.1

▶ New   → Revised   ✔ Reinstated   deleted Deleted
⊘ Special coverage instructions   ◆ Not covered or valid by Medicare   ✳ Carrier discretion

◆ **A4520** Incontinence garment, any type, (e.g. brief, diaper), each

Bill DME/MAC

IOM: 100-03, 4, 280.1

⊘ **A4550** Surgical trays

Bill local carrier

No longer payable by Medicare; included in practice expense for procedures. Some private payers may pay, most private payers follow Medicare guidelines

IOM: 100-04, 12, 20.3, 30.4

◆ **A4554** Disposable underpads, all sizes

Bill DME/MAC

IOM: 100-02, 15, 120; 100-03, 4, 280.1

✳ **A4556** Electrodes, (e.g., apnea monitor), per pair

If "incident to" a physician's service, do not bill; otherwise, bill DME/MAC.

✳ **A4557** Lead wires, (e.g., apnea monitor), per pair

If "incident to" a physician's service, do not bill; otherwise, bill DME/MAC.

✳ **A4558** Conductive gel or paste, for use with electrical device (e.g., TENS, NMES), per oz

If "incident to" a physician's service, do not bill; otherwise, bill DME/MAC.

✳ **A4559** Coupling gel or paste, for use with ultrasound device, per oz

If "incident to" a physician's service, do not bill; otherwise, bill DME/MAC.

✳ **A4561** Pessary, rubber, any type

Bill local carrier

✳ **A4562** Pessary, non rubber, any type

Bill local carrier

✳ **A4565** Slings

Bill local carrier

▶◆ **A4566** Shoulder sling or vest design, abduction restrainer, with or without swathe control, prefabricated, includes fitting and adjustment

◆ **A4570** Splint

Bill local carrier

IOM: 100-02, 6, 10; 100-02, 15, 100; 100-04, 4, 240

◆ **A4575** Topical hyperbaric oxygen chamber, disposable

Bill DME/MAC

IOM: 100-03, 1, 20.29

◆ **A4580** Cast supplies (e.g. plaster)

Bill local carrier

IOM: 100-02, 6, 10; 100-02, 15, 100; 100-04, 4, 240

◆ **A4590** Special casting material (e.g. fiberglass)

Bill local carrier

IOM: 100-02, 6, 10; 100-02, 15, 100; 100-04, 4, 240

⊘ **A4595** Electrical stimulator supplies, 2 lead, per month, (e.g. TENS, NMES)

If "incident to" a physician's service, do not bill; otherwise, bill DME/MAC.

IOM: 100-03, 2, 160.13

✳ **A4600** Sleeve for intermittent limb compression device, replacement only, each

Bill DME/MAC

✳ **A4601** Lithium ion battery for non-prosthetic use, replacement

Bill DME/MAC

✳ **A4604** Tubing with integrated heating element for use with positive airway pressure device

Bill DME/MAC

✳ **A4605** Tracheal suction catheter, closed system, each

Bill DME/MAC

✳ **A4606** Oxygen probe for use with oximeter device, replacement

Bill DME/MAC

✳ **A4608** Transtracheal oxygen catheter, each

Bill DME/MAC

Supplies for Respiratory and Oxygen Equipment

✳ **A4611** Battery, heavy duty; replacement for patient owned ventilator

Bill DME/MAC

✳ **A4612** Battery cables; replacement for patient-owned ventilator

Bill DME/MAC

✳ **A4613** Battery charger; replacement for patient-owned ventilator

Bill DME/MAC

✳ **A4614** Peak expiratory flow rate meter, hand held

If "incident to" a physician's service, do not bill; otherwise, bill DME/MAC.

▶ New	→ Revised	✔ Reinstated	deleted Deleted
⊘ Special coverage instructions		◆ Not covered or valid by Medicare	✳ Carrier discretion

⚙ **A4615** Cannula, nasal

If "incident to" a physician's service, do not bill; otherwise, bill DME/MAC.

IOM: 100-03, 2, 160.6; 100-04, 20, 100.2

⚙ **A4616** Tubing (oxygen), per foot

If "incident to" a physician's service, do not bill; otherwise, bill DME/MAC.

IOM: 100-03, 2, 160.6; 100-04, 20, 100.2

⚙ **A4617** Mouth piece

If "incident to" a physician's service, do not bill; otherwise, bill DME/MAC.

IOM: 100-03, 2, 160.6; 100-04, 20, 100.2

⚙ **A4618** Breathing circuits

If "incident to" a physician's service, do not bill; otherwise, bill DME/MAC.

IOM: 100-03, 2, 160.6; 100-04, 20, 100.2

→ ⚙ **A4619** Face tent

If "incident to" a physician's service, do not bill; otherwise, bill DME/MAC.

IOM: 100-03, 2, 160.6; 100-04, 20, 100.2

⚙ **A4620** Variable concentration mask

If "incident to" a physician's service, do not bill; otherwise, bill DME/MAC.

IOM: 100-03, 2, 160.6; 100-04, 20, 100.2

⚙ **A4623** Tracheostomy, inner cannula

If "incident to" a physician's service, do not bill; otherwise, bill DME/MAC.

IOM: 100-02, 15, 120; 100-03, 1, 20.9

✳ **A4624** Tracheal suction catheter, any type, other than closed system, each

If "incident to" a physician's service, do not bill; otherwise, bill DME/MAC.

Sterile suction catheters are medically necessary only for tracheostomy suctioning. Limitations include three suction catheters per day when covered for medically necessary tracheostomy suctioning. Assign DX V44.0 or V55.0 on the claim form. (CMS Manual System, Pub. 100-3, NCD manual, Chapter 1, Section 280-1)

⚙ **A4625** Tracheostomy care kit for new tracheostomy

If "incident to" a physician's service, do not bill; otherwise, bill DME/MAC.

Dressings used with tracheostomies are included in the allowance for the code. This starter kit is covered after a surgical tracheostomy. (https://www.noridianmedicare.com/dme/coverage/docs/lcds/current_lcds/tracheostomy_care_supplies.htm)

IOM: 100-02, 15, 120

⚙ **A4626** Tracheostomy cleaning brush, each

If "incident to" a physician's service, do not bill; otherwise, bill DME/MAC.

IOM: 100-02, 15, 120

◆ **A4627** Spacer, bag, or reservoir, with or without mask, for use with metered dose inhaler

If "incident to" a physician's service, do not bill; otherwise, bill DME/MAC.

IOM: 100-02, 15, 110

✳ **A4628** Oropharyngeal suction catheter, each

If "incident to" a physician's service, do not bill; otherwise, bill DME/MAC.

No more than three catheters per week are covered for medically necessary oropharyngeal suctioning because the catheters can be reused if cleansed and disinfected. (MS Manual System, Pub. 100-3, NCD manual, Chapter 1, Section 280-1

⚙ **A4629** Tracheostomy care kit for established tracheostomy

If "incident to" a physician's service, do not bill; otherwise, bill DME/MAC.

IOM: 100-02, 15, 120

Supplies for Other Durable Medical Equipment

A4630-A4640: Bill DME/MAC

⚙ **A4630** Replacement batteries, medically necessary, transcutaneous electrical stimulator, owned by patient

IOM: 100-03, 3, 160.7

✳ **A4633** Replacement bulb/lamp for ultraviolet light therapy system, each

✳ **A4634** Replacement bulb for therapeutic light box, tabletop model

⚙ **A4635** Underarm pad, crutch, replacement, each

IOM: 100-03, 4, 280.1

▶ New   → Revised   ✔ Reinstated   deleted Deleted
⚙ Special coverage instructions   ◆ Not covered or valid by Medicare   ✳ Carrier discretion

⊛ **A4636** Replacement, handgrip, cane, crutch, or walker, each

IOM: 100-03, 4, 280.1

⊛ **A4637** Replacement, tip, cane, crutch, walker, each

IOM: 100-03, 4, 280.1

✳ **A4638** Replacement battery for patient-owned ear pulse generator, each

✳ **A4639** Replacement pad for infrared heating pad system, each

⊛ **A4640** Replacement pad for use with medically necessary alternating pressure pad owned by patient

IOM: 100-03, 4, 280.1; 100-08, 5, 5.2.3

Supplies for Radiological Procedures

✳ **A4641** Radiopharmaceutical, diagnostic, not otherwise classified

Bill local carrier. Is not an applicable tracer for PET scans.

✳ **A4642** Indium In-111 satumomab pendetide, diagnostic, per study dose, up to 6 millicuries

Bill local carrier

Miscellaneous Supplies

✳ **A4648** Tissue marker, implantable, any type, each

Bill local carrier

✳ **A4649** Surgical supply; miscellaneous

Bill local carrier if incident to a physician's service (not separately payable) or if supply for implanted prosthetic device or implanted DME. If other, bill DME/MAC.

✳ **A4650** Implantable radiation dosimeter, each

Bill local carrier

⊛ **A4651** Calibrated microcapillary tube, each

Bill DME/MAC

IOM: 100-04, 3, 40.3

⊛ **A4652** Microcapillary tube sealant

Bill DME/MAC

IOM: 100-04, 3, 40.3

Supplies for Dialysis

A4653-A4932: Bill DME/MAC

✳ **A4653** Peritoneal dialysis catheter anchoring device, belt, each

⊛ **A4657** Syringe, with or without needle, each

IOM: 100-04, 8, 90.3.2

⊛ **A4660** Sphygmomanometer/blood pressure apparatus with cuff and stethoscope

IOM: 100-04, 8, 90.3.2

⊛ **A4663** Blood pressure cuff only

IOM: 100-04, 8, 90.3.2

◆ **A4670** Automatic blood pressure monitor

IOM: 100-04, 8, 90.3.2

⊛ **A4671** Disposable cycler set used with cycler dialysis machine, each

IOM: 100-04, 8, 90.3.2

⊛ **A4672** Drainage extension line, sterile, for dialysis, each

IOM: 100-04, 8, 90.3.2

⊛ **A4673** Extension line with easy lock connectors, used with dialysis

IOM: 100-04, 8, 90.3.2

⊛ **A4674** Chemicals/antiseptics solution used to clean/sterilize dialysis equipment, per 8 oz

IOM: 100-04, 8, 90.3.2

⊛ **A4680** Activated carbon filters for hemodialysis, each

IOM: 100-04, 8, 90.3.2

⊛ **A4690** Dialyzers (artificial kidneys), all types, all sizes, for hemodialysis, each

IOM: 100-04, 8, 90.3.2

⊛ **A4706** Bicarbonate concentrate, solution, for hemodialysis, per gallon

IOM: 100-04, 8, 90.3.2

⊛ **A4707** Bicarbonate concentrate, powder, for hemodialysis, per packet

IOM: 100-04, 8, 90.3.2

⊛ **A4708** Acetate concentrate solution, for hemodialysis, per gallon

IOM: 100-04, 8, 90.3.2

⊛ **A4709** Acid concentrate, solution, for hemodialysis, per gallon

IOM: 100-04, 8, 90.3.2

⊛ **A4714** Treated water (deionized, distilled, or reverse osmosis) for peritoneal dialysis, per gallon

IOM: 100-03, 4, 230.7; 100-04, 3, 40.3

▶ New → Revised ✔ Reinstated deleted Deleted

⊛ Special coverage instructions ◆ Not covered or valid by Medicare ✳ Carrier discretion

⚙ **A4719** "Y set" tubing for peritoneal dialysis

IOM: 100-04, 8, 90.3.2

⚙ **A4720** Dialysate solution, any concentration of dextrose, fluid volume greater than 249cc, but less than or equal to 999cc, for peritoneal dialysis

Do not use AX modifier

IOM: 100-04, 8, 90.3.2

⚙ **A4721** Dialysate solution, any concentration of dextrose, fluid volume greater than 999cc but less than or equal to 1999cc, for peritoneal dialysis

IOM: 100-04, 8, 90.3.2

⚙ **A4722** Dialysate solution, any concentration of dextrose, fluid volume greater than 1999cc but less than or equal to 2999cc, for peritoneal dialysis

IOM: 100-04, 8, 90.3.2

⚙ **A4723** Dialysate solution, any concentration of dextrose, fluid volume greater than 2999cc but less than or equal to 3999cc, for peritoneal dialysis

IOM: 100-04, 8, 90.3.2

⚙ **A4724** Dialysate solution, any concentration of dextrose, fluid volume greater than 3999cc but less than or equal to 4999cc for peritoneal dialysis

IOM: 100-04, 8, 90.3.2

⚙ **A4725** Dialysate solution, any concentration of dextrose, fluid volume greater than 4999cc but less than or equal to 5999cc, for peritoneal dialysis

IOM: 100-04, 8, 90.3.2

⚙ **A4726** Dialysate solution, any concentration of dextrose, fluid volume greater than 5999cc, for peritoneal dialysis

IOM: 100-04, 8, 90.3.2

✳ **A4728** Dialysate solution, non-dextrose containing, 500 ml

⚙ **A4730** Fistula cannulation set for hemodialysis, each

IOM: 100-04, 8, 90.3.2

⚙ **A4736** Topical anesthetic, for dialysis, per gram

IOM: 100-04, 8, 90.3.2

⚙ **A4737** Injectable anesthetic, for dialysis, per 10 ml

IOM: 100-04, 8, 90.3.2

⚙ **A4740** Shunt accessory, for hemodialysis, any type, each

IOM: 100-04, 8, 90.3.2

⚙ **A4750** Blood tubing, arterial or venous, for hemodialysis, each

IOM: 100-04, 8, 90.3.2

⚙ **A4755** Blood tubing, arterial and venous combined, for hemodialysis, each

IOM: 100-04, 8, 90.3.2

⚙ **A4760** Dialysate solution test kit, for peritoneal dialysis, any type, each

IOM: 100-04, 8, 90.3.2

⚙ **A4765** Dialysate concentrate, powder, additive for peritoneal dialysis, per packet

IOM: 100-04, 8, 90.3.2

⚙ **A4766** Dialysate concentrate, solution, additive for peritoneal dialysis, per 10 ml

IOM: 100-04, 8, 90.3.2

⚙ **A4770** Blood collection tube, vacuum, for dialysis, per 50

IOM: 100-04, 8, 90.3.2

⚙ **A4771** Serum clotting time tube, for dialysis, per 50

IOM: 100-04, 8, 90.3.2

⚙ **A4772** Blood glucose test strips, for dialysis, per 50

IOM: 100-04, 8, 90.3.2

⚙ **A4773** Occult blood test strips, for dialysis, per 50

IOM: 100-04, 8, 90.3.2

⚙ **A4774** Ammonia test strips, for dialysis, per 50

IOM: 100-04, 8, 90.3.2

⚙ **A4802** Protamine sulfate, for hemodialysis, per 50 mg

IOM: 100-04, 8, 90.3.2

⚙ **A4860** Disposable catheter tips for peritoneal dialysis, per 10

IOM: 100-04, 8, 90.3.2

⚙ **A4870** Plumbing and/or electrical work for home hemodialysis equipment

IOM: 100-04, 8, 90.3.2

⚙ **A4890** Contracts, repair and maintenance, for hemodialysis equipment

IOM: 100-02, 15, 110.2

⚙ **A4911** Drain bag/bottle, for dialysis, each

⚙ **A4913** Miscellaneous dialysis supplies, not otherwise specified

Items not related to dialysis must not be billed with the miscellaneous codes A4913 or E1699.

⚙ **A4918** Venous pressure clamp, for hemodialysis, each

▶ New → Revised ✔ Reinstated ~~deleted~~ Deleted

⚙ Special coverage instructions ◆ Not covered or valid by Medicare ✳ Carrier discretion

⚙ **A4927**   Gloves, non-sterile, per 100

⚙ **A4928**   Surgical mask, per 20

⚙ **A4929**   Tourniquet for dialysis, each

⚙ **A4930**   Gloves, sterile, per pair

✳ **A4931**   Oral thermometer, reusable, any type, each

✳ **A4932**   Rectal thermometer, reusable, any type, each

Additional Ostomy Supplies

A5051-A5093:   If provided in the physician's office for a temporary condition, the item is incident to the physician's service and billed to the local carrier. If provided in the physician's office or other place of service for a permanent condition, the item is a prosthetic device and billed to the DME/MAC.

⚙ **A5051**   Ostomy pouch, closed; with barrier attached (1 piece), each

IOM: 100-02, 15, 120

⚙ **A5052**   Ostomy pouch, closed; without barrier attached (1 piece), each

IOM: 100-02, 15, 120

⚙ **A5053**   Ostomy pouch, closed; for use on faceplate, each

IOM: 100-02, 15, 120

⚙ **A5054**   Ostomy pouch, closed; for use on barrier with flange (2 piece), each

IOM: 100-02, 15, 120

⚙ **A5055**   Stoma cap

IOM: 100-02, 15, 120

▶ ✳ **A5056**   Ostomy pouch, drainable, with extended wear barrier attached, with filter, (1 piece), each

IOM: 100-02, 15, 120

▶ ✳ **A5057**   Ostomy pouch, drainable, with extended wear barrier attached, with built in convexity, with filter, (1 piece), each

IOM: 100-02, 15, 120

✳ **A5061**   Ostomy pouch, drainable; with barrier attached, (1 piece), each

IOM: 100-02, 15, 120

⚙ **A5062**   Ostomy pouch, drainable; without barrier attached (1 piece), each

IOM: 100-02, 15, 120

⚙ **A5063**   Ostomy pouch, drainable; for use on barrier with flange (2 piece system), each

IOM: 100-02, 15, 120

⚙ **A5071**   Ostomy pouch, urinary; with barrier attached (1 piece), each

IOM: 100-02, 15, 120

⚙ **A5072**   Ostomy pouch, urinary; without barrier attached (1 piece), each

IOM: 100-02, 15, 120

⚙ **A5073**   Ostomy pouch, urinary; for use on barrier with flange (2 piece), each

IOM: 100-02, 15, 120

⚙ **A5081**   Continent device; plug for continent stoma

IOM: 100-02, 15, 120

⚙ **A5082**   Continent device; catheter for continent stoma

IOM: 100-02, 15, 120

✳ **A5083**   Continent device, stoma absorptive cover for continent stoma

⚙ **A5093**   Ostomy accessory; convex insert

IOM: 100-02, 15, 120

Additional Incontinence Appliances/Supplies

A5102-A5114:   If provided in the physician's office for a temporary condition, the item is incident to the physician's service and billed to the local carrier. If provided in the physician's office or other place of service for a permanent condition, the item is a prosthetic device and billed to the DME/MAC.

⚙ **A5102**   Bedside drainage bottle with or without tubing, rigid or expandable, each

IOM: 100-02, 15, 120

⚙ **A5105**   Urinary suspensory, with leg bag, with or without tube, each

IOM: 100-02, 15, 120

→ ⚙ **A5112**   Urinary drainage bag, leg bag, leg or abdomen, latex, with or without tube, with straps, each

IOM: 100-02, 15, 120

⚙ **A5113**   Leg strap; latex, replacement only, per set

IOM: 100-02, 15, 120

⚙ **A5114**   Leg strap; foam or fabric, replacement only, per set

IOM: 100-02, 15, 120

▶ New   → Revised   ✔ Reinstated   ~~deleted~~ Deleted
⚙ Special coverage instructions   ◆ Not covered or valid by Medicare   ✳ Carrier discretion

Supplies for Either Incontinence or Ostomy Appliances

A5120-A5200: If provided in the physician's office for a temporary condition, the item is incident to the physician's service and billed to the local carrier. If provided in the physician's office or other place of service for a permanent condition, the item is a prosthetic device and billed to the DME/MAC.

⚙ **A5120** Skin barrier, wipes or swabs, each
IOM: 100-02, 15, 120

⚙ **A5121** Skin barrier; solid, 6 × 6 or equivalent, each
IOM: 100-02, 15, 120

⚙ **A5122** Skin barrier; solid, 8 × 8 or equivalent, each
IOM: 100-02, 15, 120

⚙ **A5126** Adhesive or non-adhesive; disk or foam pad
IOM: 100-02, 15, 120

⚙ **A5131** Appliance cleaner, incontinence and ostomy appliances, per 16 oz
IOM: 100-02, 15, 120

⚙ **A5200** Percutaneous catheter/tube anchoring device, adhesive skin attachment
IOM: 100-02, 15, 120

Diabetic Shoes, Fitting, and Modifications

A5500-A5513: Bill DME/MAC

⚙ **A5500** For diabetics only, fitting (including follow-up), custom preparation and supply of off-the-shelf depth-inlay shoe manufactured to accommodate multi-density insert(s), per shoe
IOM: 100-02, 15, 140

⚙ **A5501** For diabetics only, fitting (including follow-up), custom preparation and supply of shoe molded from cast(s) of patient's foot (custom-molded shoe), per shoe
Covered when patient has foot deformity that cannot be accommodated by depth shoe
IOM: 100-02, 15, 140

⚙ **A5503** For diabetics only, modification (including fitting) of off-the-shelf depth-inlay shoe or custom-molded shoe with roller or rigid rocker bottom, per shoe
IOM: 100-02, 15, 140

⚙ **A5504** For diabetics only, modification (including fitting) of off-the-shelf depth-inlay shoe or custom-molded shoe with wedge(s), per shoe
IOM: 100-02, 15, 140

⚙ **A5505** For diabetics only, modification (including fitting) of off-the-shelf depth-inlay shoe or custom-molded shoe with metatarsal bar, per shoe
IOM: 100-02, 15, 140

⚙ **A5506** For diabetics only, modification (including fitting) of off-the-shelf depth-inlay shoe or custom-molded shoe with off-set heel(s), per shoe
IOM: 100-02, 15, 140

⚙ **A5507** For diabetics only, not otherwise specified modification (including fitting) of off-the-shelf depth-inlay shoe or custom-molded shoe, per shoe
Only used for not otherwise specified therapeutic modifications to shoe or for repairs to a diabetic shoe(s)
IOM: 100-02, 15, 140

⚙ **A5508** For diabetics only, deluxe feature of off-the-shelf depth-inlay shoe or custom-molded shoe, per shoe

⚙ **A5510** For diabetics only, direct formed, compression molded to patient's foot without external heat source, multiple-density insert(s) prefabricated, per shoe
IOM: 100-02, 15, 140

✳ **A5512** For diabetics only, multiple density insert, direct formed, molded to foot after external heat source of 230 degrees Fahrenheit or higher, total contact with patient's foot, including arch, base layer minimum of 1/4 inch material of shore a 35 durometer or 3/16 inch material of shore a 40 durometer (or higher), prefabricated, each

---

▶ New   → Revised   ✔ Reinstated   ~~deleted~~ Deleted
⚙ Special coverage instructions   ◆ Not covered or valid by Medicare   ✳ Carrier discretion

✳ **A5513** For diabetics only, multiple density insert, custom molded from model of patient's foot, total contact with patient's foot, including arch, base layer minimum of 3/16 inch material of shore a 35 durometer (or higher), includes arch filler and other shaping material, custom fabricated, each

Dressings

A6010-A6512: Bill local carrier if incident to a physician's service (not separately payable) or if supply for implanted prosthetic device or implanted DME. If other, bill DME/MAC.

◆ **A6000** Non-contact wound warming wound cover for use with the non-contact wound warming device and warming card

Bill DME/MAC

IOM: 100-02, 16, 20

✪ **A6010** Collagen based wound filler, dry form, sterile, per gram of collagen

IOM: 100-02, 15, 100

→ ✪ **A6011** Collagen based wound filler, gel/paste, per gram of collagen

IOM: 100-02, 15, 100

✪ **A6021** Collagen dressing, sterile, pad size 16 sq. in. or less, each

IOM: 100-02, 15, 100

✪ **A6022** Collagen dressing, sterile, pad size more than 16 sq. in. but less than or equal to 48 sq. in., each

IOM: 100-02, 15, 100

✪ **A6023** Collagen dressing, sterile, pad size more than 48 sq. in., each

IOM: 100-02, 15, 100

✪ **A6024** Collagen dressing wound filler, sterile, per 6 inches

IOM: 100-02, 15, 100

✳ **A6025** Gel sheet for dermal or epidermal application, (e.g., silicone, hydrogel, other), each

Only for gel sheets for treatment of keloids or other scars

If used for the treatment of keloids or other scars, a silicone gel sheet will not meet the definition of the surgical dressing benefit and will be denied as noncovered.

✪ **A6154** Wound pouch, each

Waterproof collection device with drainable port that adheres to skin around wound. Usual dressing change is up to 3 × per week.

IOM: 100-02, 15, 100

✪ **A6196** Alginate or other fiber gelling dressing, wound cover, sterile, pad size 16 sq. in. or less, each dressing

IOM: 100-02, 15, 100

✪ **A6197** Alginate or other fiber gelling dressing, wound cover, sterile, pad size more than 16 sq. in., but less than or equal to 48 sq. in., each dressing

IOM: 100-02, 15, 100

✪ **A6198** Alginate or other fiber gelling dressing, wound cover, sterile, pad size more than 48 sq. in., each dressing

IOM: 100-02, 15, 100

✪ **A6199** Alginate or other fiber gelling dressing, wound filler, sterile, per 6 inches

IOM: 100-02, 15, 100

✪ **A6203** Composite dressing, sterile, pad size 16 sq. in. or less, with any size adhesive border, each dressing

Usual composite dressing change is up to 3 times per week, one wound cover per dressing change.

IOM: 100-02, 15, 100

✪ **A6204** Composite dressing, sterile, pad size more than 16 sq. in. but less than or equal to 48 sq. in., with any size adhesive border, each dressing

Usual composite dressing change is up to 3 times per week, one wound cover per dressing change.

IOM: 100-02, 15, 100

✪ **A6205** Composite dressing, sterile, pad size more than 48 sq. in., with any size adhesive border, each dressing

Usual composite dressing change is up to 3 times per week, one wound cover per dressing change.

IOM: 100-02, 15, 100

✪ **A6206** Contact layer, sterile, 16 sq. in. or less, each dressing

Contact layers are porous to allow wound fluid to pass through for absorption by separate overlying dressing and are not intended to be changed with each dressing change. Usual dressing change is up to once per week.

IOM: 100-02, 15, 100

▶ New	→ Revised	✔ Reinstated	~~deleted~~ Deleted
✪ Special coverage instructions		◆ Not covered or valid by Medicare	✳ Carrier discretion

⊛ **A6207** Contact layer, sterile, more than 16 sq. in. but less than or equal to 48 sq. in., each dressing

Contact layer dressings are used to line the entire wound; they are not intended to be changed with each dressing change. Usual dressing change is up to once per week.

IOM: 100-02, 15, 100

⊛ **A6208** Contact layer, sterile, more than 48 sq. in., each dressing

Contact layer dressings are used to line the entire wound; they are not intended to be changed with each dressing change. Usual dressing change is up to once per week.

IOM: 100-02, 15, 100

⊛ **A6209** Foam dressing, wound cover, sterile, pad size 16 sq. in. or less, without adhesive border, each dressing

Made of open cell, medical grade expanded polymer; with nonadherent property over wound site

IOM: 100-02, 15, 100

⊛ **A6210** Foam dressing, wound cover, sterile, pad size more than 16 sq. in. but less than or equal to 48 sq. in., without adhesive border, each dressing

Foam dressings are covered items when used on full thickness wounds (e.g., stage III or IV ulcers) with moderate to heavy exudates. Usual dressing change for a foam wound cover when used as primary dressing is up to 3 times per week. When foam wound cover is used as a secondary dressing for wounds with very heavy exudates, dressing change may be up to 3 times per week. Usual dressing change for foam wound fillers is up to once per day (A6209-A6215).

IOM: 100-02, 15, 100

⊛ **A6211** Foam dressing, wound cover, sterile, pad size more than 48 sq. in., without adhesive border, each dressing

IOM: 100-02, 15, 100

⊛ **A6212** Foam dressing, wound cover, sterile, pad size 16 sq. in. or less, with any size adhesive border, each dressing

IOM: 100-02, 15, 100

⊛ **A6213** Foam dressing, wound cover, sterile, pad size more than 16 sq. in. but less than or equal to 48 sq. in., with any size adhesive border, each dressing

IOM: 100-02, 15, 100

⊛ **A6214** Foam dressing, wound cover, sterile, pad size more than 48 sq. in., with any size adhesive border, each dressing

IOM: 100-02, 15, 100

⊛ **A6215** Foam dressing, wound filler, sterile, per gram

IOM: 100-02, 15, 100

⊛ **A6216** Gauze, non-impregnated, non-sterile, pad size 16 sq. in. or less, without adhesive border, each dressing

IOM: 100-02, 15, 100

⊛ **A6217** Gauze, non-impregnated, non-sterile, pad size more than 16 sq. in. but less than or equal to 48 sq. in., without adhesive border, each dressing

IOM: 100-02, 15, 100

⊛ **A6218** Gauze, non-impregnated, non-sterile, pad size more than 48 sq. in., without adhesive border, each dressing

IOM: 100-02, 15, 100

⊛ **A6219** Gauze, non-impregnated, sterile, pad size 16 sq. in. or less, with any size adhesive border, each dressing

IOM: 100-02, 15, 100

⊛ **A6220** Gauze, non-impregnated, sterile, pad size more than 16 sq. in. but less than or equal to 48 sq. in., with any size adhesive border, each dressing

IOM: 100-02, 15, 100

⊛ **A6221** Gauze, non-impregnated, sterile, pad size more than 48 sq. in., with any size adhesive border, each dressing

IOM: 100-02, 15, 100

⊛ **A6222** Gauze, impregnated with other than water, normal saline, or hydrogel, sterile, pad size 16 sq. in. or less, without adhesive border, each dressing

Substances may have been incorporated into dressing material (i.e., iodinated agents, petrolatum, zinc paste, crystalline sodium chloride, chlorhexadine gluconate [CHG], bismuth tribromophenate [BTP], water, aqueous saline, hydrogel, or agents)

IOM: 100-02, 15, 100

▶ New   → Revised   ✔ Reinstated   ~~deleted~~ Deleted
⊛ Special coverage instructions   ◆ Not covered or valid by Medicare   ✳ Carrier discretion

⊛ **A6223** Gauze, impregnated with other than water, normal saline, or hydrogel, sterile, pad size more than 16 sq. in. but less than or equal to 48 sq. in., without adhesive border, each dressing

IOM: 100-02, 15, 100

⊛ **A6224** Gauze, impregnated with other than water, normal saline, or hydrogel, sterile, pad size more than 48 square inches, without adhesive border, each dressing

IOM: 100-02, 15, 100

⊛ **A6228** Gauze, impregnated, water or normal saline, sterile, pad size 16 sq. in. or less, without adhesive border, each dressing

IOM: 100-02, 15, 100

⊛ **A6229** Gauze, impregnated, water or normal saline, sterile, pad size more than 16 sq. in. but less than or equal to 48 sq. in., without adhesive border, each dressing

IOM: 100-02, 15, 100

⊛ **A6230** Gauze, impregnated, water or normal saline, sterile, pad size more than 48 sq. in., without adhesive border, each dressing

IOM: 100-02, 15, 100

⊛ **A6231** Gauze, impregnated, hydrogel, for direct wound contact, sterile, pad size 16 sq. in. or less, each dressing

IOM: 100-02, 15, 100

⊛ **A6232** Gauze, impregnated, hydrogel, for direct wound contact, sterile, pad size greater than 16 sq. in., but less than or equal to 48 sq. in., each dressing

IOM: 100-02, 15, 100

⊛ **A6233** Gauze, impregnated, hydrogel, for direct wound contact, sterile, pad size more than 48 sq. in., each dressing

IOM: 100-02, 15, 100

⊛ **A6234** Hydrocolloid dressing, wound cover, sterile, pad size 16 sq. in. or less, without adhesive border, each dressing

This type of dressing is usually used on wounds with light to moderate exudate with an average of three dressing changes a week.

IOM: 100-02, 15, 100

⊛ **A6235** Hydrocolloid dressing, wound cover, sterile, pad size more than 16 sq. in. but less than or equal to 48 sq. in., without adhesive border, each dressing

IOM: 100-02, 15, 100

⊛ **A6236** Hydrocolloid dressing, wound cover, sterile, pad size more than 48 sq. in., without adhesive border, each dressing

IOM: 100-02, 15, 100

⊛ **A6237** Hydrocolloid dressing, wound cover, sterile, pad size 16 sq. in. or less, with any size adhesive border, each dressing

IOM: 100-02, 15, 100

⊛ **A6238** Hydrocolloid dressing, wound cover, sterile, pad size more than 16 sq. in. but less than or equal to 48 sq. in., with any size adhesive border, each dressing

IOM: 100-02, 15, 100

⊛ **A6239** Hydrocolloid dressing, wound cover, sterile, pad size more than 48 sq. in., with any size adhesive border, each dressing

IOM: 100-02, 15, 100

⊛ **A6240** Hydrocolloid dressing, wound filler, paste, sterile, per ounce

IOM: 100-02, 15, 100

⊛ **A6241** Hydrocolloid dressing, wound filler, dry form, sterile, per gram

IOM: 100-02, 15, 100

⊛ **A6242** Hydrogel dressing, wound cover, sterile, pad size 16 sq. in. or less, without adhesive border, each dressing

Considered medically necessary when used on full thickness wounds with minimal or no exudate (e.g., stage III or IV ulcers)

Usually up to one dressing change per day is considered medically necessary, but if well documented and medically necessary, the payer may allow more frequent dressing changes.

IOM: 100-02, 15, 100

⊛ **A6243** Hydrogel dressing, wound cover, sterile, pad size more than 16 sq. in. but less than or equal to 48 sq. in., without adhesive border, each dressing

IOM: 100-02, 15, 100

⊛ **A6244** Hydrogel dressing, wound cover, sterile, pad size more than 48 sq. in., without adhesive border, each dressing

IOM: 100-02, 15, 100

⊛ **A6245** Hydrogel dressing, wound cover, sterile, pad size 16 sq. in. or less, with any size adhesive border, each dressing

Coverage of a non-elastic gradient compression wrap is limited to one per 6 months per leg.

IOM: 100-02, 15, 100

▶ **New** → **Revised** ✔ **Reinstated** ~~deleted~~ **Deleted**
⊛ **Special coverage instructions** ◆ **Not covered or valid by Medicare** ✳ **Carrier discretion**

⊛ **A6246** Hydrogel dressing, wound cover, sterile, pad size more than 16 sq. in. but less than or equal to 48 sq. in., with any size adhesive border, each dressing

IOM: 100-02, 15, 100

⊛ **A6247** Hydrogel dressing, wound cover, sterile, pad size more than 48 sq. in., with any size adhesive border, each dressing

IOM: 100-02, 15, 100

→ ⊛ **A6248** Hydrogel dressing, wound filler, gel, per fluid ounce

IOM: 100-02, 15, 100

⊛ **A6250** Skin sealants, protectants, moisturizers, ointments, any type, any size

IOM: 100-02, 15, 100

⊛ **A6251** Specialty absorptive dressing, wound cover, sterile, pad size 16 sq. in. or less, without adhesive border, each dressing

IOM: 100-02, 15, 100

⊛ **A6252** Specialty absorptive dressing, wound cover, sterile, pad size more than 16 sq. in. but less than or equal to 48 sq. in., without adhesive border, each dressing

IOM: 100-02, 15, 100

⊛ **A6253** Specialty absorptive dressing, wound cover, sterile, pad size more than 48 sq. in., without adhesive border, each dressing

IOM: 100-02, 15, 100

⊛ **A6254** Specialty absorptive dressing, wound cover, sterile, pad size 16 sq. in. or less, with any size adhesive border, each dressing

IOM: 100-02, 15, 100

⊛ **A6255** Specialty absorptive dressing, wound cover, sterile, pad size more than 16 sq. in. but less than or equal to 48 sq. in., with any size adhesive border, each dressing

IOM: 100-02, 15, 100

⊛ **A6256** Specialty absorptive dressing, wound cover, sterile, pad size more than 48 sq. in., with any size adhesive border, each dressing

Considered medically necessary when used for moderately or highly exudative wounds (e.g., stage III or IV ulcers)

IOM: 100-02, 15, 100

⊛ **A6257** Transparent film, sterile, 16 sq. in. or less, each dressing

Considered medically necessary when used on open partial thickness wounds with minimal exudate or closed wounds

IOM: 100-02, 15, 100

⊛ **A6258** Transparent film, sterile, more than 16 sq. in. but less than or equal to 48 sq. in., each dressing

IOM: 100-02, 15, 100

⊛ **A6259** Transparent film, sterile, more than 48 sq. in., each dressing

IOM: 100-02, 15, 100

→ ⊛ **A6260** Wound cleansers, any type, any size

IOM: 100-02, 15, 100

→ ⊛ **A6261** Wound filler, gel/paste, per fluid ounce, not otherwise specified

Units of service for wound fillers are 1 gram, 1 fluid ounce, 6 inch length, or 1 yard depending on product

IOM: 100-02, 15, 100

→ ⊛ **A6262** Wound filler, dry form, per gram, not otherwise specified

Dry forms (e.g., powder, granules, beads) are used to eliminate dead space in an open wound.

IOM: 100-02, 15, 100

⊛ **A6266** Gauze, impregnated, other than water, normal saline, or zinc paste, sterile, any width, per linear yard

IOM: 100-02, 15, 100

⊛ **A6402** Gauze, non-impregnated, sterile, pad size 16 sq. in. or less, without adhesive border, each dressing

IOM: 100-02, 15, 100

⊛ **A6403** Gauze, non-impregnated, sterile, pad size more than 16 sq. in., less than or equal to 48 sq. in., without adhesive border, each dressing

IOM: 100-02, 15, 100

⊛ **A6404** Gauze, non-impregnated, sterile, pad size more than 48 sq. in., without adhesive border, each dressing

IOM: 100-02, 15, 100

✳ **A6407** Packing strips, non-impregnated, sterile, up to 2 inches in width, per linear yard

IOM: 100-02, 15, 100

⊛ **A6410** Eye pad, sterile, each

IOM: 100-02, 15, 100

▶ New   → Revised   ✔ Reinstated   ~~deleted~~ Deleted

⊛ Special coverage instructions   ◆ Not covered or valid by Medicare   ✳ Carrier discretion

◎ **A6411** Eye pad, non-sterile, each
IOM: 100-02, 15, 100

✳ **A6412** Eye patch, occlusive, each

◆ **A6413** Adhesive bandage, first-aid type, any size, each

First aid type bandage is a wound cover with a pad size of less than 4 square inches.
Medicare Statute 1861(s)(5)

✳ **A6441** Padding bandage, non-elastic, non-woven/non-knitted, width greater than or equal to three inches and less than five inches, per yard

✳ **A6442** Conforming bandage, non-elastic, knitted/woven, non-sterile, width less than three inches, per yard

Non-elastic, moderate or high compression that is typically sustained for one week

✳ **A6443** Conforming bandage, non-elastic, knitted/woven, non-sterile, width greater than or equal to three inches and less than five inches, per yard

✳ **A6444** Conforming bandage, non-elastic, knitted/woven, non-sterile, width greater than or equal to five inches, per yard

✳ **A6445** Conforming bandage, non-elastic, knitted/woven, sterile, width less than three inches, per yard

✳ **A6446** Conforming bandage, non-elastic, knitted/woven, sterile, width greater than or equal to three inches and less than five inches, per yard

✳ **A6447** Conforming bandage, non-elastic, knitted/woven, sterile, width greater than or equal to five inches, per yard

✳ **A6448** Light compression bandage, elastic, knitted/woven, width less than three inches, per yard

Used to hold wound cover dressings in place over a wound. Example is an ACE type elastic bandages.

✳ **A6449** Light compression bandage, elastic, knitted/woven, width greater than or equal to three inches and less than five inches, per yard

✳ **A6450** Light compression bandage, elastic, knitted/woven, width greater than or equal to five inches, per yard

✳ **A6451** Moderate compression bandage, elastic, knitted/woven, load resistance of 1.25 to 1.34 foot pounds at 50% maximum stretch, width greater than or equal to three inches and less than five inches, per yard

Elastic bandages that produce moderate compression that is typically sustained for one week

Medicare considers coverage if part of a multi-layer compression bandage system for the treatment of a venous stasis ulcer. Do not assign for strains or sprains.

✳ **A6452** High compression bandage, elastic, knitted/woven, load resistance greater than or equal to 1.35 foot pounds at 50% maximum stretch, width greater than or equal to three inches and less than five inches, per yard

Elastic bandages that produce high compression that is typically sustained for one week

✳ **A6453** Self-adherent bandage, elastic, non-knitted/non-woven, width less than three inches, per yard

✳ **A6454** Self-adherent bandage, elastic, non-knitted/non-woven, width greater than or equal to three inches and less than five inches, per yard

✳ **A6455** Self-adherent bandage, elastic, non-knitted/non-woven, width greater than or equal to five inches, per yard

✳ **A6456** Zinc paste impregnated bandage, non-elastic, knitted/woven, width greater than or equal to three inches and less than five inches, per yard

✳ **A6457** Tubular dressing with or without elastic, any width, per linear yard

◎ **A6501** Compression burn garment, bodysuit (head to foot), custom fabricated   A

Garments used to reduce hypertrophic scarring and joint contractures following burn injury
IOM: 100-02, 15, 100

◎ **A6502** Compression burn garment, chin strap, custom fabricated
IOM: 100-02, 15, 100

◎ **A6503** Compression burn garment, facial hood, custom fabricated
IOM: 100-02, 15, 100

◎ **A6504** Compression burn garment, glove to wrist, custom fabricated
IOM: 100-02, 15, 100

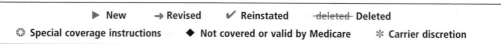

▶ New   → Revised   ✔ Reinstated   deleted Deleted
◎ Special coverage instructions   ◆ Not covered or valid by Medicare   ✳ Carrier discretion

☼ **A6505** Compression burn garment, glove to elbow, custom fabricated

IOM: 100-02, 15, 100

☼ **A6506** Compression burn garment, glove to axilla, custom fabricated

IOM: 100-02, 15, 100

☼ **A6507** Compression burn garment, foot to knee length, custom fabricated

IOM: 100-02, 15, 100

☼ **A6508** Compression burn garment, foot to thigh length, custom fabricated

IOM: 100-02, 15, 100

☼ **A6509** Compression burn garment, upper trunk to waist including arm openings (vest), custom fabricated

IOM: 100-02, 15, 100

☼ **A6510** Compression burn garment, trunk, including arms down to leg openings (leotard), custom fabricated

IOM: 100-02, 15, 100

☼ **A6511** Compression burn garment, lower trunk including leg openings (panty), custom fabricated

IOM: 100-02, 15, 100

☼ **A6512** Compression burn garment, not otherwise classified

IOM: 100-02, 15, 100

✳ **A6513** Compression burn mask, face and/or neck, plastic or equal, custom fabricated

Bill DME/MAC

GRADIENT COMPRESSION STOCKINGS (A6530-A6549)

A6530-A6549: Bill DME/MAC

→ ◆ **A6530** Gradient compression stocking, below knee, 18–30 mmHg, each

IOM: 100-03, 4, 280.1

☼ **A6531** Gradient compression stocking, below knee, 30–40 mmHg, each

Covered when used in treatment of open venous stasis ulcer. Modifiers A1-A9 are not assigned. Must be billed with AW, RT, or LT

IOM: 100-02, 15, 100

☼ **A6532** Gradient compression stocking, below knee, 40–50 mmHg, each

Covered when used in treatment of open venous stasis ulcer. Modifiers A1-A9 are not assigned. Must be billed with AW, RT, or LT

IOM: 100-02, 15, 100

→ ◆ **A6533** Gradient compression stocking, thigh length, 18–30 mmHg, each

IOM: 100-02, 15, 130; 100-03, 4, 280.1

→ ◆ **A6534** Gradient compression stocking, thigh length, 30–40 mmHg, each

IOM: 100-02, 15, 130; 100-03, 4, 280.1

→ ◆ **A6535** Gradient compression stocking, thigh length, 40–50 mmHg, each

IOM: 100-02, 15, 130; 100-03, 4, 280.1

→ ◆ **A6536** Gradient compression stocking, full length/chap style, 18–30 mmHg, each

IOM: 100-02, 15, 130; 100-03, 4, 280.1

→ ◆ **A6537** Gradient compression stocking, full length/chap style, 30–40 mmHg, each

IOM: 100-02, 15, 130; 100-03, 4, 280.1

→ ◆ **A6538** Gradient compression stocking, full length/chap style, 40–50 mmHg, each

IOM: 100-02, 15, 130; 100-03, 4, 280.1

→ ◆ **A6539** Gradient compression stocking, waist length, 18–30 mmHg, each

IOM: 100-02, 15, 130; 100-03, 4, 280.1

→ ◆ **A6540** Gradient compression stocking, waist length, 30–40 mmHg, each

IOM: 100-02, 15, 130; 100-03, 4, 280.1

→ ◆ **A6541** Gradient compression stocking, waist length, 40–50 mmHg, each

IOM: 100-02, 15, 130; 100-03, 4, 280.1

→ ◆ **A6544** Gradient compression stocking, garter belt

IOM: 100-02, 15, 130; 100-03, 4, 280.1

→ ☼ **A6545** Gradient compression wrap, non-elastic, below knee, 30-50 mm hg, each

Modifiers -RT and/or -LT must be appended. When assigned for bilateral items (left/right) on the same date of service, bill both items on the same claim line using -RT/-LT modifiers and 2 units of service.

IOM: 10-02, 15, 100

→ ◆ **A6549** Gradient compression stocking/sleeve, not otherwise specified

IOM: 100-02, 15, 130; 100-03, 4, 280.1

▶ New → Revised ✔ Reinstated ~~deleted~~ Deleted
☼ Special coverage instructions ◆ Not covered or valid by Medicare ✳ Carrier discretion

WOUND CARE (A6550)

* **A6550** Wound care set, for negative pressure wound therapy electrical pump, includes all supplies and accessories

  Bill DME/MAC

RESPIRATORY DURABLE MEDICAL EQUIPMENT, INEXPENSIVE AND ROUTINELY PURCHASED (A7000-A7509)

* **A7000** Canister, disposable, used with suction pump, each

  Bill DME/MAC

* **A7001** Canister, non-disposable, used with suction pump, each

  Bill DME/MAC

* **A7002** Tubing, used with suction pump, each

  Bill DME/MAC

* **A7003** Administration set, with small volume nonfiltered pneumatic nebulizer, disposable

  Bill DME/MAC

* **A7004** Small volume nonfiltered pneumatic nebulizer, disposable

  Bill DME/MAC

* **A7005** Administration set, with small volume nonfiltered pneumatic nebulizer, non-disposable

  Bill DME/MAC

* **A7006** Administration set, with small volume filtered pneumatic nebulizer

  Bill DME/MAC

* **A7007** Large volume nebulizer, disposable, unfilled, used with aerosol compressor

  Bill DME/MAC

* **A7008** Large volume nebulizer, disposable, prefilled, used with aerosol compressor

  Bill DME/MAC

* **A7009** Reservoir bottle, nondisposable, used with large volume ultrasonic nebulizer

  Bill DME/MAC

* **A7010** Corrugated tubing, disposable, used with large volume nebulizer, 100 feet

  Bill DME/MAC

* **A7011** Corrugated tubing, non-disposable, used with large volume nebulizer, 10 feet

  Bill DME/MAC

* **A7012** Water collection device, used with large volume nebulizer

  Bill DME/MAC

→ * **A7013** Filter, disposable, used with aerosol compressor or ultrasonic generator

  Bill DME/MAC

* **A7014** Filter, non-disposable, used with aerosol compressor or ultrasonic generator

  Bill DME/MAC

* **A7015** Aerosol mask, used with DME nebulizer

  Bill DME/MAC

* **A7016** Dome and mouthpiece, used with small volume ultrasonic nebulizer

  Bill DME/MAC

☺ **A7017** Nebulizer, durable, glass or autoclavable plastic, bottle type, not used with oxygen

  Bill DME/MAC

  IOM: 100-03, 4, 280.1

* **A7018** Water, distilled, used with large volume nebulizer, 1000 ml

  Bill DME/MAC

▶ * **A7020** Interface for cough stimulating device, includes all components, replacement only

  Bill DME/MAC

* **A7025** High frequency chest wall oscillation system vest, replacement for use with patient owned equipment, each

  Bill DME/MAC

* **A7026** High frequency chest wall oscillation system hose, replacement for use with patient owned equipment, each

  Bill DME/MAC

* **A7027** Combination oral/nasal mask, used with continuous positive airway pressure device, each

  Bill DME/MAC

* **A7028** Oral cushion for combination oral/nasal mask, replacement only, each

  Bill DME/MAC

| ▶ New | → Revised | ✔ Reinstated | -deleted- Deleted |

☺ Special coverage instructions   ◆ Not covered or valid by Medicare   * Carrier discretion

* **A7029** Nasal pillows for combination oral/nasal mask, replacement only, pair

Bill DME/MAC

* **A7030** Full face mask used with positive airway pressure device, each

Bill DME/MAC

* **A7031** Face mask interface, replacement for full face mask, each

Bill DME/MAC

* **A7032** Cushion for use on nasal mask interface, replacement only, each

Bill DME/MAC

* **A7033** Pillow for use on nasal cannula type interface, replacement only, pair

Bill DME/MAC

* **A7034** Nasal interface (mask or cannula type) used with positive airway pressure device, with or without head strap

Bill DME/MAC

* **A7035** Headgear used with positive airway pressure device

Bill DME/MAC

* **A7036** Chinstrap used with positive airway pressure device

Bill DME/MAC

* **A7037** Tubing used with positive airway pressure device

Bill DME/MAC

* **A7038** Filter, disposable, used with positive airway pressure device

Bill DME/MAC

* **A7039** Filter, non disposable, used with positive airway pressure device

Bill DME/MAC

* **A7040** One way chest drain valve

Bill local carrier

* **A7041** Water seal drainage container and tubing for use with implanted chest tube

Bill local carrier

* **A7042** Implanted pleural catheter, each

Bill local carrier

* **A7043** Vacuum drainage bottle and tubing for use with implanted catheter

Bill local carrier

* **A7044** Oral interface used with positive airway pressure device, each

Bill DME/MAC

☺ **A7045** Exhalation port with or without swivel used with accessories for positive airway devices, replacement only

Bill DME/MAC

IOM: 100-03, 4, 230.17

☺ **A7046** Water chamber for humidifier, used with positive airway pressure device, replacement, each

Bill DME/MAC

IOM: 100-03, 4, 230.17

☺ **A7501** Tracheostoma valve, including diaphragm, each

Bill DME/MAC

IOM: 100-02, 15, 120

☺ **A7502** Replacement diaphragm/faceplate for tracheostoma valve, each

Bill DME/MAC

IOM: 100-02, 15, 120

☺ **A7503** Filter holder or filter cap, reusable, for use in a tracheostoma heat and moisture exchange system, each

Bill DME/MAC

IOM: 100-02, 15, 120

☺ **A7504** Filter for use in a tracheostoma heat and moisture exchange system, each

Bill DME/MAC

IOM: 100-02, 15, 120

☺ **A7505** Housing, reusable without adhesive, for use in a heat and moisture exchange system and/or with a tracheostoma valve, each

Bill DME/MAC

IOM: 100-02, 15, 120

☺ **A7506** Adhesive disc for use in a heat and moisture exchange system and/or with tracheostoma valve, any type, each

Bill DME/MAC

IOM: 100-02, 15, 120

☺ **A7507** Filter holder and integrated filter without adhesive, for use in a tracheostoma heat and moisture exchange system, each

Bill DME/MAC

IOM: 100-02, 15, 120

▶ **New** → **Revised** ✔ **Reinstated** ~~deleted~~ **Deleted**

☺ **Special coverage instructions** ◆ **Not covered or valid by Medicare** * **Carrier discretion**

© **A7508**   Housing and integrated adhesive, for use in a tracheostoma heat and moisture exchange system and/or with a tracheostoma valve, each

Bill DME/MAC

IOM: 100-02, 15, 120

© **A7509**   Filter holder and integrated filter housing, and adhesive, for use as a tracheostoma heat and moisture exchange system, each

Bill DME/MAC

IOM: 100-02, 15, 120

✳ **A7520**   Tracheostomy/laryngectomy tube, non-cuffed, polyvinylchloride (PVC), silicone or equal, each

Bill DME/MAC

✳ **A7521**   Tracheostomy/laryngectomy tube, cuffed, polyvinylchloride (PVC), silicone or equal, each

Bill DME/MAC

✳ **A7522**   Tracheostomy/laryngectomy tube, stainless steel or equal (sterilizable and reusable), each

Bill DME/MAC

✳ **A7523**   Tracheostomy shower protector, each

Bill DME/MAC

✳ **A7524**   Tracheostoma stent/stud/button, each

Bill DME/MAC

✳ **A7525**   Tracheostomy mask, each

Bill DME/MAC

✳ **A7526**   Tracheostomy tube collar/holder, each

Bill DME/MAC

✳ **A7527**   Tracheostomy/laryngectomy tube plug/stop, each

Bill DME/MAC

HELMETS (A8000-A8004)

A8000-A8004:   Bill DME/MAC

✳ **A8000**   Helmet, protective, soft, prefabricated, includes all components and accessories

✳ **A8001**   Helmet, protective, hard, prefabricated, includes all components and accessories

✳ **A8002**   Helmet, protective, soft, custom fabricated, includes all components and accessories

✳ **A8003**   Helmet, protective, hard, custom fabricated, includes all components and accessories

✳ **A8004**   Soft interface for helmet, replacement only

ADMINISTRATIVE, MISCELLANEOUS, AND INVESTIGATIONAL (A9000-A9999)

NOTE: The following codes do not imply that codes in other sections are necessarily covered.

© **A9150**   Non-prescription drugs

Bill local carrier

IOM: 100-02, 15, 50

◆ **A9152**   Single vitamin/mineral/trace element, oral, per dose, not otherwise specified

Bill local carrier

◆ **A9153**   Multiple vitamins, with or without minerals and trace elements, oral, per dose, not otherwise specified

Bill local carrier

✳ **A9155**   Artificial saliva, 30 ml

Bill local carrier

◆ **A9180**   Pediculosis (lice infestation) treatment, topical, for administration by patient/caretaker

Bill local carrier

◆ **A9270**   Non-covered item or service

Bill DME/MAC

IOM: 100-02, 16, 20

▶ ◆ **A9272**   Mechanical wound suction, disposable, includes dressing, all accessories and components, each

▶ ◆ **A9273**   Hot water bottle, ice cap or collar, heat and/or cold wrap, any type

◆ **A9274**   External ambulatory insulin delivery system, disposable, each, includes all supplies and accessories

Bill DME/MAC

◆ **A9275**   Home glucose disposable monitor, includes test strips

Bill DME/MAC

◆ **A9276**   Sensor; invasive (e.g. subcutaneous), disposable, for use with interstitial continuous glucose monitoring system, one unit = 1 day supply

Bill DME/MAC

Medicare Statute 1861(n)

▶ New   → Revised   ✔ Reinstated   ~~deleted~~ Deleted

© Special coverage instructions   ◆ Not covered or valid by Medicare   ✳ Carrier discretion

◆ **A9277** Transmitter; external, for use with interstitial continuous glucose monitoring system

Bill DME/MAC

Medicare Statute 1861(n)

◆ **A9278** Receiver (monitor); external, for use with interstitial continuous glucose monitoring system

Bill DME/MAC

Medicare Statute 1861(n)

◆ **A9279** Monitoring feature/device, stand-alone or integrated, any type, includes all accessories, components and electronics, not otherwise classified

Bill DME/MAC

◆ **A9280** Alert or alarm device, not otherwise classified

Bill DME/MAC

Medicare Statute 1861

◆ **A9281** Reaching/grabbing device, any type, any length, each

Bill DME/MAC

Medicare Statute 1862 SSA

◆ **A9282** Wig, any type, each

Bill DME/MAC

Medicare Statute 1862 SSA

◆ **A9283** Foot pressure off loading/supportive device, any type, each

Bill DME/MAC

Medicare Statute 1862A(i)13

◎ **A9284** Spirometer, non-electronic, includes all accessories

Bill DME/MAC

◆ **A9300** Exercise equipment

Bill DME/MAC

IOM: 100-02, 15, 110.1; 100-03, 4, 280.1

Supplies for Radiology Procedures (Radiopharmaceuticals)

A9500-A9700: Bill local carrier

✳ **A9500** Technetium Tc-99m sestamibi, diagnostic, per study dose

Should be filed on same claim as procedure code reporting radiopharmaceutical. Verify with payer definition of a "study."

✳ **A9501** Technetium Tc-99m teboroxime, diagnostic, per study dose

✳ **A9502** Technetium Tc-99m tetrofosmin, diagnostic, per study dose

✳ **A9503** Technetium Tc-99m medronate, diagnostic, per study dose, up to 30 millicuries

✳ **A9504** Technetium Tc-99m apcitide, diagnostic, per study dose, up to 20 millicuries

✳ **A9505** Thallium Tl-201 thallous chloride, diagnostic, per millicurie

✳ **A9507** Indium In-111 capromab pendetide, diagnostic, per study dose, up to 10 millicuries

✳ **A9508** Iodine I-131 iobenguane sulfate, diagnostic, per 0.5 millicurie

✳ **A9509** Iodine I-123 sodium iodide, diagnostic, per millicurie

✳ **A9510** Technetium Tc-99m disofenin, diagnostic, per study dose, up to 15 millicuries

✳ **A9512** Technetium Tc-99m pertechnetate, diagnostic, per millicurie

✳ **A9516** Iodine I-123 sodium iodide, diagnostic, per 100 microcuries, up to 999 microcuries

✳ **A9517** Iodine I-131 sodium iodide capsule(s), therapeutic, per millicurie

✳ **A9521** Technetium Tc-99m exametazime, diagnostic, per study dose, up to 25 millicuries

✳ **A9524** Iodine I-131 iodinated serum albumin, diagnostic, per 5 microcuries

✳ **A9526** Nitrogen N-13 ammonia, diagnostic, per study dose, up to 40 millicuries

✳ **A9527** Iodine I-125, sodium iodide solution, therapeutic, per millicurie

✳ **A9528** Iodine I-131 sodium iodide capsule(s), diagnostic, per millicurie

✳ **A9529** Iodine I-131 sodium iodide solution, diagnostic, per millicurie

✳ **A9530** Iodine I-131 sodium iodide solution, therapeutic, per millicurie

✳ **A9531** Iodine I-131 sodium iodide, diagnostic, per microcurie (up to 100 microcuries)

✳ **A9532** Iodine I-125 serum albumin, diagnostic, per 5 microcuries

✳ **A9536** Technetium Tc-99m depreotide, diagnostic, per study dose, up to 35 millicuries

✳ **A9537** Technetium Tc-99m mebrofenin, diagnostic, per study dose, up to 15 millicuries

---

▶ New → Revised ✔ Reinstated ~~deleted~~ Deleted
◎ Special coverage instructions ◆ Not covered or valid by Medicare ✳ Carrier discretion

* **A9538** Technetium Tc-99m pyrophosphate, diagnostic, per study dose, up to 25 millicuries

* **A9539** Technetium Tc-99m pentetate, diagnostic, per study dose, up to 25 millicuries

* **A9540** Technetium Tc-99m macroaggregated albumin, diagnostic, per study dose, up to 10 millicuries

* **A9541** Technetium Tc-99m sulfur colloid, diagnostic, per study dose, up to 20 millicuries

* **A9542** Indium In-111 ibritumomab tiuxetan, diagnostic, per study dose, up to 5 millicuries

    Specifically for diagnostic use.

* **A9543** Yttrium Y-90 ibritumomab tiuxetan, therapeutic, per treatment dose, up to 40 millicuries

    Specifically for therapeutic use.

* **A9544** Iodine I-131 tositumomab, diagnostic, per study dose

* **A9545** Iodine I-131 tositumomab, therapeutic, per treatment dose

* **A9546** Cobalt Co-57/58, cyanocobalamin, diagnostic, per study dose, up to 1 microcurie

* **A9547** Indium In-111 oxyquinoline, diagnostic, per 0.5 millicurie

* **A9548** Indium In-111 pentetate, diagnostic, per 0.5 millicurie

* **A9550** Technetium Tc-99m sodium gluceptate, diagnostic, per study dose, up to 25 millicuries

* **A9551** Technetium Tc-99m succimer, diagnostic, per study dose, up to 10 millicuries

* **A9552** Fluorodeoxyglucose F-18 FDG, diagnostic, per study dose, up to 45 millicuries

* **A9553** Chromium Cr-51 sodium chromate, diagnostic, per study dose, up to 250 microcuries

* **A9554** Iodine I-125 sodium Iothalamate, diagnostic, per study dose, up to 10 microcuries

* **A9555** Rubidium Rb-82, diagnostic, per study dose, up to 60 millicuries

* **A9556** Gallium Ga-67 citrate, diagnostic, per millicurie

* **A9557** Technetium Tc-99m bicisate, diagnostic, per study dose, up to 25 millicuries

* **A9558** Xenon Xe-133 gas, diagnostic, per 10 millicuries

* **A9559** Cobalt Co-57 cyanocobalamin, oral, diagnostic, per study dose, up to 1 microcurie

* **A9560** Technetium Tc-99m labeled red blood cells, diagnostic, per study dose, up to 30 millicuries

* **A9561** Technetium Tc-99m oxidronate, diagnostic, per study dose, up to 30 millicuries

* **A9562** Technetium Tc-99m mertiatide, diagnostic, per study dose, up to 15 millicuries

* **A9563** Sodium phosphate P-32, therapeutic, per millicurie

* **A9564** Chromic phosphate P-32 suspension, therapeutic, per millicurie

* **A9566** Technetium Tc-99m fanolesomab, diagnostic, per study dose, up to 25 millicuries

* **A9567** Technetium Tc-99m pentetate, diagnostic, aerosol, per study dose, up to 75 millicuries

* **A9568** Technetium TC-99m arcitumomab, diagnostic, per study dose, up to 45 millicuries

* **A9569** Technetium Tc-99m exametazime labeled autologous white blood cells, diagnostic, per study dose

* **A9570** Indium In-111 labeled autologous white blood cells, diagnostic, per study dose

* **A9571** Indium In-111 labeled autologous platelets, diagnostic, per study dose

* **A9572** Indium In-111 pentetreotide, diagnostic, per study dose, up to 6 millicuries

* **A9576** Injection, gadoteridol, (ProHance Multipack), per ml

* **A9577** Injection, gadobenate dimeglumine (MultiHance), per ml

* **A9578** Injection, gadobenate dimeglumine (MultiHance Multipack), per ml

* **A9579** Injection, gadolinium-based magnetic resonance contrast agent, not otherwise specified (NOS), per ml

    NDC: Magnevist, Omniscan, Optimark, Prohance

* **A9580** Sodium fluoride F-18, diagnostic, per study dose, up to 30 millicuries

▶ New   → Revised   ✔ Reinstated   ~~deleted~~ Deleted
☼ Special coverage instructions   ◆ Not covered or valid by Medicare   * Carrier discretion

* **A9581**   Injection, gadoxetate disodium, 1 ml

Local Medicare contractors may require the use of modifier JW to identify unused product from single-dose vials that are appropriately discarded.

* **A9582**   Iodine I-123 iobenguane, diagnostic, per study dose, up to 15 millicuries

Molecular imaging agent that assists in the identification of rare neuroendocrine tumors.

* **A9583**   Injection, gadofosveset trisodium, 1 ml

NDC: Ablavar

▶ * **A9584**   Iodine 1-123 ioflupane, diagnostic, per study dose, up to 5 millicuries

▶ * **A9585**   Injection, gadobutrol, 0.1 ml

* **A9600**   Strontium Sr-89 chloride, therapeutic, per millicurie

* **A9604**   Samarium SM-153 lexidronam, therapeutic, per treatment dose, up to 150 millicuries

✪ **A9698**   Non-radioactive contrast imaging material, not otherwise classified, per study

IOM: 100-04, 12, 70; 100-04, 13, 20

* **A9699**   Radiopharmaceutical, therapeutic, not otherwise classified

✪ **A9700**   Supply of injectable contrast material for use in echocardiography, per study

Bill local carrier

IOM: 100-04, 12, 30.4

Miscellaneous Service Component

* **A9900**   Miscellaneous DME supply, accessory, and/or service component of another HCPCS code

Local carrier if used with implanted DME. If other, bill DME/MAC.

On DMEPOS fee schedule as a payable replacement for miscellaneous implanted or non-implanted items.

* **A9901**   DME delivery, set up, and/or dispensing service component of another HCPCS code

Bill DME/MAC

* **A9999**   Miscellaneous DME supply or accessory, not otherwise specified

Local carrier if used with implanted DME. If other, bill DME/MAC.

On DMEPOS fee schedule as a payable replacement for miscellaneous implanted or non-implanted items.

▶ New   → Revised   ✔ Reinstated   ~~deleted~~ Deleted

✪ Special coverage instructions   ◆ Not covered or valid by Medicare   * Carrier discretion

ENTERAL AND PARENTERAL THERAPY (B4000-B9999)

Enteral Formulae and Enteral Medical Supplies

B4034-B4162: Bill DME/MAC

→ ⊛ **B4034** Enteral feeding supply kit; syringe fed, per day, includes but not limited to feeding/flushing syringe, administration set tubing, dressings, tape

Dressings used with gastrostomy tubes for enteral nutrition (covered under the prosthetic device benefit) are included in the payment.

IOM: 100-02, 15, 120; 100-03, 3, 180.2; 100-04, 20, 100.2.2

→ ⊛ **B4035** Enteral feeding supply kit; pump fed, per day, includes but not limited to feeding/flushing syringe, administration set tubing, dressings, tape

IOM: 100-02, 15, 120; 100-03, 3, 180.2; 100-04, 20, 100.2.2

→ ⊛ **B4036** Enteral feeding supply kit; gravity fed, per day, includes but not limited to feeding/flushing syringe, administration set tubing, dressings, tape

IOM: 100-02, 15, 120; 100-03, 3, 180.2; 100-04, 20, 100.2.2

⊛ **B4081** Nasogastric tubing with stylet

More than 3 nasogastric tubes (B4081-B4083), or 1 gastrostomy/jejunostomy tube (B4087-B4088) every three months is rarely medically necessary

IOM: 100-02, 15, 120; 100-03, 3, 180.2; 100-04, 20, 100.2.2

⊛ **B4082** Nasogastric tubing without stylet

IOM: 100-02, 15, 120; 100-03, 3, 180.2; 100-04, 20, 100.2.2

⊛ **B4083** Stomach tube - Levine type

IOM: 100-02, 15, 120; 100-03, 3, 180.2; 100-04, 20, 100.2.2

✳ **B4087** Gastrostomy/jejunostomy tube, standard, any material, any type, each

✳ **B4088** Gastrostomy/jejunostomy tube, low-profile, any material, any type, each

◆ **B4100** Food thickener, administered orally, per ounce

⊛ **B4102** Enteral formula, for adults, used to replace fluids and electrolytes (e.g. clear liquids), 500 ml = 1 unit

IOM: 100-03, 3, 180.2

⊛ **B4103** Enteral formula, for pediatrics, used to replace fluids and electrolytes (e.g. clear liquids), 500 ml = 1 unit

IOM: 100-03, 3, 180.2

⊛ **B4104** Additive for enteral formula (e.g. fiber)

IOM: 100-03, 3, 180.2

⊛ **B4149** Enteral formula, manufactured blenderized natural foods with intact nutrients, includes proteins, fats, carbohydrates, vitamins and minerals, may include fiber, administered through an enteral feeding tube, 100 calories = 1 unit

Produced to meet unique nutrient needs for specific disease conditions; medical record must document specific condition and need for special nutrient

IOM: 100-02, 15, 120; 100-03, 3, 180.2; 100-04, 20, 100.2.2

⊛ **B4150** Enteral formulae, nutritionally complete with intact nutrients, includes proteins, fats, carbohydrates, vitamins, and minerals, may include fiber, administered through an enteral feeding tube, 100 calories = 1 unit

IOM: 100-02, 15, 120; 100-03, 3, 180.2; 100-04, 20, 100.2.2

⊛ **B4152** Enteral formula, nutritionally complete, calorically dense (equal to or greater than 1.5 kcal/ml) with intact nutrients, includes proteins, fats, carbohydrates, vitamins and minerals, may include fiber, administered through an enteral feeding tube, 100 calories = 1 unit

IOM: 100-02, 15, 120; 100-03, 3, 180.2; 100-04, 20, 100.2.2

⊛ **B4153** Enteral formula, nutritionally complete, hydrolyzed proteins (amino acids and peptide chain), includes fats, carbohydrates, vitamins and minerals, may include fiber, administered through an enteral feeding tube, 100 calories = 1 unit

If 2 enteral nutrition products described by same HCPCS code and provided at same time billed on single claim line with units of service reflecting total calories of both nutrients

IOM: 100-02, 15, 120; 100-03, 3, 180.2; 100-04, 20, 100.2.2

▶ New   → Revised   ✔ Reinstated   ~~deleted~~ Deleted

⊛ Special coverage instructions   ◆ Not covered or valid by Medicare   ✳ Carrier discretion

⊕ **B4154** Enteral formula, nutritionally complete, for special metabolic needs, excludes inherited disease of metabolism, includes altered composition of proteins, fats, carbohydrates, vitamins and/or minerals, may include fiber, administered through an enteral feeding tube, 100 calories = 1 unit

IOM: 100-02, 15, 120; 100-03, 3, 180.2; 100-04, 20, 100.2.2

⊕ **B4155** Enteral formula, nutritionally incomplete/modular nutrients, includes specific nutrients, carbohydrates (e.g. glucose polymers), proteins/amino acids (e.g. glutamine, arginine), fat (e.g. medium chain triglycerides) or combination, administered through an enteral feeding tube, 100 calories = 1 unit

IOM: 100-02, 15, 120; 100-03, 3, 180.2; 100-04, 20, 100.2.2

⊕ **B4157** Enteral formula, nutritionally complete, for special metabolic needs for inherited disease of metabolism, includes proteins, fats, carbohydrates, vitamins and minerals, may include fiber, administered through an enteral feeding tube, 100 calories = 1 unit

IOM: 100-03, 3, 180.2

⊕ **B4158** Enteral formula, for pediatrics, nutritionally complete with intact nutrients, includes proteins, fats, carbohydrates, vitamins and minerals, may include fiber and/or iron, administered through an enteral feeding tube, 100 calories = 1 unit

IOM: 100-03, 3, 180.2

⊕ **B4159** Enteral formula, for pediatrics, nutritionally complete soy based with intact nutrients, includes proteins, fats, carbohydrates, vitamins and minerals, may include fiber and/or iron, administered through an enteral feeding tube, 100 calories = 1 unit

IOM: 100-03, 3, 180.2

⊕ **B4160** Enteral formula, for pediatrics, nutritionally complete calorically dense (equal to or greater than 0.7 kcal/ml) with intact nutrients, includes proteins, fats, carbohydrates, vitamins and minerals, may include fiber, administered through an enteral feeding tube, 100 calories = 1 unit

IOM: 100-03, 3, 180.2

⊕ **B4161** Enteral formula, for pediatrics, hydrolyzed/amino acids and peptide chain proteins, includes fats, carbohydrates, vitamins and minerals, may include fiber, administered through an enteral feeding tube, 100 calories = 1 unit

IOM: 100-03, 3, 180.2

⊕ **B4162** Enteral formula, for pediatrics, special metabolic needs for inherited disease of metabolism, includes proteins, fats, carbohydrates, vitamins and minerals, may include fiber, administered through an enteral feeding tube, 100 calories = 1 unit

IOM: 100-03, 3, 180.2

Parenteral Nutritional Solutions and Supplies

B4164-B5200: Bill DME/MAC

⊕ **B4164** Parenteral nutrition solution: carbohydrates (dextrose), 50% or less (500 ml = 1 unit) - homemix

IOM: 100-02, 15, 120; 100-03, 3, 180.2; 100-04, 20, 100.2.2

⊕ **B4168** Parenteral nutrition solution; amino acid, 3.5%, (500 ml = 1 unit) - homemix

IOM: 100-02, 15, 120; 100-03, 3, 180.2; 100-04, 20, 100.2.2

⊕ **B4172** Parenteral nutrition solution; amino acid, 5.5% through 7%, (500 ml = 1 unit) - homemix

IOM: 100-02, 15, 120; 100-03, 3, 180.2; 100-04, 20, 100.2.2

⊕ **B4176** Parenteral nutrition solution; amino acid, 7% through 8.5%, (500 ml = 1 unit) - homemix

IOM: 100-02, 15, 120; 100-03, 3, 180.2; 100-04, 20, 100.2.2

⊕ **B4178** Parenteral nutrition solution: amino acid, greater than 8.5%, (500 ml = 1 unit) - homemix

IOM: 100-02, 15, 120; 100-03, 3, 180.2; 100-04, 20, 100.2.2

⊕ **B4180** Parenteral nutrition solution; carbohydrates (dextrose), greater than 50% (500 ml = 1 unit) - home mix

IOM: 100-02, 15, 120; 100-03, 3, 180.2; 100-04, 20, 100.2.2

▶ New	→ Revised	✔ Reinstated	deleted Deleted
⊕ Special coverage instructions	◆ Not covered or valid by Medicare	✳ Carrier discretion	

⚙ **B4185** Parenteral nutrition solution, per 10 grams lipids

⚙ **B4189** Parenteral nutrition solution; compounded amino acid and carbohydrates with electrolytes, trace elements, and vitamins, including preparation, any strength, 10 to 51 grams of protein - premix

IOM: 100-02, 15, 120; 100-03, 3, 180.2; 100-04, 20, 100.2.2

⚙ **B4193** Parenteral nutrition solution; compounded amino acid and carbohydrates with electrolytes, trace elements, and vitamins, including preparation, any strength, 52 to 73 grams of protein - premix

IOM: 100-02, 15, 120; 100-03, 3, 180.2; 100-04, 20, 100.2.2

⚙ **B4197** Parenteral nutrition solution; compounded amino acid and carbohydrates with electrolytes, trace elements and vitamins, including preparation, any strength, 74 to 100 grams of protein - premix

IOM: 100-02, 15, 120; 100-03, 3, 180.2; 100-04, 20, 100.2.2

⚙ **B4199** Parenteral nutrition solution; compounded amino acid and carbohydrates with electrolytes, trace elements and vitamins, including preparation, any strength, over 100 grams of protein - premix

IOM: 100-02, 15, 120; 100-03, 3, 180.2; 100-04, 20, 100.2.2

⚙ **B4216** Parenteral nutrition; additives (vitamins, trace elements, heparin, electrolytes) homemix per day

IOM: 100-02, 15, 120; 100-03, 3, 180.2; 100-04, 20, 100.2.2

⚙ **B4220** Parenteral nutrition supply kit; premix, per day

IOM: 100-02, 15, 120; 100-03, 3, 180.2; 100-04, 20, 100.2.2

⚙ **B4222** Parenteral nutrition supply kit; home mix, per day

IOM: 100-02, 15, 120; 100-03, 3, 180.2; 100-04, 20, 100.2.2

⚙ **B4224** Parenteral nutrition administration kit, per day

Dressings used with parenteral nutrition (covered under the prosthetic device benefit) are included in the payment. (www.cms.gov/medicare-coverage-database/)

IOM: 100-02, 15, 120; 100-03, 3, 180.2; 100-04, 20, 100.2.2

⚙ **B5000** Parenteral nutrition solution: compounded amino acid and carbohydrates with electrolytes, trace elements, and vitamins, including preparation, any strength, renal - Amirosyn-RF, NephrAmine, RenAmine - premix

IOM: 100-02, 15, 120; 100-03, 3, 180.2; 100-04, 20, 100.2.2

⚙ **B5100** Parenteral nutrition solution: compounded amino acid and carbohydrates with electrolytes, trace elements, and vitamins, including preparation, any strength, hepatic - FreAmine HBC, HepatAmine - premix

IOM: 100-02, 15, 120; 100-03, 3, 180.2; 100-04, 20, 100.2.2

⚙ **B5200** Parenteral nutrition solution; compounded amino acid and carbohydrates with electrolytes, trace elements, and vitamins, including preparation, any strength, stress - branch chain amino acids - premix

IOM: 100-02, 15, 120; 100-03, 3, 180.2; 100-04, 20, 100.2.2

Enteral and Parenteral Pumps

B9000-B9999: Bill DME/MAC

⚙ **B9000** Enteral nutrition infusion pump - without alarm

Pump will be denied as not medically necessary if medical necessity of pump is not documented

IOM: 100-02, 15, 120; 100-03, 3, 180.2; 100-04, 20, 100.2.2

⚙ **B9002** Enteral nutrition infusion pump - with alarm

IOM: 100-02, 15, 120; 100-03, 3, 180.2; 100-04, 20, 100.2.2

▶ New   → Revised   ✔ Reinstated   ~~deleted~~ Deleted
⚙ Special coverage instructions   ◆ Not covered or valid by Medicare   ✳ Carrier discretion

⊛ **B9004** Parenteral nutrition infusion pump, portable

IOM: 100-02, 15, 120; 100-03, 3, 180.2; 100-04, 20, 100.2.2

⊛ **B9006** Parenteral nutrition infusion pump, stationary

IOM: 100-02, 15, 120; 100-03, 3, 180.2; 100-04, 20, 100.2.2

⊛ **B9998** NOC for enteral supplies

IOM: 100-02, 15, 120; 100-03, 3, 180.2; 100-04, 20, 100.2.2

⊛ **B9999** NOC for parenteral supplies

Determine if an alternative HCPCS Level II or a CPT code better describes the service being reported. This code should be reported only if a more specific code is unavailable.

IOM: 100-02, 15, 120; 100-03, 3, 180.2; 100-04, 20, 100.2.2

CMS HOSPITAL OUTPATIENT PAYMENT SYSTEM (C1000-C9999)

NOTE: C codes are used ONLY as a part of Hospital Outpatient Prospective Payment System (OPPS) and are not to be used to report other services. C codes are updated quarterly by the Centers for Medicare and Medicaid Services.

⊛ **C1300**   Hyperbaric oxygen under pressure, full body chamber, per 30-minute interval

Medicare Statute 1833(t)

⊛ **C1713**   Anchor/Screw for opposing bone-to-bone or soft tissue-to-bone (implantable)

Medicare Statute 1833(t)

⊛ **C1714**   Catheter, transluminal atherectomy, directional

Medicare Statute 1833(t)

⊛ **C1715**   Brachytherapy needle

Medicare Statute 1833(t)

⊛ **C1716**   Brachytherapy source, non-stranded, gold-198, per source

Medicare Statute 1833(t)

⊛ **C1717**   Brachytherapy source, non-stranded, high dose rate iridium 192, per source

Medicare Statute 1833(t)

⊛ **C1719**   Brachytherapy source, non-stranded, non-high dose rate iridium-192, per source

Medicare Statute 1833(t)

⊛ **C1721**   Cardioverter-defibrillator, dual chamber (implantable)

Related CPT codes: 33224, 33240, 33249.

Medicare Statute 1833(t)

⊛ **C1722**   Cardioverter-defibrillator, single chamber (implantable)

Related CPT codes: 33240, 33249.

Medicare Statute 1833(t)

⊛ **C1724**   Catheter, transluminal atherectomy, rotational

Medicare Statute 1833(t)

⊛ **C1725**   Catheter, transluminal angioplasty, non-laser (may include guidance, infusion/perfusion capability)

Medicare Statute 1833(t)

⊛ **C1726**   Catheter, balloon dilatation, non-vascular

Medicare Statute 1833(t)

⊛ **C1727**   Catheter, balloon tissue dissector, non-vascular (insertable)

Medicare Statute 1833(t)

⊛ **C1728**   Catheter, brachytherapy seed administration

Medicare Statute 1833(t)

⊛ **C1729**   Catheter, drainage

Medicare Statute 1833(t)

⊛ **C1730**   Catheter, electrophysiology, diagnostic, other than 3D mapping (19 or fewer electrodes)

Medicare Statute 1833(t)

⊛ **C1731**   Catheter, electrophysiology, diagnostic, other than 3D mapping (20 or more electrodes)

Medicare Statute 1833(t)

⊛ **C1732**   Catheter, electrophysiology, diagnostic/ablation, 3D or vector mapping

Medicare Statute 1833(t)

⊛ **C1733**   Catheter, electrophysiology, diagnostic/ablation, other than 3D or vector mapping, other than cool-tip

Medicare Statute 1833(t)

▶ ⊛ **C1749**   Endoscope, retrograde imaging/illumination colonoscope device (implantable)

Medicare Statute 1833(t)

⊛ **C1750**   Catheter, hemodialysis/peritoneal, long-term

Medicare Statute 1833(t)

⊛ **C1751**   Catheter, infusion, inserted peripherally, centrally, or midline (other than hemodialysis)

Medicare Statute 1833(t)

⊛ **C1752**   Catheter, hemodialysis/peritoneal, short-term

Medicare Statute 1833(t)

⊛ **C1753**   Catheter, intravascular ultrasound

Medicare Statute 1833(t)

⊛ **C1754**   Catheter, intradiscal

Medicare Statute 1833(t)

⊛ **C1755**   Catheter, instraspinal

Medicare Statute 1833(t)

⊛ **C1756**   Catheter, pacing, transesophageal

Medicare Statute 1833(t)

▶ New   → Revised   ✔ Reinstated   ~~deleted~~ Deleted

⊛ Special coverage instructions   ◆ Not covered or valid by Medicare   ✳ Carrier discretion

✿ **C1757** Catheter, thrombectomy/embolectomy
Medicare Statute 1833(t)

✿ **C1758** Catheter, ureteral
Medicare Statute 1833(t)

✿ **C1759** Catheter, intracardiac echocardiography
Medicare Statute 1833(t)

✿ **C1760** Closure device, vascular (implantable/insertable)
Medicare Statute 1833(t)

✿ **C1762** Connective tissue, human (includes fascia lata)
Medicare Statute 1833(t)

✿ **C1763** Connective tissue, non-human (includes synthetic)
Medicare Statute 1833(t)

✿ **C1764** Event recorder, cardiac (implantable)
Medicare Statute 1833(t)

✿ **C1765** Adhesion barrier
Medicare Statute 1833(t)

✿ **C1766** Introducer/sheath, guiding, intracardiac electrophysiological, steerable, other than peel-away
Medicare Statute 1833(t)

✿ **C1767** Generator, neurostimulator (implantable), nonrechargeable
Related CPT codes: 61885, 61886, 63685, 64590.
Medicare Statute 1833(t)

✿ **C1768** Graft, vascular
Medicare Statute 1833(t)

✿ **C1769** Guide wire
Medicare Statute 1833(t)

✿ **C1770** Imaging coil, magnetic reasonance (insertable)
Medicare Statute 1833(t)

✿ **C1771** Repair device, urinary, incontinence, with sling graft
Medicare Statute 1833(t)

✿ **C1772** Infusion pump, programmable (implantable)
Medicare Statute 1833(t)

✿ **C1773** Retrieval device, insertable (used to retrieve fractured medical devices)
Medicare Statute 1833(t)

✿ **C1776** Joint device (implantable)
Medicare Statute 1833(t)

✿ **C1777** Lead, cardioverter-defibrillator, endocardial single coil (implantable)
Related CPT codes: 33216, 33217, 33249.
Medicare Statute 1833(t)

✿ **C1778** Lead, neurostimulator (implantable)
Related CPT codes: 43647, 63650, 63655, 63663, 63664, 64553, 64555, 64560, 64561, 64565, 64573, 64575, 64577, 64580, 64581.
Medicare Statute 1833(t)

✿ **C1779** Lead, pacemaker, trasvenous VDD single pass
Related CPT codes: 33206, 33207, 33208, 33210, 33211, 33214, 33216, 33217, 33249.
Medicare Statute 1833(t)

✿ **C1780** Lens, intraocular (new technology)
Medicare Statute 1833(t)

✿ **C1781** Mesh (implantable)
Medicare Statute 1833(t)

✿ **C1782** Morcellator
Medicare Statute 1833(t)

✿ **C1783** Ocular implant, aqueous drainage assist device
Medicare Statute 1833(t)

✿ **C1784** Ocular device, intraoperative, detached retina
Medicare Statute 1833(t)

✿ **C1785** Pacemaker, dual chamber, rate-responsive (implantable)
Related CPT codes: 33206, 33207, 33208, 33213, 33214, 33224.
Medicare Statute 1833(t)

✿ **C1786** Pacemaker, single chamber, rate-responsive (implantable)
Related CPT codes: 33206, 33207, 33212.
Medicare Statute 1833(t)

✿ **C1787** Patient programmer, neurostimulator
Medicare Statute 1833(t)

✿ **C1788** Port, indwelling (implantable)
Medicare Statute 1833(t)

✿ **C1789** Prosthesis, breast (implantable)
Medicare Statute 1833(t)

▶ New → Revised ✔ Reinstated ~~deleted~~ Deleted
✿ Special coverage instructions ◆ Not covered or valid by Medicare ✳ Carrier discretion

⊗ **C1813**   Prosthesis, penile, inflatable

Medicare Statute 1833(t)

⊗ **C1814**   Retinal tamponade device, silicone oil

Medicare Statute 1833(t)

⊗ **C1815**   Prosthesis, urinary sphincter (implantable)

Medicare Statute 1833(t)

⊗ **C1816**   Receiver and/or transmitter, neurostimulator (implantable)

Medicare Statute 1833(t)

⊗ **C1817**   Septal defect implant system, intracardiac

Medicare Statute 1833(t)

⊗ **C1818**   Integrated keratoprosthesic

Medicare Statute 1833(t)

⊗ **C1819**   Surgical tissue localization and excision device (implantable)

Medicare Statute 1833(t)

⊗ **C1820**   Generator, neurostimulator (implantable), with rechargeable battery and charging system

Related CPT codes: 61885, 61886, 63685, 64590.

Medicare Statute 1833(t)

⊗ **C1821**   Interspinous process distraction device (implantable)

Medicare Statute 1833(t)

▶ ⊗ **C1830**   Powered bone marrow biopsy needle

Medicare Statute 1833(t)

▶ ⊗ **C1840**   Lens, intraocular (telescopic)

Medicare Statute 1833(t)

⊗ **C1874**   Stent, coated/covered, with delivery system

Medicare Statute 1833(t)

⊗ **C1875**   Stent, coated/covered, without delivery system

Medicare Statute 1833(t)

⊗ **C1876**   Stent, non-coated/non-covered, with delivery system

Medicare Statute 1833(t)

⊗ **C1877**   Stent, non-coated/non-covered, without delivery system

Medicare Statute 1833(t)

⊗ **C1878**   Material for vocal cord medialization, synthetic (implantable)

Medicare Statute 1833(t)

⊗ **C1879**   Tissue marker (implantable)

Medicare Statute 1833(t)

⊗ **C1880**   Vena cava filter

Medicare Statute 1833(t)

⊗ **C1881**   Dialysis access system (implantable)

Medicare Statute 1833(t)

⊗ **C1882**   Cardioverter-defibrillator, other than single or dual chamber (implantable)

Related CPT codes: 33224, 33240, 33249.

Medicare Statute 1833(t)

⊗ **C1883**   Adaptor/Extension, pacing lead or neurostimulator lead (implantable)

Medicare Statute 1833(t)

⊗ **C1884**   Embolization protective system

Medicare Statute 1833(t)

⊗ **C1885**   Catheter, transluminal angioplasty, laser

Medicare Statute 1833(t)

▶ ⊗ **C1886**   Catheter, extravascular tissue ablation, any modality (insertable)

Medicare Statute 1833(t)

⊗ **C1887**   Catheter, guiding (may include infusion/perfusion capability)

Medicare Statute 1833(t)

⊗ **C1888**   Catheter, ablation, non-cardiac, endovascular (implantable)

Medicare Statute 1833(t)

⊗ **C1891**   Infusion pump, non-programmable, permanent (implantable)

Medicare Statute 1833(t)

⊗ **C1892**   Introducer/sheath, guiding, intracardiac electrophysiological, fixed-curve, peel-away

Medicare Statute 1833(t)

⊗ **C1893**   Introducer/sheath, guiding, intracardiac electrophysiological, fixed-curve, other than peel-away

Medicare Statute 1833(t)

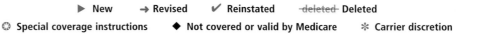

▶ New   → Revised   ✔ Reinstated   ~~deleted~~ Deleted
⊗ Special coverage instructions   ◆ Not covered or valid by Medicare   ✳ Carrier discretion

120

⊛ **C1894** Introducer/sheath, other than guiding, other than intracardiac electrophysiological, non-laser

Medicare Statute 1833(t)

⊛ **C1895** Lead, cardioverter-defibrillator, endocardial dual coil (implantable)

Related CPT codes: 33216, 33217, 33249.

Medicare Statute 1833(t)

⊛ **C1896** Lead, cardioverter-defibrillator, other than endocardial single or dual coil (implantable)

Related CPT codes: 33216, 33217, 33249.

Medicare Statute 1833(t)

⊛ **C1897** Lead, neurostimulator test kit (implantable)

Related CPT codes: 43647, 63650, 63655, 63663, 63664, 64553, 64555, 64560, 64561, 64565, 64575, 64577, 64580, 64581.

Medicare Statute 1833(t)

⊛ **C1898** Lead, pacemaker, other than transvenous VDD single pass

Related CPT codes: 33206, 33207, 33208, 33210, 33211, 33214, 33216, 33217, 33249.

Medicare Statute 1833(t)

⊛ **C1899** Lead, pacemaker/cardioverter-defibrillator combination (implantable)

Related CPT codes: 33216, 33217, 33249.

Medicare Statute 1833(t)

⊛ **C1900** Lead, left ventricular coronary venous system

Related CPT codes: 33224, 33225.

Medicare Statute 1833(t)

⊛ **C2614** Probe, percutaneous lumbar discectomy

Medicare Statute 1833(t)

⊛ **C2615** Sealant, pulmonary, liquid

Medicare Statute 1833(t)

⊛ **C2616** Brachytherapy source, non-stranded, yttrium-90, per source

Medicare Statute 1833(t)

⊛ **C2617** Stent, non-coronary, temporary, without delivery system

Medicare Statute 1833(t)

⊛ **C2618** Probe, cryoablation

Medicare Statute 1833(t)

⊛ **C2619** Pacemaker, dual chamber, non rate-responsive (implantable)

Related CPT codes: 33206, 33207, 33208, 33213, 33214, 33224.

Medicare Statute 1833(t)

⊛ **C2620** Pacemaker, single chamber, non rate-responsive (implantable)

Related CPT codes: 33206, 33207, 33212, 33224.

Medicare Statute 1833(t)

⊛ **C2621** Pacemaker, other than single or dual chamber (implantable)

Related CPT codes: 33206, 33207, 33208, 33212, 33213, 33214, 33224.

Medicare Statute 1833(t)

⊛ **C2622** Prosthesis, penile, non-inflatable

Medicare Statute 1833(t)

⊛ **C2625** Stent, non-coronary, temporary, with delivery system

Medicare Statute 1833(t)

⊛ **C2626** Infusion pump, non-programmable, temporary (implantable)

Medicare Statute 1833(t)

⊛ **C2627** Catheter, suprapubic/cystoscopic

Medicare Statute 1833(t)

⊛ **C2628** Catheter, occlusion

Medicare Statute 1833(t)

⊛ **C2629** Introducer/Sheath, other than guiding, intracardiac electrophysiological, laser

Medicare Statute 1833(t)

⊛ **C2630** Catheter, electrophysiology, diagnostic/ablation, other than 3D or vector mapping, cool-tip

Medicare Statute 1833(t)

⊛ **C2631** Repair device, urinary, incontinence, without sling graft

Medicare Statute 1833(t)

⊛ **C2634** Brachytherapy source, non-stranded, high activity, iodine-125, greater than 1.01 mci (NIST), per source

Medicare Statute 1833(t)

⊛ **C2635** Brachytherapy source, non-stranded, high activity, paladium-103, greater than 2.2 mci (NIST), per source

Medicare Statute 1833(t)

▶ New   → Revised   ✔ Reinstated   ~~deleted~~ Deleted
⊛ Special coverage instructions   ◆ Not covered or valid by Medicare   ＊ Carrier discretion

◎ **C2636** Brachytherapy linear source, non-stranded, paladium-103, per 1 mm

◎ **C2637** Brachytherapy source, non-stranded, Ytterbium-169, per source
Medicare Statute 1833(t)

◎ **C2638** Brachytherapy source, stranded, iodine-125, per source
Medicare Statute 1833(t)(2)

◎ **C2639** Brachytherapy source, non-stranded, iodine-125, per source
Medicare Statute 1833(t)(2)

◎ **C2640** Brachytherapy source, stranded, palladium-103, per source
Medicare Statute 1833(t)(2)

◎ **C2641** Brachytherapy source, non-stranded, palladium-103, per source
Medicare Statute 1833(t)(2)

◎ **C2642** Brachytherapy source, stranded, cesium-131, per source
Medicare Statute 1833(t)(2)

◎ **C2643** Brachytherapy source, non-stranded, cesium-131, per source
Medicare Statute 1833(t)(2)

◎ **C2698** Brachytherapy source, stranded, not otherwise specified, per source
Medicare Statute 1833(t)(2)

◎ **C2699** Brachytherapy source, non-stranded, not otherwise specified, per source
Medicare Statute 1833(t)(2)

◎ **C8900** Magnetic resonance angiography with contrast, abdomen
Medicare Statute 1833(t)(2)

◎ **C8901** Magnetic resonance angiography without contrast, abdomen
Medicare Statute 1833(t)(2)

◎ **C8902** Magnetic resonance angiography without contrast followed by with contrast, abdomen
Medicare Statute 1833(t)(2)

◎ **C8903** Magnetic resonance imaging with contrast, breast; unilateral
Medicare Statute 1833(t)(2)

◎ **C8904** Magnetic resonance imaging without contrast, breast; unilateral
Medicare Statute 1833(t)(2)

◎ **C8905** Magnetic resonance imaging without contrast followed by with contrast, breast; unilateral
Medicare Statute 1833(t)(2)

◎ **C8906** Magnetic resonance imaging with contrast, breast; bilateral
Medicare Statute 1833(t)(2)

◎ **C8907** Magnetic resonance imaging without contrast, breast; bilateral
Medicare Statute 1833(t)(2)

◎ **C8908** Magnetic resonance imaging without contrast followed by with contrast, breast; bilateral
Medicare Statute 1833(t)(2)

◎ **C8909** Magnetic resonance angiography with contrast, chest (excluding myocardium)
Medicare Statute 1833(t)(2)

◎ **C8910** Magnetic resonance angiography without contrast, chest (excluding myocardium)
Medicare Statute 1833(t)(2)

◎ **C8911** Magnetic resonance angiography without contrast followed by with contrast, chest (excluding myocardium)
Medicare Statute 1833(t)(2)

◎ **C8912** Magnetic resonance angiography with contrast, lower extremity
Medicare Statute 1833(t)(2)

◎ **C8913** Magnetic resonance angiography without contrast, lower extremity
Medicare Statute 1833(t)(2)

◎ **C8914** Magnetic resonance angiography without contrast followed by with contrast, lower extremity
Medicare Statute 1833(t)(2)

◎ **C8918** Magnetic resonance angiography with contrast, pelvis
Medicare Statute 1833(t)(2)

◎ **C8919** Magnetic resonance angiography without contrast, pelvis
Medicare Statute 1833(t)(2)

◎ **C8920** Magnetic resonance angiography without contrast followed by with contrast, pelvis
Medicare Statute 1833(t)(2)

◎ **C8921** Transthoracic echocardiography with contrast, or without contrast followed by with contrast, for congenital cardiac anomalies; complete
Medicare Statute 1833(t)(2)

▶ New   → Revised   ✔ Reinstated   ~~deleted~~ Deleted

◎ Special coverage instructions   ◆ Not covered or valid by Medicare   ✳ Carrier discretion

✪ **C8922** Transthoracic echocardiography with contrast, or without contrast followed by with contrast, for congenital cardiac anomalies; follow-up or limited study

Medicare Statute 1833(t)(2)

✪ **C8923** Transthoracic echocardiography with contrast, or without contrast followed by with contrast, real-time with image documentation (2D), includes M-mode recording, when performed, complete, without spectral or color Doppler echocardiography

Medicare Statute 1833(t)(2)

✪ **C8924** Transthoracic echocardiography with contrast, or without contrast followed by with contrast, real-time with image documentation (2D), includes M-mode recording, when performed, follow-up or limited study

Medicare Statute 1833(t)(2)

✪ **C8925** Transesophageal echocardiography (TEE) with contrast, or without contrast followed by with contrast, real time with image documentation (2D) (with or without M-mode recording); including probe placement, image acquisition, interpretation and report

Medicare Statute 1833(t)(2)

✪ **C8926** Transesophageal echocardiography (TEE) with contrast, or without contrast followed by with contrast, for congenital cardiac anomalies; including probe placement, image acquisition, interpretation and report

Medicare Statute 1833(t)(2)

✪ **C8927** Transesophageal echocardiography (TEE) with contrast, or without contrast followed by with contrast, for monitoring purposes, including probe placement, real time 2-dimensional image acquisition and interpretation leading to ongoing (continuous) assessment of (dynamically changing) cardiac pumping function and to therapeutic measures on an immediate time basis

Medicare Statute 1833(t)(2)

✪ **C8928** Transthoracic echocardiography with contrast, or without contrast followed by with contrast, real-time with image documentation (2D), includes M-mode recording, when performed, during rest and cardiovascular stress test using treadmill, bicycle exercise and/or pharmacologically induced stress, with interpretation and report

Medicare Statute 1833(t)(2)

✪ **C8929** Transthoracic echocardiography with contrast, or without contrast followed by with contrast, real-time with image documentation (2D), includes M-mode recording, when performed, complete, with spectral Doppler echocardiography, and with color flow Doppler echocardiography

Medicare Statute 1833(t)(2)

✪ **C8930** Transthoracic echocardiography, with contrast, or without contrast followed by with contrast, real-time with image documentation (2D), includes M-mode recording, when performed, during rest and cardiovascular stress test using treadmill, bicycle exercise and/or pharmacologically induced stress, with interpretation and report; including performance of continuous electrocardiographic monitoring, with physician supervision

Medicare Statute 1833(t)(2)

▶ ✪ **C8931** Magnetic resonance angiography with contrast, spinal canal and contents

Medicare Statute 1833(t)

▶ ✪ **C8932** Magnetic resonance angiography without contrast, spinal canal and contents

Medicare Statute 1833(t)

▶ ✪ **C8933** Magnetic resonance angiography without contrast followed by with contrast, spinal canal and contents

Medicare Statute 1833(t)

▶ ✪ **C8934** Magnetic resonance angiography with contrast, upper extremity

Medicare Statute 1833(t)

▶ ✪ **C8935** Magnetic resonance angiography without contrast, upper extremity

Medicare Statute 1833(t)

▶ ✪ **C8936** Magnetic resonance angiography without contrast followed by with contrast, upper extremity

Medicare Statute 1833(t)

✪ **C8957** Intravenous infusion for therapy/diagnosis; initiation of prolonged infusion (more than 8 hours), requiring use of portable or implantable pump

Medicare Statute 1833(t)

✪ **C9113** Injection, pantoprazole sodium, per vial

Medicare Statute 1833(t)

✪ **C9121** Injection, argatroban, per 5 mg

Medicare Statute 1833(t)

▶ New → Revised ✔ Reinstated deleted Deleted
✪ Special coverage instructions ◆ Not covered or valid by Medicare ✳ Carrier discretion

✳ **C9248** Injection, clevidipine butyrate, 1 mg

Medicare Statute 1833(t)

✿ **C9250** Human plasma fibrin sealant, vapor-heated, solvent-detergent (ARTISS), 2ml

Example of diagnosis codes to be reported with C9250: 941.00–949.5.

621MMA

✿ **C9254** Injection, lacosamide, 1 mg

621MMA

✿ **C9257** Injection, bevacizumab, 0.25 mg

Medicare Statute 1833(t)

~~C9270~~ ~~Injection, immune globulin (Gammaplex), intravenous, non-lyophilized (e.g. liquid), 500 mg~~ ✖

~~Medicare Statute 1833(t)~~

~~C9272~~ ~~Injection, denosumab, 1 mg~~ ✖

~~Medicare Statute 1833(t)~~

~~C9273~~ ~~Sipuleucel-T, minimum of 50 million autologous CD54+ cells activated with PAP-GM-CSF, including leukapheresis and all other preparatory procedures, per infusion~~ ✖

~~Medicare Statute 1833(t)~~

~~C9274~~ ~~Crotalidae polyvalent immune fab (Ovine), 1 vial~~ ✖

~~Medicare Statute 1833(t)~~

▶ ✿ **C9275** Injection, hexaminolevulinate hydrochloride, 100 mg, per study dose

Medicare Statute 1833(t)

~~C9276~~ ~~Injection, cabazitaxel, 1 mg~~ ✖

~~Medicare Statute 1833(t)~~

~~C9277~~ ~~Injection, alglucosidase alfa (Lumizyme), 1 mg~~ ✖

~~Medicare Statute 1833(t)~~

~~C9278~~ ~~Injection, incobotulinumtoxin a, 1 unit~~ ✖

~~Medicare Statute 1833(t)~~

▶ ✿ **C9279** Injection, ibuprofen, 100 mg

Medicare Statute 1833(t)

~~C9280~~ ~~Injection, eribulin mesylate, 1 mg~~ ✖

~~C9281~~ ~~Injection, pegloticase, 1 mg~~ ✖

~~C9282~~ ~~Injection, ceftaroline fosamil, 10 mg~~ ✖

~~C9283~~ ~~Injection, acetaminophen, 10 mg~~ ✖

~~C9284~~ ~~Injection, ipilimumab, 1 mg~~ ✖

▶ ✿ **C9285** Lidocaine 70 mg/tetracaine 70 mg, per patch

Medicare Statute 1833(t)

▶ ✿ **C9286** Injection, betacept, 1 mg

Medicare Statute 1833(t)

▶ ✿ **C9287** Injection, brentuximab vedotin, 1 mg

Medicare Statute 1833(t)

✿ **C9352** Microporous collagen implantable tube (NeuraGen Nerve Guide), per centimeter length

621MMA

✿ **C9353** Microporous collagen implantable slit tube (NeuraWrap Nerve Protector), per centimeter length

621MMA

✿ **C9354** Acellular pericardial tissue matrix of non-human origin (Veritas), per square centimeter

621MMA

✿ **C9355** Collagen nerve cuff (NeuroMatrix), per 0.5 centimeter length

621MMA

✿ **C9356** Tendon, porous matrix of cross-linked collagen and glycosaminoglycan matrix (TenoGlide Tendon Protector Sheet), per square centimeter

621MMA

✿ **C9358** Dermal substitute, native, non-denatured collagen, fetal bovine origin (SurgiMend Collagen Matrix), per 0.5 square centimeters

621MMA

✿ **C9359** Porous purified collagen matrix bone void filler (Integra Mozaik Osteoconductive Scaffold Putty, Integra OS Osteoconductive Scaffold Putty), per 0.5 cc

Medicare Statute 1833(t)

✿ **C9360** Dermal substitute, native, non-denatured collagen, neonatal bovine origin (SurgiMend Collagen Matrix), per 0.5 square centimeters

621MMA

✿ **C9361** Collagen matrix nerve wrap (NeuroMend Collagen Nerve Wrap), per 0.5 centimeter length

621MMA

✿ **C9362** Porous purified collagen matrix bone void filler (Integra Mozaik Osteoconductive Scaffold Strip), per 0.5 cc

621MMA

▶ New   → Revised   ✔ Reinstated   ~~deleted~~ Deleted

✿ Special coverage instructions   ◆ Not covered or valid by Medicare   ✳ Carrier discretion

⊕ **C9363** Skin substitute, Integra Meshed Bilayer Wound Matrix, per square centimeter

621MMA

⊕ **C9364** Porcine implant, Permacol, per square centimeter

621MMA

~~C9365~~ ~~Oasis ultra tri-layer matrix, per square centimeter~~ ✖

▶ ⊕ **C9366** Epifix, per square centimeter

Medicare Statute 1833(t)

▶ ⊕ **C9367** Skin substitute, endoform dermal template, per square centimeter

Medicare Statute 1833(t)(6)

⊕ **C9399** Unclassified drugs or biologicals

621MMA

~~C9406~~ ~~Iodine i 123 ioflupane, diagnostic, per study dose, up to 5 millicuries~~ ✖

⊕ **C9716** Creations of thermal anal lesions by radiofrequency energy

Medicare Statute 1833(t)

⊕ **C9724** Endoscopic full-thickness plication in the gastric cardia using endoscopic plication system (EPS); includes endoscopy

Medicare Statute 1833(t)

⊕ **C9725** Placement of endorectal intracavitary applicator for high intensity brachytherapy

Medicare Statute 1833(t)

⊕ **C9726** Placement and removal (if performed) of applicator into breast for radiation therapy

Medicare Statute 1833(t)

⊕ **C9727** Insertion of implants into the soft palate; minimum of three implants

Medicare Statute 1833(t)

✳ **C9728** Placement of interstitial device(s) for radiation therapy/surgery guidance (e.g., fiducial markers, dosimeter), for other than the following sites (any approach): abdomen, pelvis, prostate, retroperitoneum, thorax, single or multiple

Medicare Statute 1833(t)

~~C9729~~ ~~Percutaneous laminotomy/ laminectomy (intralaminar approach) for decompression of neural elements (with ligamentous resection, discectomy, facetectomy and/or foraminotomy, when performed) any method under indirect image guidance, with the use of an endoscope when performed, single or multiple levels, unilateral or bilateral; lumbar~~ ✖

~~C9730~~ ~~Bronchoscopic bronchial thermoplasty with imaging guidance (if performed), radiofrequency ablation of airway smooth muscle, 1 lobe~~ ✖

~~C9731~~ ~~Bronchoscopic bronchial thermoplasty with imaging guidance (if performed), radiofrequency ablation of airway smooth muscle, 2 or more lobes~~ ✖

▶ ⊕ **C9732** Insertion of ocular telescope prosthesis including removal of crystalline lens

Medicare Statute 1833(t)

▶ ⊕ **C9800** Dermal injection procedure(s) for facial lipodystrophy syndrome (LDS) and provision of radiesse or sculptra dermal filler, including all items and supplies

Temporary office-based destination
Medicare Statute 1833(t)

⊕ **C9898** Radiolabeled product provided during a hospital inpatient stay

⊕ **C9899** Implanted prosthetic device, payable only for inpatients who do not have inpatient coverage

Medicare Statute 1833(t)

▶ New   → Revised   ✔ Reinstated   ~~deleted~~ Deleted

⊕ Special coverage instructions   ◆ Not covered or valid by Medicare   ✳ Carrier discretion

DURABLE MEDICAL EQUIPMENT (E0100-E9999)

Canes

E0100-E0105: Bill DME/MAC

⊛ **E0100**   Cane, includes canes of all materials, adjustable or fixed, with tip

IOM: 100-02, 15, 110.1; 100-03, 4, 280.1; 100-03, 4, 280.2

⊛ **E0105**   Cane, quad or three prong, includes canes of all materials, adjustable or fixed, with tips

IOM: 100-02, 15, 110.1; 100-03, 4, 280.1; 100-03, 4, 280.2

Crutches

E0110-E0118: Bill DME/MAC

⊛ **E0110**   Crutches, forearm, includes crutches of various materials, adjustable or fixed, pair, complete with tips and handgrips

Crutches are covered when prescribed for a patient who is normally ambulatory but suffers from a condition that impairs ambulation. Provides minimal to moderate weight support while ambulating.

IOM: 100-02, 15, 110.1; 100-03, 4, 280.1

⊛ **E0111**   Crutch forearm, includes crutches of various materials, adjustable or fixed, each, with tips and handgrips

IOM: 100-02, 15, 110.1; 100-03, 4, 280.1

⊛ **E0112**   Crutches, underarm, wood, adjustable or fixed, pair, with pads, tips, and handgrips

IOM: 100-02, 15, 110.1; 100-03, 4, 280.1

⊛ **E0113**   Crutch underarm, wood, adjustable or fixed, each, with pad, tip, and handgrip

IOM: 100-02, 15, 110.1; 100-03, 4, 280.1

⊛ **E0114**   Crutches, underarm, other than wood, adjustable or fixed, pair, with pads, tips and handgrips

IOM: 100-02, 15, 110.1; 100-03, 4, 280.1

⊛ **E0116**   Crutch, underarm, other than wood, adjustable or fixed, with pad, tip, handgrip, with or without shock absorber, each

IOM: 100-02, 15, 110.1; 100-03, 4, 280.1

⊛ **E0117**   Crutch, underarm, articulating, spring assisted, each

IOM: 100-02, 15, 110.1

✻ **E0118**   Crutch substitute, lower leg platform, with or without wheels, each

Walkers

E0130-E0155: Bill DME/MAC

⊛ **E0130**   Walker, rigid (pickup), adjustable or fixed height

Standard walker criteria for payment: Individual has a mobility limitation that significantly impairs ability to participate in mobility-related activities of daily living that cannot be adequately or safely addressed by a cane. The patient is able to use the walker safely; the functional mobility deficit can be resolved with use of a standard walker.

IOM: 100-02, 15, 110.1; 100-03, 4, 280.1

⊛ **E0135**   Walker, folding (pickup), adjustable or fixed height

IOM: 100-02, 15, 110.1; 100-03, 4, 280.1

⊛ **E0140**   Walker, with trunk support, adjustable or fixed height, any type

IOM: 100-02, 15, 110.1; 100-03, 4, 280.1

⊛ **E0141**   Walker, rigid, wheeled, adjustable or fixed height

IOM: 100-02, 15, 110.1; 100-03, 4, 280.1

⊛ **E0143**   Walker, folding, wheeled, adjustable or fixed height

IOM: 100-02, 15, 110.1; 100-03, 4, 280.1

⊛ **E0144**   Walker, enclosed, four sided framed, rigid or folding, wheeled, with posterior seat

IOM: 100-02, 15, 110.1; 100-03, 4, 280.1

⊛ **E0147**   Walker, heavy duty, multiple braking system, variable wheel resistance

IOM: 100-02, 15, 110.1; 100-03, 4, 280.1

✻ **E0148**   Walker, heavy duty, without wheels, rigid or folding, any type, each

Heavy-duty walker is labeled as capable of supporting more than 300 pounds

✻ **E0149**   Walker, heavy duty, wheeled, rigid or folding, any type

Heavy-duty walker is labeled as capable of supporting more than 300 pounds

✻ **E0153**   Platform attachment, forearm crutch, each

✻ **E0154**   Platform attachment, walker, each

▶ New   → Revised   ✔ Reinstated   ~~deleted~~ Deleted

⊛ Special coverage instructions   ◆ Not covered or valid by Medicare   ✻ Carrier discretion

* **E0155** Wheel attachment, rigid pick-up walker, per pair

Attachments

E0156-E0159: Bill DME/MAC

* **E0156** Seat attachment, walker

* **E0157** Crutch attachment, walker, each

* **E0158** Leg extensions for walker, per set of four (4)

   Leg extensions are considered medically necessary DME for patients 6 feet tall or more

* **E0159** Brake attachment for wheeled walker, replacement, each

Commodes

E0160-E0175: Bill DME/MAC

☺ **E0160** Sitz type bath or equipment, portable, used with or without commode

   IOM: 100-03, 4, 280.1

☺ **E0161** Sitz type bath or equipment, portable, used with or without commode, with faucet attachment/s

   IOM: 100-03, 4, 280.1

☺ **E0162** Sitz bath chair

   IOM: 100-03, 4, 280.1

☺ **E0163** Commode chair, mobile or stationary, with fixed arms

   IOM: 100-02, 15, 110.1; 100-03, 4, 280.1

☺ **E0165** Commode chair, mobile or stationary, with detachable arms

   IOM: 100-02, 15, 110.1; 100-03, 4, 280.1

☺ **E0167** Pail or pan for use with commode chair, replacement only

   IOM: 100-03, 4, 280.1

* **E0168** Commode chair, extra wide and/or heavy duty, stationary or mobile, with or without arms, any type, each

* **E0170** Commode chair with integrated seat lift mechanism, electric, any type

* **E0171** Commode chair with integrated seat lift mechanism, non-electric, any type

◆ **E0172** Seat lift mechanism placed over or on top of toilet, any type

   Medicare Statute 1861 SSA

* **E0175** Foot rest, for use with commode chair, each

Decubitus Care Equipment

E0181-E0199: Bill DME/MAC

☺ **E0181** Powered pressure reducing mattress overlay/pad, alternating, with pump, includes heavy duty

   Requires the provider to determine medical necessity compliance. To demonstrate the requirements in the medical policy were met, attach -KX.

   IOM: 100-03, 4, 280.1; 100-08, 5, 5.2.3

☺ **E0182** Pump for alternating pressure pad, for replacement only

   IOM: 100-03, 4, 280.1; 100-08, 5, 5.2.3

☺ **E0184** Dry pressure mattress

   IOM: 100-03, 4, 280.1; 100-08, 5, 5.2.3

☺ **E0185** Gel or gel-like pressure pad for mattress, standard mattress length and width

   IOM: 100-03, 4, 280.1; 100-08, 5, 5.2.3

☺ **E0186** Air pressure mattress

   IOM: 100-03, 4, 280.1

☺ **E0187** Water pressure mattress

   IOM: 100-03, 4, 280.1

☺ **E0188** Synthetic sheepskin pad

   IOM: 100-03, 4, 280.1; 100-08, 5, 5.2.3

☺ **E0189** Lambswool sheepskin pad, any size

   IOM: 100-03, 4, 280.1; 100-08, 5, 5.2.3

☺ **E0190** Positioning cushion/pillow/wedge, any shape or size, includes all components and accessories

   IOM: 100-02, 15, 110.1

* **E0191** Heel or elbow protector, each

* **E0193** Powered air flotation bed (low air loss therapy)

☺ **E0194** Air fluidized bed

   IOM: 100-03, 4, 280.1

☺ **E0196** Gel pressure mattress

   IOM: 100-03, 4, 280.1

☺ **E0197** Air pressure pad for mattress, standard mattress length and width

   IOM: 100-03, 4, 280.1

☺ **E0198** Water pressure pad for mattress, standard mattress length and width

   IOM: 100-03, 4, 280.1

☺ **E0199** Dry pressure pad for mattress, standard mattress length and width

   IOM: 100-03, 4, 280.1

▶ New → Revised ✔ Reinstated ~~deleted~~ Deleted
☺ Special coverage instructions ◆ Not covered or valid by Medicare * Carrier discretion

Heat/Cold Application

E0200-E0239: Bill DME/MAC

☺ **E0200** Heat lamp, without stand (table model), includes bulb, or infrared element
Covered when medical review determines patient's medical condition is one for which application of heat by heat lamp is therapeutically effective
IOM: 100-02, 15, 110.1; 100-03, 4, 280.1

✳ **E0202** Phototherapy (bilirubin) light with photometer

◆ **E0203** Therapeutic lightbox, minimum 10,000 lux, table top model
IOM: 100-03, 4, 280.1

☺ **E0205** Heat lamp, with stand, includes bulb, or infrared element
IOM: 100-02, 15, 110.1; 100-03, 4, 280.1

☺ **E0210** Electric heat pad, standard
Flexible device containing electric resistive elements producing heat; has fabric cover to prevent burns; with or without timing devices for automatic shut-off
IOM: 100-03, 4, 280.1

☺ **E0215** Electric heat pad, moist
Flexible device containing electric resistive elements producing heat. Must have component that will absorb and retain liquid (water)
IOM: 100-03, 4, 280.1

☺ **E0217** Water circulating heat pad with pump
Consists of flexible pad containing series of channels through which water is circulated by means of electrical pumping mechanism and heated in external reservoir
IOM: 100-03, 4, 280.1

☺ **E0218** Water circulating cold pad with pump
IOM: 100-03, 4, 280.1

✳ **E0221** Infrared heating pad system

☺ **E0225** Hydrocollator unit, includes pads
IOM: 100-02, 15, 230; 100-03, 4, 280.1

◆ **E0231** Non-contact wound warming device (temperature control unit, AC adapter and power cord) for use with warming card and wound cover
IOM: 100-02, 16, 20

◆ **E0232** Warming card for use with the non-contact wound warming device and non-contact wound warming wound cover
IOM: 100-02, 16, 20

☺ **E0235** Paraffin bath unit, portable (see medical supply code A4265 for paraffin)
Ordered by physician and patient's condition expected to be relieved by long term use of modality
IOM: 100-02, 15, 230; 100-03, 4, 280.1

☺ **E0236** Pump for water circulating pad
IOM: 100-03, 4, 280.1

☺ **E0239** Hydrocollator unit, portable
IOM: 100-02, 15, 230; 100-03, 4, 280.1

Bath and Toilet Aids

E0240-E0249: Bill DME/MAC

◆ **E0240** Bath/shower chair, with or without wheels, any size
IOM: 100-03, 4, 280.1

◆ **E0241** Bath tub wall rail, each
IOM: 100-02, 15, 110.1; 100-03, 4, 280.1

◆ **E0242** Bath tub rail, floor base
IOM: 100-02, 15, 110.1; 100-03, 4, 280.1

◆ **E0243** Toilet rail, each
IOM: 100-02, 15, 110.1; 100-03, 4, 280.1

◆ **E0244** Raised toilet seat
IOM: 100-03, 4, 280.1

◆ **E0245** Tub stool or bench
IOM: 100-03, 4, 280.1

✳ **E0246** Transfer tub rail attachment

☺ **E0247** Transfer bench for tub or toilet with or without commode opening
IOM: 100-03, 4, 280.1

☺ **E0248** Transfer bench, heavy duty, for tub or toilet with or without commode opening
IOM: 100-03, 4, 280.1

✳ **E0249** Pad for water circulating heat unit, for replacement only
Describes durable replacement pad used with water circulating heat pump system
IOM: 100-03, 4, 280.1

▶ New → Revised ✔ Reinstated ~~deleted~~ Deleted
☺ Special coverage instructions ◆ Not covered or valid by Medicare ✳ Carrier discretion

Hospital Beds and Accessories

E0250-E0373: Bill DME/MAC

☼ **E0250** Hospital bed, fixed height, with any type side rails, with mattress
IOM: 100-02, 15, 110.1; 100-03, 4, 280.7

☼ **E0251** Hospital bed, fixed height, with any type side rails, without mattress
IOM:100-02, 15, 110.1; 100-03, 4, 280.7

☼ **E0255** Hospital bed, variable height, hi-lo, with any type side rails, with mattress
IOM: 100-02, 15, 110.1; 100-03, 4, 280.7

☼ **E0256** Hospital bed, variable height, hi-lo, with any type side rails, without mattress
IOM: 100-02, 15, 110.1; 100-03, 4, 280.7

☼ **E0260** Hospital bed, semi-electric (head and foot adjustment), with any type side rails, with mattress
IOM: 100-02, 15, 110.1; 100-03, 4, 280.7

☼ **E0261** Hospital bed, semi-electric (head and foot adjustment), with any type side rails, without mattress
IOM: 100-02, 15, 110.1; 100-03, 4, 280.7

☼ **E0265** Hospital bed, total electric (head, foot and height adjustments), with any type side rails, with mattress
IOM: 100-02, 15, 110.1; 100-03, 4, 280.7

☼ **E0266** Hospital bed, total electric (head, foot and height adjustments), with any type side rails, without mattress
IOM: 100-02, 15, 110.1; 100-03, 4, 280.7

◆ **E0270** Hospital bed, institutional type includes: oscillating, circulating and Stryker frame, with mattress
IOM: 100-03, 4, 280.1

☼ **E0271** Mattress, innerspring
IOM: 100-03, 4, 280.1; 100-03, 4, 280.7

☼ **E0272** Mattress, foam rubber
IOM: 100-03, 4, 280.1; 100-03, 4, 280.7

◆ **E0273** Bed board
IOM: 100-03, 4, 280.1

◆ **E0274** Over-bed table
IOM: 100-03, 4, 280.1

☼ **E0275** Bed pan, standard, metal or plastic
IOM: 100-03, 4, 280.1

☼ **E0276** Bed pan, fracture, metal or plastic
IOM: 100-03, 4, 280.1

☼ **E0277** Powered pressure-reducing air mattress
IOM: 100-03, 4, 280.1

✳ **E0280** Bed cradle, any type

☼ **E0290** Hospital bed, fixed height, without side rails, with mattress
IOM: 100-02, 15, 110.1; 100-03, 4, 280.7

☼ **E0291** Hospital bed, fixed height, without side rails, without mattress
IOM: 100-02, 15, 110.1; 100-03, 4, 280.7

☼ **E0292** Hospital bed, variable height, hi-lo, without side rails, with mattress
IOM: 100-02, 15, 110.1; 100-03, 4, 280.7

☼ **E0293** Hospital bed, variable height, hi-lo, without side rails, without mattress
IOM: 100-02, 15, 110.1; 100-03, 4, 280.7

☼ **E0294** Hospital bed, semi-electric (head and foot adjustment), without side rails, with mattress
IOM: 100-02, 15, 110.1; 100-03, 4, 280.7

☼ **E0295** Hospital bed, semi-electric (head and foot adjustment), without side rails, without mattress
IOM: 100-02, 15, 110.1; 100-03, 4, 280.7

☼ **E0296** Hospital bed, total electric (head, foot and height adjustments). Without side rails, with mattress
IOM: 100-02, 15, 110.1; 100-03, 4, 280.7

☼ **E0297** Hospital bed, total electric (head, foot and height adjustments), without side rails, without mattress
IOM: 100-02, 15, 110.1; 100-03, 4, 280.7

✳ **E0300** Pediatric crib, hospital grade, fully enclosed

☼ **E0301** Hospital bed, heavy duty, extra wide, with weight capacity greater than 350 pounds, but less than or equal to 600 pounds, with any type side rails, without mattress
IOM: 100-03, 4, 280.7

☼ **E0302** Hospital bed, extra heavy duty, extra wide, with weight capacity greater than 600 pounds, with any type side rails, without mattress
IOM: 100-03, 4, 280.7

☼ **E0303** Hospital bed, heavy duty, extra wide, with weight capacity greater than 350 pounds, but less than or equal to 600 pounds, with any type side rails, with mattress
IOM: 100-03, 4, 280.7

▶ New → Revised ✔ Reinstated ~~deleted~~ Deleted
☼ Special coverage instructions ◆ Not covered or valid by Medicare ✳ Carrier discretion

⊛ **E0304** Hospital bed, extra heavy duty, extra wide, with weight capacity greater than 600 pounds, with any type side rails, with mattress

IOM: 100-03, 4, 280.7

⊛ **E0305** Bed side rails, half length

IOM: 100-03, 4, 280.7

⊛ **E0310** Bed side rails, full length

IOM: 100-03, 4, 280.7

◆ **E0315** Bed accessory: board, table, or support device, any type

IOM: 100-03, 4, 280.1

∗ **E0316** Safety enclosure frame/canopy for use with hospital bed, any type

⊛ **E0325** Urinal; male, jug-type, any material

IOM: 100-03, 4, 280.1

⊛ **E0326** Urinal; female, jug-type, any material

IOM: 100-03, 4, 280.1

∗ **E0328** Hospital bed, pediatric, manual, 360 degree side enclosures, top of headboard, footboard and side rails up to 24 inches above the spring, includes mattress

∗ **E0329** Hospital bed, pediatric, electric or semi-electric, 360 degree side enclosures, top of headboard, footboard and side rails up to 24 inches above the spring, includes mattress

∗ **E0350** Control unit for electronic bowel irrigation/evacuation system

Pulsed Irrigation Enhanced Evacuation (PIEE) is pulsed irrigation of severely impacted fecal material and may be necessary for patients who have not responded to traditional bowel program.

∗ **E0352** Disposable pack (water reservoir bag, speculum, valving mechanism and collection bag/box) for use with the electronic bowel irrigation/evacuation system

Therapy kit includes 1 B-Valve circuit, 2 containment bags, 1 lubricating jelly, 1 bed pad, 1 tray liner-waste disposable bag, and 2 hose clamps

∗ **E0370** Air pressure elevator for heel

∗ **E0371** Non powered advanced pressure reducing overlay for mattress, standard mattress length and width

Patient has at least one large Stage III or Stage IV pressure sore (greater than 2 × 2 cm.) on trunk, with only two turning surfaces on which to lie

∗ **E0372** Powered air overlay for mattress, standard mattress length and width

∗ **E0373** Non powered advanced pressure reducing mattress

Oxygen and Related Respiratory Equipment

E0424-E0487: Bill DME/MAC

⊛ **E0424** Stationary compressed gaseous oxygen system, rental; includes container, contents, regulator, flowmeter, humidifier, nebulizer, cannula or mask, and tubing

IOM: 100-03, 4, 280.1; 100-04, 20, 30.6

⊛ **E0425** Stationary compressed gas system, purchase; includes regulator, flowmeter, humidifier, nebulizer, cannula or mask, and tubing

IOM: 100-03, 4, 280.1; 100-04, 20, 30.6

⊛ **E0430** Portable gaseous oxygen system, purchase; includes regulator, flowmeter, humidifier, cannula or mask, and tubing

IOM: 100-03, 4, 280.1; 100-04, 20, 30.6

⊛ **E0431** Portable gaseous oxygen system, rental; includes portable container, regulator, flowmeter, humidifier, cannula or mask, and tubing

IOM: 100-03, 4, 280.1; 100-04, 20, 30.6

∗ **E0433** Portable liquid oxygen system, rental; home liquefier used to fill portable liquid oxygen containers, includes portable containers, regulator, flowmeter, humidifier, cannula or mask and tubing, with or without supply reservoir and contents gauge

⊛ **E0434** Portable liquid oxygen system, rental; includes portable container, supply reservoir, humidifier, flowmeter, refill adaptor, contents gauge, cannula or mask, and tubing

Fee schedule payments for stationary oxygen system rentals are all-inclusive and represent monthly allowance for beneficiary. Non-Medicare payers may rent device to beneficiaries, or arrange for purchase of device

IOM: 100-03, 4, 280.1; 100-04, 20, 30.6

⊛ **E0435** Portable liquid oxygen system, purchase; includes portable container, supply reservoir, flowmeter, humidifier, contents gauge, cannula or mask, tubing and refill adaptor

IOM: 100-03, 4, 280.1; 100-04, 20, 30.6

▶ New   → Revised   ✔ Reinstated   ~~deleted~~ Deleted

⊛ Special coverage instructions   ◆ Not covered or valid by Medicare   ∗ Carrier discretion

✿ **E0439** Stationary liquid oxygen system, rental; includes container, contents, regulator, flowmeter, humidifier, nebulizer, cannula or mask, & tubing

This allowance includes payment for equipment, contents, and accessories furnished during rental month

IOM: 100-03, 4, 280.1; 100-04, 20, 30.6

✿ **E0440** Stationary liquid oxygen system, purchase; includes use of reservoir, contents indicator, regulator, flowmeter, humidifier, nebulizer, cannula or mask, and tubing

IOM: 100-03, 4, 280.1; 100-04, 20, 30.6

✳ **E0441** Stationary oxygen contents, gaseous, 1 month's supply = 1 unit

IOM: 100-03, 4, 280.1; 100-04, 20, 30.6

✳ **E0442** Stationary oxygen contents, liquid, 1 month's supply = 1 unit

IOM: 100-03, 4, 280.1; 100-04, 20, 30.6

✳ **E0443** Portable oxygen contents, gaseous, 1 month's supply = 1 unit

IOM: 100-03, 4, 280.1; 100-04, 20, 30.6

✳ **E0444** Portable oxygen contents, liquid, 1 month's supply = 1 unit

IOM: 100-03, 4, 280.1; 100-04, 20, 30.6

✳ **E0445** Oximeter device for measuring blood oxygen levels non-invasively

▶ ◆ **E0446** Topical oxygen delivery system, not otherwise specified, includes all supplies and accessories

✿ **E0450** Volume control ventilator, without pressure support mode, may include pressure control mode, used with invasive interface (e.g., tracheostomy tube)

Patient confined to wheelchair during day may receive reimbursement for 2 ventilators. One ventilator is mounted to wheelchair and second used while in bed

IOM: 100-03, 4, 280.1

✿ **E0455** Oxygen tent, excluding croup or pediatric tents

IOM: 100-03, 4, 280.1; 100-04, 20, 30.6

✳ **E0457** Chest shell (cuirass)

✳ **E0459** Chest wrap

✿ **E0460** Negative pressure ventilator; portable or stationary

Noninvasive device, generates airflow into lungs by creating negative pressure around chest by means of interface

IOM: 100-03, 4, 240.2

✿ **E0461** Volume control ventilator, without pressure support mode, may include pressure control mode, used with non-invasive interface (e.g. mask)

IOM: 100-03, 4, 240.2

✳ **E0462** Rocking bed with or without side rails

✳ **E0463** Pressure support ventilator with volume control mode, may include pressure control mode, used with invasive interface (e.g., tracheostomy tube)

✳ **E0464** Pressure support ventilator with volume control mode, may include pressure control mode, used with non-invasive interface (e.g., mask)

✿ **E0470** Respiratory assist device, bi-level pressure capability, without backup rate feature, used with noninvasive interface, e.g., nasal or facial mask (intermittent assist device with continuous positive airway pressure device)

IOM: 100-03, 4, 240.2

✿ **E0471** Respiratory assist device, bi-level pressure capability, with back-up rate feature, used with noninvasive interface, e.g., nasal or facial mask (intermittent assist device with continuous positive airway pressure device)

IOM: 100-03, 4, 240.2

✿ **E0472** Respiratory assist device, bi-level pressure capability, with backup rate feature, used with invasive interface, e.g., tracheostomy tube (intermittent assist device with continuous positive airway pressure device)

IOM: 100-03, 4, 240.2

✿ **E0480** Percussor, electric or pneumatic, home model

IOM: 100-03, 4, 240.2

◆ **E0481** Intrapulmonary percussive ventilation system and related accessories

IOM: 100-03, 4, 240.2

✳ **E0482** Cough stimulating device, alternating positive and negative airway pressure

✳ **E0483** High frequency chest wall oscillation air-pulse generator system, (includes hoses and vest), each

✳ **E0484** Oscillatory positive expiratory pressure device, non-electric, any type, each

---

▶ New   → Revised   ✔ Reinstated   deleted Deleted

✿ Special coverage instructions   ◆ Not covered or valid by Medicare   ✳ Carrier discretion

* **E0485** Oral device/appliance used to reduce upper airway collapsibility, adjustable or non-adjustable, prefabricated, includes fitting and adjustment

* **E0486** Oral device/appliance used to reduce upper airway collapsibility, adjustable or non-adjustable, custom fabricated, includes fitting and adjustment

⊛ **E0487** Spirometer, electronic, includes all accessories

IPPB Machines

⊛ **E0500** IPPB machine, all types, with built-in nebulization; manual or automatic valves; internal or external power source

Bill DME/MAC

IOM: 100-03, 4, 240.2

Humidifiers/Nebulizers/Compressors for Use with Oxygen IPPB Equipment

E0550-E0585: Bill DME/MAC

⊛ **E0550** Humidifier, durable for extensive supplemental humidification during IPPB treatments or oxygen delivery

IOM: 100-03, 4, 240.2

⊛ **E0555** Humidifier, durable, glass or autoclavable plastic bottle type, for use with regulator or flowmeter

IOM: 100-03, 4, 280.1; 100-04, 20, 30.6

⊛ **E0560** Humidifier, durable for supplemental humidification during IPPB treatment or oxygen delivery

IOM: 100-03, 4, 280.1

* **E0561** Humidifier, non-heated, used with positive airway pressure device

* **E0562** Humidifier, heated, used with positive airway pressure device

* **E0565** Compressor, air power source for equipment which is not self-contained or cylinder driven

⊛ **E0570** Nebulizer, with compressor

IOM: 100-03, 4, 240.2; 100-03, 4, 280.1

E0571 ~~Aerosol compressor, battery powered, for use with small volume nebulizer~~ ✖

~~*IOM: 100-03, 4, 240.2*~~

* **E0572** Aerosol compressor, adjustable pressure, light duty for intermittent use

* **E0574** Ultrasonic/electronic aerosol generator with small volume nebulizer

⊛ **E0575** Nebulizer, ultrasonic, large volume

IOM: 100-03, 4, 240.2

⊛ **E0580** Nebulizer, durable, glass or autoclavable plastic, bottle type, for use with regulator or flowmeter

IOM: 100-03, 4, 240.2; 100-03, 4, 280.1

⊛ **E0585** Nebulizer, with compressor and heater

IOM: 100-03, 4, 240.2; 100-03, 4, 280.1

Suction Pump/Room Vaporizers

E0600-E0606: Bill DME/MAC

⊛ **E0600** Respiratory suction pump, home model, portable or stationary, electric

IOM: 100-03, 4, 240.2

⊛ **E0601** Continuous airway pressure (CPAP) device

IOM: 100-03, 4, 240.4

* **E0602** Breast pump, manual, any type

Bill either manual breast pump or breast pump kit

* **E0603** Breast pump, electric (AC and/or DC), any type

* **E0604** Breast pump, hospital grade, electric (AC and/or DC), any type

⊛ **E0605** Vaporizer, room type

IOM: 100-03, 4, 240.2

⊛ **E0606** Postural drainage board

IOM: 100-03, 4, 240.2

Monitoring Equipment

⊛ **E0607** Home blood glucose monitor

Bill DME/MAC

Document recipient or caregiver is competent to monitor equipment and that device is designed for home rather than clinical use

IOM: 100-03, 4, 280.1; 100-03, 1, 40.2

Pacemaker Monitor

☼ **E0610** Pacemaker monitor, self-contained, (checks battery depletion, includes audible and visible check systems)

Bill DME/MAC

IOM: 100-03, 1, 20.8

☼ **E0615** Pacemaker monitor, self-contained, checks battery depletion and other pacemaker components, includes digital/visible check systems

Bill DME/MAC

IOM: 100-03, 1, 20.8

✱ **E0616** Implantable cardiac event recorder with memory, activator and programmer

Bill local carrier

Assign when two 30-day pre-symptom external loop recordings fail to establish a definitive diagnosis. Bill to local carrier.

✱ **E0617** External defibrillator with integrated electrocardiogram analysis

Bill DME/MAC

✱ **E0618** Apnea monitor, without recording feature

Bill DME/MAC

✱ **E0619** Apnea monitor, with recording feature

Bill DME/MAC

✱ **E0620** Skin piercing device for collection of capillary blood, laser, each

Bill DME/MAC

Patient Lifts

E0621-E0642: Bill DME/MAC

☼ **E0621** Sling or seat, patient lift, canvas or nylon

IOM: 100-03, 4, 240.2, 280.4

◆ **E0625** Patient lift, bathroom or toilet, not otherwise classified

IOM: 100-03, 4, 240.2

☼ **E0627** Seat lift mechanism incorporated into a combination lift-chair mechanism

IOM: 100-03, 4, 280.4; 100-04, 4, 20

Cross Reference Q0080

☼ **E0628** Separate seat lift mechanism for use with patient owned furniture - electric

IOM: 100-03, 4, 280.4; 100-04, 4, 20

Cross Reference Q0078

☼ **E0629** Separate seat lift mechanism for use with patient owned furniture - non-electric

IOM: 100-04, 4, 20

Cross Reference Q0079

☼ **E0630** Patient lift, hydraulic or mechanical, includes any seat, sling, strap(s) or pad(s)

IOM: 100-03, 4, 240.2

☼ **E0635** Patient lift, electric, with seat or sling

IOM: 100-03, 4, 240.2

✱ **E0636** Multipositional patient support system, with integrated lift, patient accessible controls

→ ◆ **E0637** Combination sit to stand frame/table system, any size including pediatric, with seat lift feature, with or without wheels

IOM: 100-03, 4, 240.2

→ ◆ **E0638** Standing frame/table system, one position (e.g. upright, supine or prone stander), any size including pediatric, with or without wheels

IOM: 100-03, 4, 240.2

✱ **E0639** Patient lift, moveable from room to room with disassembly and reassembly, includes all components/accessories

✱ **E0640** Patient lift, fixed system, includes all components/accessories

→ ◆ **E0641** Standing frame/table system, multi-position (e.g. three-way stander), any size including pediatric, with or without wheels

IOM: 100-03, 4, 240.2

→ ◆ **E0642** Standing frame/table system, mobile (dynamic stander), any size including pediatric

IOM: 100-03, 4, 240.2

▶ New   → Revised   ✔ Reinstated   ~~deleted~~ Deleted

☼ Special coverage instructions   ◆ Not covered or valid by Medicare   ✱ Carrier discretion

Pneumatic Compressor and Appliances

E0650-E0676: Bill DME/MAC

⚙ **E0650** Pneumatic compressor, non-segmental home model

Lymphedema pumps are classified as segmented or nonsegmented, depending on whether distinct segments of devices can be inflated sequentially

IOM: 100-03, 4, 280.6

⚙ **E0651** Pneumatic compressor, segmental home model without calibrated gradient pressure

IOM: 100-03, 4, 280.6

⚙ **E0652** Pneumatic compressor, segmental home model with calibrated gradient pressure

IOM: 100-03, 4, 280.6

⚙ **E0655** Non-segmental pneumatic appliance for use with pneumatic compressor, half arm

IOM: 100-03, 4, 280.6

⚙ **E0656** Segmental pneumatic appliance for use with pneumatic compressor, trunk

⚙ **E0657** Segmental pneumatic appliance for use with pneumatic compressor, chest

⚙ **E0660** Non-segmental pneumatic appliance for use with pneumatic compressor, full leg

IOM: 100-03, 4, 280.6

⚙ **E0665** Non-segmental pneumatic appliance for use with pneumatic compressor, full arm

IOM: 100-03, 4, 280.6

⚙ **E0666** Non-segmental pneumatic appliance for use with pneumatic compressor, half leg

IOM: 100-03, 4, 280.6

⚙ **E0667** Segmental pneumatic appliance for use with pneumatic compressor, full leg

IOM: 100-03, 4, 280.6

⚙ **E0668** Segmental pneumatic appliance for use with pneumatic compressor, full arm

IOM: 100-03, 4, 280.6

⚙ **E0669** Segmental pneumatic appliance for use with pneumatic compressor, half leg

IOM: 100-03, 4, 280.6

⚙ **E0671** Segmental gradient pressure pneumatic appliance, full leg

IOM: 100-03, 4, 280.6

⚙ **E0672** Segmental gradient pressure pneumatic appliance, full arm

IOM: 100-03, 4, 280.6

⚙ **E0673** Segmental gradient pressure pneumatic appliance, half leg

IOM: 100-03, 4, 280.6

✳ **E0675** Pneumatic compression device, high pressure, rapid inflation/deflation cycle, for arterial insufficiency (unilateral or bilateral system)

✳ **E0676** Intermittent limb compression device (includes all accessories), not otherwise specified

Ultraviolet Cabinet

E0691-E0694: Bill DME/MAC

→ ✳ **E0691** Ultraviolet light therapy system, includes bulbs/lamps, timer and eye protection; treatment area 2 square feet or less

✳ **E0692** Ultraviolet light therapy system panel, includes bulbs/lamps, timer and eye protection, 4 foot panel

✳ **E0693** Ultraviolet light therapy system panel, includes bulbs/lamps, timer and eye protection, 6 foot panel

✳ **E0694** Ultraviolet multidirectional light therapy system in 6 foot cabinet, includes bulbs/lamps, timer and eye protection

Safety Equipment

E0700-E0705: Bill DME/MAC

✳ **E0700** Safety equipment, device or accessory, any type

⚙ **E0705** Transfer device, any type, each

Restraints

✳ **E0710** Restraints, any type (body, chest, wrist or ankle)

Bill DME/MAC

▶ New   → Revised   ✔ Reinstated   ~~deleted~~ Deleted
⚙ Special coverage instructions   ◆ Not covered or valid by Medicare   ✳ Carrier discretion

Transcutaneous and/or Neuromuscular Electrical Nerve Stimulators (TENS)

⊛ **E0720** Transcutaneous electrical nerve stimulation (TENS) device, two lead, localized stimulation

Bill DME/MAC

A Certificate of Medical Necessity (CMN) is not needed for a TENS rental, but is needed purchase.

IOM: 100-03, 2, 160.2; 100-03, 4, 280.1

⊛ **E0730** Transcutaneous electrical nerve stimulation (TENS) device, four or more leads, for multiple nerve stimulation

Bill DME/MAC

IOM: 100-03, 2, 160.2; 100-03, 4, 280.1

⊛ **E0731** Form fitting conductive garment for delivery of TENS or NMES (with conductive fibers separated from the patient's skin by layers of fabric)

Bill DME/MAC

IOM: 100-03, 2, 160.13

⊛ **E0740** Incontinence treatment system, pelvic floor stimulator, monitor, sensor and/or trainer

Bill DME/MAC

IOM: 100-03, 4, 230.8

✳ **E0744** Neuromuscular stimulator for scoliosis

Bill DME/MAC

⊛ **E0745** Neuromuscular stimulator, electronic shock unit

Bill DME/MAC

IOM: 100-03, 2, 160.12

⊛ **E0746** Electromyography (EMG), biofeedback device

Bill local carrier

IOM: 100-03, 1, 30.1

⊛ **E0747** Osteogenesis stimulator, electrical, non-invasive, other than spinal applications

Bill DME/MAC

Devices are composed of two basic parts: Coils that wrap around cast and pulse generator that produces electric current

⊛ **E0748** Osteogenesis stimulator, electrical, non-invasive, spinal applications

Bill DME/MAC

Device should be applied within 30 days as adjunct to spinal fusion surgery

⊛ **E0749** Osteogenesis stimulator, electrical, surgically implanted

Bill local carrier

✳ **E0755** Electronic salivary reflex stimulator (intra-oral/non-invasive)

Bill DME/MAC

✳ **E0760** Osteogenesis stimulator, low intensity ultrasound, non-invasive

Bill DME/MAC

Ultrasonic osteogenesis stimulator may not be used concurrently with other noninvasive stimulators

⊛ **E0761** Non-thermal pulsed high frequency radiowaves, high peak power electromagnetic energy treatment device

Bill DME/MAC

✳ **E0762** Transcutaneous electrical joint stimulation device system, includes all accessories

Bill DME/MAC

⊛ **E0764** Functional neuromuscular stimulator, transcutaneous stimulation of sequential muscle groups of ambulation with computer control, used for walking by spinal cord injured, entire system, after completion of training program

Bill DME/MAC

IOM: 100-03, 2, 160.12

→ ✳ **E0765** FDA approved nerve stimulator, with replaceable batteries, for treatment of nausea and vomiting

Bill DME/MAC

⊛ **E0769** Electrical stimulation or electromagnetic wound treatment device, not otherwise classified

Bill DME/MAC

IOM: 100-04, 32, 11.1

⊛ **E0770** Functional electrical stimulator, transcutaneous stimulation of nerve and/or muscle groups, any type, complete system, not otherwise specified

Bill DME/MAC

Infusion Supplies

✳ **E0776** IV pole

Bill DME/MAC

▶ New   → Revised   ✔ Reinstated   deleted Deleted

⊛ Special coverage instructions   ◆ Not covered or valid by Medicare   ✳ Carrier discretion

* **E0779**   Ambulatory infusion pump, mechanical, reusable, for infusion 8 hours or greater

Bill DME/MAC

Requires prior authorization and copy of invoice

This is a capped rental infusion pump modifier. The correct monthly modifier (-KH, -KI, -KJ) is used to indicate which month the rental is for (i.e. -KH month 1; -KI, months 2 and 3; -KJ, months 4 through 13).

* **E0780**   Ambulatory infusion pump, mechanical, reusable, for infusion less than 8 hours

Bill DME/MAC

Requires prior authorization and copy of invoice

☺ **E0781**   Ambulatory infusion pump, single or multiple channels, electric or battery operated with administrative equipment, worn by patient

Billable to both the local carrier and the DME/MAC. This item may be billed to the DME/MAC whenever the infusion is initiated in the physician's office but the patient does not return during the same business day.

IOM: 100-03, 1, 50.3

☺ **E0782**   Infusion pump, implantable, non-programmable (includes all components, e.g., pump, catheter, connectors, etc.)

Bill local carrier

IOM: 100-03, 1, 50.3

☺ **E0783**   Infusion pump system, implantable, programmable (includes all components, e.g., pump, catheter, connectors, etc.)

Bill local carrier

IOM: 100-03, 1, 50.3

☺ **E0784**   External ambulatory infusion pump, insulin

Bill DME/MAC

IOM: 100-03, 4, 280.14

☺ **E0785**   Implantable intraspinal (epidural/intrathecal) catheter used with implantable infusion pump, replacement

Bill local carrier

IOM: 100-03, 1, 50.3

☺ **E0786**   Implantable programmable infusion pump, replacement (excludes implantable intraspinal catheter)

Bill local carrier

IOM: 100-03, 1, 50.3

☺ **E0791**   Parenteral infusion pump, stationary, single or multi-channel

Bill DME/MAC

IOM: 100-02, 15, 120; 100-03, 3, 180.2; 100-04, 20, 100.2.2

Traction Equipment: All Types and Cervical

E0830-E0856:   Bill DME/MAC

☺ **E0830**   Ambulatory traction device, all types, each

IOM: 100-03, 4, 280.1

☺ **E0840**   Traction frame, attached to headboard, cervical traction

IOM: 100-03, 4, 280.1

* **E0849**   Traction equipment, cervical, free-standing stand/frame, pneumatic, applying traction force to other than mandible

☺ **E0850**   Traction stand, free standing, cervical traction

IOM: 100-03, 4, 280.1

* **E0855**   Cervical traction equipment not requiring additional stand or frame

* **E0856**   Cervical traction device, cervical collar with inflatable air bladder

Traction: Overdoor

☺ **E0860**   Traction equipment, overdoor, cervical

Bill DME/MAC

IOM: 100-03, 4, 280.1

Traction: Extremity

E0870-E0880:   Bill DME/MAC

☺ **E0870**   Traction frame, attached to footboard, extremity traction, (e.g., Buck's)

IOM: 100-03, 4, 280.1

☺ **E0880**   Traction stand, free standing, extremity traction, (e.g., Buck's)

IOM: 100-03, 4, 280.1

▶ New   → Revised   ✔ Reinstated   ~~deleted~~ Deleted

☺ Special coverage instructions   ◆ Not covered or valid by Medicare   * Carrier discretion

Traction: Pelvic

E0890-E0900: Bill DME/MAC

- ⚙ **E0890** Traction frame, attached to footboard, pelvic traction
  IOM: 100-03, 4, 280.1
- ⚙ **E0900** Traction stand, free standing, pelvic traction, (e.g., Buck's)
  IOM: 100-03, 4, 280.1

Trapeze Equipment, Fracture Frame, and Other Orthopedic Devices

E0910-E0948: Bill DME/MAC

- ⚙ **E0910** Trapeze bars, A/K/A patient helper, attached to bed, with grab bar
  IOM: 100-03, 4, 280.1
- ⚙ **E0911** Trapeze bar, heavy duty, for patient weight capacity greater than 250 pounds, attached to bed, with grab bar
  IOM: 100-03, 4, 280.1
- ⚙ **E0912** Trapeze bar, heavy duty, for patient weight capacity greater than 250 pounds, free standing, complete with grab bar
  IOM: 100-03, 4, 280.1
- ⚙ **E0920** Fracture frame, attached to bed, includes weights
  IOM: 100-03, 4, 280.1
- ⚙ **E0930** Fracture frame, free standing, includes weights
  IOM: 100-03, 4, 280.1
- ⚙ **E0935** Continuous passive motion exercise device for use on knee only
  To qualify for coverage, use of device must commence within two days following surgery
  IOM: 100-03, 4, 280.1
- ◆ **E0936** Continuous passive motion exercise device for use other than knee
- ⚙ **E0940** Trapeze bar, free standing, complete with grab bar
  IOM: 100-03, 4, 280.1
- ⚙ **E0941** Gravity assisted traction device, any type
  IOM: 100-03, 4, 280.1
- ✳ **E0942** Cervical head harness/halter
- ✳ **E0944** Pelvic belt/harness/boot
- ✳ **E0945** Extremity belt/harness

- ⚙ **E0946** Fracture, frame, dual with cross bars, attached to bed, (e.g. Balken, 4 poster)
  IOM: 100-03, 4, 280.1
- ⚙ **E0947** Fracture frame, attachments for complex pelvic traction
  IOM: 100-03, 4, 280.1
- ⚙ **E0948** Fracture frame, attachments for complex cervical traction
  IOM: 100-03, 4, 280.1

Wheelchair Accessories

E0950-E1030: Bill DME/MAC

- ⚙ **E0950** Wheelchair accessory, tray, each
  IOM: 100-03, 4, 280.1
- ✳ **E0951** Heel loop/holder, any type, with or without ankle strap, each
- ⚙ **E0952** Toe loop/holder, any type, each
  IOM: 100-03, 4, 280.1
- ✳ **E0955** Wheelchair accessory, headrest, cushioned, any type, including fixed mounting hardware, each
- ✳ **E0956** Wheelchair accessory, lateral trunk or hip support, any type, including fixed mounting hardware, each
- ✳ **E0957** Wheelchair accessory, medial thigh support, any type, including fixed mounting hardware, each
- ⚙ **E0958** Manual wheelchair accessory, one-arm drive attachment, each
  IOM: 100-03, 4, 280.1
- ✳ **E0959** Manual wheelchair accessory, adapter for amputee, each
  IOM: 100-03, 4, 280.1
- ✳ **E0960** Wheelchair accessory, shoulder harness/straps or chest strap, including any type mounting hardware
- ✳ **E0961** Manual wheelchair accessory, wheel lock brake extension (handle), each
  IOM: 100-03, 4, 280.1
- ✳ **E0966** Manual wheelchair accessory, headrest extension, each
  IOM: 100-03, 4, 280.1
- ⚙ **E0967** Manual wheelchair accessory, hand rim with projections, any type, each
  IOM: 100-03, 4, 280.1
- ⚙ **E0968** Commode seat, wheelchair
  IOM: 100-03, 4, 280.1

▶ New → Revised ✔ Reinstated deleted Deleted
⚙ Special coverage instructions ◆ Not covered or valid by Medicare ✳ Carrier discretion

⊙ **E0969**   Narrowing device, wheelchair

IOM: 100-03, 4, 280.1

◆ **E0970**   No.2 footplates, except for elevating leg rest

IOM: 100-03, 4, 280.1

Cross Reference CPT K0037, K0042

∗ **E0971**   Manual wheelchair accessory, anti-tipping device, each

IOM: 100-03, 4, 280.1

Cross Reference CPT K0021

⊙ **E0973**   Wheelchair accessory, adjustable height, detachable armrest, complete assembly, each

IOM: 100-03, 4, 280.1

⊙ **E0974**   Manual wheelchair accessory, anti-rollback device, each

IOM: 100-03, 4, 280.1

→ ∗ **E0978**   Wheelchair accessory, positioning belt/safety belt/pelvic strap, each

∗ **E0980**   Safety vest, wheelchair

∗ **E0981**   Wheelchair accessory, seat upholstery, replacement only, each

∗ **E0982**   Wheelchair accessory, back upholstery, replacement only, each

∗ **E0983**   Manual wheelchair accessory, power add-on to convert manual wheelchair to motorized wheelchair, joystick control

∗ **E0984**   Manual wheelchair accessory, power add-on to convert manual wheelchair to motorized wheelchair, tiller control

∗ **E0985**   Wheelchair accessory, seat lift mechanism

∗ **E0986**   Manual wheelchair accessory, push activated power assist, each

▶ ∗ **E0988**   Manual wheelchair accessory, lever-activated, wheel drive, pair

∗ **E0990**   Wheelchair accessory, elevating leg rest, complete assembly, each

IOM: 100-03, 4, 280.1

∗ **E0992**   Manual wheelchair accessory, solid seat insert

⊙ **E0994**   Arm rest, each

IOM: 100-03, 4, 280.1

∗ **E0995**   Wheelchair accessory, calf rest/pad, each

IOM: 100-03, 4, 280.1

∗ **E1002**   Wheelchair accessory, power seating system, tilt only

∗ **E1003**   Wheelchair accessory, power seating system, recline only, without shear reduction

∗ **E1004**   Wheelchair accessory, power seating system, recline only, with mechanical shear reduction

∗ **E1005**   Wheelchair accessory, power seating system, recline only, with power shear reduction

∗ **E1006**   Wheelchair accessory, power seating system, combination tilt and recline, without shear reduction

∗ **E1007**   Wheelchair accessory, power seating system, combination tilt and recline, with mechanical shear reduction

∗ **E1008**   Wheelchair accessory, power seating system, combination tilt and recline, with power shear reduction

∗ **E1009**   Wheelchair accessory, addition to power seating system, mechanically linked leg elevation system, including pushrod and leg rest, each

∗ **E1010**   Wheelchair accessory, addition to power seating system, power leg elevation system, including leg rest, pair

⊙ **E1011**   Modification to pediatric size wheelchair, width adjustment package (not to be dispensed with initial chair)

IOM: 100-03, 4, 280.1

⊙ **E1014**   Reclining back, addition to pediatric size wheelchair

IOM: 100-03, 4, 280.1

⊙ **E1015**   Shock absorber for manual wheelchair, each

IOM: 100-03, 4, 280.1

⊙ **E1016**   Shock absorber for power wheelchair, each

IOM: 100-03, 4, 280.1

⊙ **E1017**   Heavy duty shock absorber for heavy duty or extra heavy duty manual wheelchair, each

IOM: 100-03, 4, 280.1

⊙ **E1018**   Heavy duty shock absorber for heavy duty or extra heavy duty power wheelchair, each

IOM: 100-03, 4, 280.1

▶ New   → Revised   ✔ Reinstated   ~~deleted~~ Deleted

⊙ Special coverage instructions   ◆ Not covered or valid by Medicare   ∗ Carrier discretion

⊙ **E1020** Residual limb support system for wheelchair

IOM: 100-03, 3, 280.3

* **E1028** Wheelchair accessory, manual swingaway, retractable or removable mounting hardware for joystick, other control interface or positioning accessory

* **E1029** Wheelchair accessory, ventilator tray, fixed

* **E1030** Wheelchair accessory, ventilator tray, gimbaled

Rollabout Chair and Transfer System

E1031-E1039: Bill DME/MAC

⊙ **E1031** Rollabout chair, any and all types with castors 5" or greater

IOM: 100-03, 4, 280.1

* **E1035** Multi-positional patient transfer system, with integrated seat, operated by care giver, patient weight capacity up to and including 300 lbs

IOM: 100-02, 15, 110

* **E1036** Multi-positional patient transfer system, extra-wide, with integrated seat, operated by caregiver, patient weight capacity greater than 300 lbs

⊙ **E1037** Transport chair, pediatric size

IOM: 100-03, 4, 280.1

⊙ **E1038** Transport chair, adult size, patient weight capacity up to and including 300 pounds

IOM: 100-03, 4, 280.1

* **E1039** Transport chair, adult size, heavy duty, patient weight capacity greater than 300 pounds

Wheelchair: Fully Reclining

E1050-E1093: Bill DME/MAC

⊙ **E1050** Fully-reclining wheelchair, fixed full length arms, swing away detachable elevating leg rests

IOM: 100-03, 4, 280.1

⊙ **E1060** Fully-reclining wheelchair, detachable arms, desk or full length, swing away detachable elevating legrests

IOM: 100-03, 4, 280.1

⊙ **E1070** Fully-reclining wheelchair, detachable arms (desk or full length) swing away detachable footrests

IOM: 100-03, 4, 280.1

⊙ **E1083** Hemi-wheelchair, fixed full length arms, swing away detachable elevating leg rest

IOM: 100-03, 4, 280.1

⊙ **E1084** Hemi-wheelchair, detachable arms desk or full length arms, swing away detachable elevating leg rests

IOM: 100-03, 4, 280.1

◆ **E1085** Hemi-wheelchair, fixed full length arms, swing away detachable foot rests

IOM: 100-03, 4, 280.1

Cross Reference CPT K0002

◆ **E1086** Hemi-wheelchair, detachable arms desk or full length, swing away detachable footrests

IOM: 100-03, 4, 280.1

Cross Reference CPT K0002

⊙ **E1087** High strength lightweight wheelchair, fixed full length arms, swing away detachable elevating leg rests

IOM: 100-03, 4, 280.1

⊙ **E1088** High strength lightweight wheelchair, detachable arms desk or full length, swing away detachable elevating leg rests

IOM: 100-03, 4, 280.1

◆ **E1089** High strength lightweight wheelchair, fixed length arms, swing away detachable footrest

IOM: 100-03, 4, 280.1

Cross Reference CPT K0004

◆ **E1090** High strength lightweight wheelchair, detachable arms desk or full length, swing away detachable foot rests

IOM: 100-03, 4, 280.1

Cross Reference CPT K0004

⊙ **E1092** Wide heavy duty wheelchair, detachable arms (desk or full length) swing away detachable elevating leg rests

IOM: 100-03, 4, 280.1

⊙ **E1093** Wide heavy duty wheelchair, detachable arms (desk or full length arms), swing away detachable foot rests

IOM: 100-03, 4, 280.1

▶ New   → Revised   ✔ Reinstated   ~~deleted~~ Deleted

⊙ **Special coverage instructions**   ◆ **Not covered or valid by Medicare**   * **Carrier discretion**

Wheelchair: Semi-reclining

E1100-E1110: Bill DME/MAC

⊛ **E1100** Semi-reclining wheelchair, fixed full length arms, swing away detachable elevating leg rests

IOM: 100-03, 4, 280.1

⊛ **E1110** Semi-reclining wheelchair, detachable arms (desk or full length), elevating leg rest

IOM: 100-03, 4, 280.1

Wheelchair: Standard

E1130-E1161: Bill DME/MAC

◆ **E1130** Standard wheelchair, fixed full length arms, fixed or swing away detachable footrests

IOM: 100-03, 4, 280.1

Cross Reference CPT K0001

◆ **E1140** Wheelchair, detachable arms, desk or full length, swing away detachable footrests

IOM: 100-03, 4, 280.1

Cross Reference CPT K0001

⊛ **E1150** Wheelchair, detachable arms, desk or full length, swing away detachable elevating legrests

IOM: 100-03, 4, 280.1

⊛ **E1160** Wheelchair, fixed full length arms, swing away detachable elevating legrests

IOM: 100-03, 4, 280.1

→ ✳ **E1161** Manual adult size wheelchair, includes tilt in space

Wheelchair: Amputee

E1170-E1200: Bill DME/MAC

⊛ **E1170** Amputee wheelchair, fixed full length arms, swing away detachable elevating legrests

IOM: 100-03, 4, 280.1

⊛ **E1171** Amputee wheelchair, fixed full length arms, without footrests or legrest

IOM: 100-03, 4, 280.1

⊛ **E1172** Amputee wheelchair, detachable arms (desk or full length) without footrests or legrest

IOM: 100-03, 4, 280.1

⊛ **E1180** Amputee wheelchair, detachable arms (desk or full length) swing away detachable footrests

IOM: 100-03, 4, 280.1

⊛ **E1190** Amputee wheelchair, detachable arms (desk or full length), swing away detachable elevating legrests

IOM: 100-03, 4, 280.1

⊛ **E1195** Heavy duty wheelchair, fixed full length arms, swing away detachable elevating legrests

IOM: 100-03, 4, 280.1

⊛ **E1200** Amputee wheelchair, fixed full length arms, swing away detachable footrest

IOM: 100-03, 4, 280.1

Wheelchair: Special Size

E1220-E1239: Bill DME/MAC

⊛ **E1220** Wheelchair; specially sized or constructed, (indicate brand name, model number, if any) and justification

IOM: 100-03, 4, 280.3

⊛ **E1221** Wheelchair with fixed arm, footrests

IOM: 100-03, 4, 280.3

⊛ **E1222** Wheelchair with fixed arm, elevating legrests

IOM: 100-03, 4, 280.3

⊛ **E1223** Wheelchair with detachable arms, footrests

IOM: 100-03, 4, 280.3

⊛ **E1224** Wheelchair with detachable arms, elevating legrests

IOM: 100-03, 4, 280.3

⊛ **E1225** Wheelchair accessory, manual semi-reclining back, (recline greater than 15 degrees, but less than 80 degrees), each

IOM: 100-03, 4, 280.3

⊛ **E1226** Wheelchair accessory, manual fully reclining back, (recline greater than 80 degrees), each

IOM: 100-03, 4, 280.1

⊛ **E1227** Special height arms for wheelchair

IOM: 100-03, 4, 280.3

⊛ **E1228** Special back height for wheelchair

IOM: 100-03, 4, 280.3

✳ **E1229** Wheelchair, pediatric size, not otherwise specified

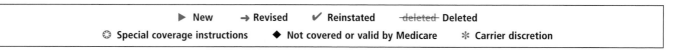

▶ New   → Revised   ✔ Reinstated   ~~deleted~~ Deleted
⊛ Special coverage instructions   ◆ Not covered or valid by Medicare   ✳ Carrier discretion

⊛ **E1230** Power operated vehicle (three or four wheel non-highway), specify brand name and model number

Patient is unable to operate manual wheelchair; patient capable of safely operating controls for scooter; patient can transfer safely in and out of scooter

IOM: 100-08, 5, 5.2.3

⊛ **E1231** Wheelchair, pediatric size, tilt-in-space, rigid, adjustable, with seating system

IOM: 100-03, 4, 280.1

⊛ **E1232** Wheelchair, pediatric size, tilt-in-space, folding, adjustable, with seating system

IOM: 100-03, 4, 280.1

⊛ **E1233** Wheelchair, pediatric size, tilt-in-space, rigid, adjustable, without seating system

IOM: 100-03, 4, 280.1

⊛ **E1234** Wheelchair, pediatric size, tilt-in-space, folding, adjustable, without seating system

IOM: 100-03, 4, 280.1

⊛ **E1235** Wheelchair, pediatric size, rigid, adjustable, with seating system

IOM: 100-03, 4, 280.1

⊛ **E1236** Wheelchair, pediatric size, folding, adjustable, with seating system

IOM: 100-03, 4, 280.1

⊛ **E1237** Wheelchair, pediatric size, rigid, adjustable, without seating system

IOM: 100-03, 4, 280.1

⊛ **E1238** Wheelchair, pediatric size, folding, adjustable, without seating system

IOM: 100-03, 4, 280.1

✳ **E1239** Power wheelchair, pediatric size, not otherwise specified

Wheelchair: Lightweight

E1240-E1270: Bill DME/MAC

⊛ **E1240** Lightweight wheelchair, detachable arms, (desk or full length) swing away detachable, elevating leg rests

IOM: 100-03, 4, 280.1

◆ **E1250** Lightweight wheelchair, fixed full length arms, swing away detachable footrest

IOM: 100-03, 4, 280.1

Cross Reference CPT K0003

◆ **E1260** Lightweight wheelchair, detachable arms (desk or full length) swing away detachable footrest

IOM: 100-03, 4, 280.1

Cross Reference CPT K0003

⊛ **E1270** Lightweight wheelchair, fixed full length arms, swing away detachable elevating legrests

IOM: 100-03, 4, 280.1

Wheelchair: Heavy Duty

E1280-E1298: Bill DME/MAC

⊛ **E1280** Heavy duty wheelchair, detachable arms (desk or full length), elevating legrests

IOM: 100-03, 4, 280.1

◆ **E1285** Heavy duty wheelchair, fixed full length arms, swing away detachable footrest

IOM: 100-03, 4, 280.1

Cross Reference CPT K0006

◆ **E1290** Heavy duty wheelchair, detachable arms (desk or full length) swing away detachable footrest

IOM: 100-03, 4, 280.1

Cross Reference CPT K0006

⊛ **E1295** Heavy duty wheelchair, fixed full length arms, elevating legrest

IOM: 100-03, 4, 280.1

⊛ **E1296** Special wheelchair seat height from floor

IOM: 100-03, 4, 280.3

⊛ **E1297** Special wheelchair seat depth, by upholstery

IOM: 100-03, 4, 280.3

⊛ **E1298** Special wheelchair seat depth and/or width, by construction

IOM: 100-03, 4, 280.3

Whirlpool Equipment

E1300-E1310: Bill DME/MAC

◆ **E1300** Whirlpool, portable (overtub type)

IOM: 100-03, 4, 280.1

⊛ **E1310** Whirlpool, non-portable (built-in type)

IOM: 100-03, 4, 280.1

▶ New   → Revised   ✔ Reinstated   ~~deleted~~ Deleted

⊛ Special coverage instructions   ◆ Not covered or valid by Medicare   ✳ Carrier discretion

Additional Oxygen Related Equipment

✿ **E1353** Regulator

Bill DME/MAC

IOM: 100-03, 4, 240.2

＊ **E1354** Oxygen accessory, wheeled cart for portable cylinder or portable concentrator, any type, replacement only, each

Bill DME/MAC

✿ **E1355** Stand/rack

Bill DME/MAC

IOM: 100-03, 4, 240.2

＊ **E1356** Oxygen accessory, battery pack/cartridge for portable concentrator, any type, replacement only, each

Bill DME/MAC

＊ **E1357** Oxygen accessory, battery charger for portable concentrator, any type, replacement only, each

Bill DME/MAC

◆ **E1358** Oxygen accessory, DC power adapter for portable concentrator, any type, replacement only, each

Bill DME/MAC

✿ **E1372** Immersion external heater for nebulizer

Bill DME/MAC

IOM: 100-03, 4, 240.2

✿ **E1390** Oxygen concentrator, single delivery port, capable of delivering 85 percent or greater oxygen concentration at the prescribed flow rate

Bill DME/MAC

IOM: 100-03, 4, 240.2

✿ **E1391** Oxygen concentrator, dual delivery port, capable of delivering 85 percent or greater oxygen concentration at the prescribed flow rate, each

Bill DME/MAC

IOM: 100-03, 4, 240.2

✿ **E1392** Portable oxygen concentrator, rental

Bill DME/MAC

IOM: 100-03, 4, 240.2

＊ **E1399** Durable medical equipment, miscellaneous

Local carrier if used with implanted DME. If other, bill DME/MAC.

Example: Therapeutic exercise putty; rubber exercise tubing; anti-vibration gloves

On DMEPOS fee schedule as a payable replacement for miscellaneous implanted or non-implanted items.

✿ **E1405** Oxygen and water vapor enriching system with heated delivery

Bill DME/MAC

IOM: 100-03, 4, 240.2

✿ **E1406** Oxygen and water vapor enriching system without heated delivery

Bill DME/MAC

IOM: 100-03, 4, 240.2

Artificial Kidney Machines and Accessories

E1500-E1699: Bill DME/MAC

✿ **E1500** Centrifuge, for dialysis

✿ **E1510** Kidney, dialysate delivery syst. kidney machine, pump recirculating, air removal syst. flowrate meter, power off, heater and temperature control with alarm, I.V. poles, pressure gauge, concentrate container

✿ **E1520** Heparin infusion pump for hemodialysis

✿ **E1530** Air bubble detector for hemodialysis, each, replacement

✿ **E1540** Pressure alarm for hemodialysis, each, replacement

✿ **E1550** Bath conductivity meter for hemodialysis, each

✿ **E1560** Blood leak detector for hemodialysis, each, replacement

✿ **E1570** Adjustable chair, for ESRD patients

✿ **E1575** Transducer protectors/fluid barriers for hemodialysis, any size, per 10

✿ **E1580** Unipuncture control system for hemodialysis

✿ **E1590** Hemodialysis machine

✿ **E1592** Automatic intermittent peritoneal dialysis system

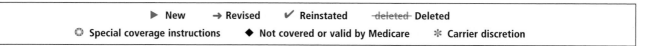

▶ **New**   → **Revised**   ✔ **Reinstated**   ~~deleted~~ **Deleted**

✿ **Special coverage instructions**   ◆ **Not covered or valid by Medicare**   ＊ **Carrier discretion**

⊛ **E1594** Cycler dialysis machine for peritoneal dialysis

⊛ **E1600** Delivery and/or installation charges for hemodialysis equipment

⊛ **E1610** Reverse osmosis water purification system, for hemodialysis

IOM: 100-03, 4, 230.7

⊛ **E1615** Deionizer water purification system, for hemodialysis

IOM: 100-03, 4, 230.7

⊛ **E1620** Blood pump for hemodialysis replacement

⊛ **E1625** Water softening system, for hemodialysis

IOM: 100-03, 4, 230.7

✳ **E1630** Reciprocating peritoneal dialysis system

⊛ **E1632** Wearable artificial kidney, each

⊛ **E1634** Peritoneal dialysis clamps, each

IOM: 100-04, 8, 60.4.2; 100-04, 8, 90.1; 100-04, 18, 80; 100-04, 18, 90

⊛ **E1635** Compact (portable) travel hemodialyzer system

⊛ **E1636** Sorbent cartridges, for hemodialysis, per 10

⊛ **E1637** Hemostats, each

⊛ **E1639** Scale, each

⊛ **E1699** Dialysis equipment, not otherwise specified

Jaw Motion Rehabilitation System and Accessories

E1700-E1702: Bill DME/MAC

✳ **E1700** Jaw motion rehabilitation system

Must be prescribed by physician

✳ **E1701** Replacement cushions for jaw motion rehabilitation system, pkg. of 6

✳ **E1702** Replacement measuring scales for jaw motion rehabilitation system, pkg. of 200

Other Orthopedic Devices

E1800-E1841: Bill DME/MAC

✳ **E1800** Dynamic adjustable elbow extension/flexion device, includes soft interface material

✳ **E1801** Static progressive stretch elbow device, extension and/or flexion, with or without range of motion adjustment, includes all components and accessories

✳ **E1802** Dynamic adjustable forearm pronation/supination device, includes soft interface material

✳ **E1805** Dynamic adjustable wrist extension/flexion device, includes soft interface material

✳ **E1806** Static progressive stretch wrist device, flexion and/or extension, with or without range of motion adjustment, includes all components and accessories

✳ **E1810** Dynamic adjustable knee extension/flexion device, includes soft interface material

✳ **E1811** Static progressive stretch knee device, extension and/or flexion, with or without range of motion adjustment, includes all components and accessories

✳ **E1812** Dynamic knee, extension/flexion device with active resistance control

✳ **E1815** Dynamic adjustable ankle extension/flexion device, includes soft interface material

✳ **E1816** Static progressive stretch ankle device, flexion and/or extension, with or without range of motion adjustment, includes all components and accessories

✳ **E1818** Static progressive stretch forearm pronation/supination device with or without range of motion adjustment, includes all components and accessories

✳ **E1820** Replacement soft interface material, dynamic adjustable extension/flexion device

✳ **E1821** Replacement soft interface material/cuffs for bi-directional static progressive stretch device

✳ **E1825** Dynamic adjustable finger extension/flexion device, includes soft interface material

✳ **E1830** Dynamic adjustable toe extension/flexion device, includes soft interface material

▶ ✳ **E1831** Static progressive stretch toe device, extension and/or flexion, with or without range of motion adjustment, includes all components and accessories

---

▶ New   → Revised   ✔ Reinstated   ~~deleted~~ Deleted

⊛ Special coverage instructions   ◆ Not covered or valid by Medicare   ✳ Carrier discretion

* **E1840** Dynamic adjustable shoulder flexion/abduction/rotation device, includes soft interface material

* **E1841** Static progressive stretch shoulder device, with or without range of motion adjustment, includes all components and accessories

MISCELLANEOUS (E1902-E2120)

* **E1902** Communication board, non-electronic augmentative or alternative communication device

    Bill DME/MAC

* **E2000** Gastric suction pump, home model, portable or stationary, electric

    Bill DME/MAC

⊚ **E2100** Blood glucose monitor with integrated voice synthesizer

    Bill DME/MAC

    IOM: 100-03, 4, 230.16

⊚ **E2101** Blood glucose monitor with integrated lancing/blood sample

    Bill DME/MAC

    IOM: 100-03, 4, 230.16

* **E2120** Pulse generator system for tympanic treatment of inner ear endolymphatic fluid

    Bill DME/MAC

Wheelchair Assessories

E2201-E2397: Bill DME/MAC

* **E2201** Manual wheelchair accessory, nonstandard seat frame, width greater than or equal to 20 inches and less than 24 inches

* **E2202** Manual wheelchair accessory, nonstandard seat frame width, 24-27 inches

* **E2203** Manual wheelchair accessory, nonstandard seat frame depth, 20 to less than 22 inches

* **E2204** Manual wheelchair accessory, nonstandard seat frame depth, 22 to 25 inches

* **E2205** Manual wheelchair accessory, handrim without projections (includes ergonomic or contoured), any type, replacement only, each

* **E2206** Manual wheelchair accessory, wheel lock assembly, complete, each

* **E2207** Wheelchair accessory, crutch and cane holder, each

* **E2208** Wheelchair accessory, cylinder tank carrier, each

* **E2209** Accessory arm trough, with or without hand support, each

* **E2210** Wheelchair accessory, bearings, any type, replacement only, each

* **E2211** Manual wheelchair accessory, pneumatic propulsion tire, any size, each

* **E2212** Manual wheelchair accessory, tube for pneumatic propulsion tire, any size, each

* **E2213** Manual wheelchair accessory, insert for pneumatic propulsion tire (removable), any type, any size, each

* **E2214** Manual wheelchair accessory, pneumatic caster tire, any size, each

* **E2215** Manual wheelchair accessory, tube for pneumatic caster tire, any size, each

* **E2216** Manual wheelchair accessory, foam filled propulsion tire, any size, each

* **E2217** Manual wheelchair accessory, foam filled caster tire, any size, each

* **E2218** Manual wheelchair accessory, foam propulsion tire, any size, each

* **E2219** Manual wheelchair accessory, foam caster tire, any size, each

* **E2220** Manual wheelchair accessory, solid (rubber/plastic) propulsion tire, any size, each

* **E2221** Manual wheelchair accessory, solid (rubber/plastic) caster tire (removable), any size, each

* **E2222** Manual wheelchair accessory, solid (rubber/plastic) caster tire with integrated wheel, any size, each

* **E2224** Manual wheelchair accessory, propulsion wheel excludes tire, any size, each

* **E2225** Manual wheelchair accessory, caster wheel excludes tire, any size, replacement only, each

* **E2226** Manual wheelchair accessory, caster fork, any size, replacement only, each

* **E2227** Manual wheelchair accessory, gear reduction drive wheel, each

* **E2228** Manual wheelchair accessory, wheel braking system and lock, complete, each

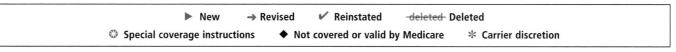

▶ New → Revised ✔ Reinstated ~~deleted~~ Deleted
⊚ Special coverage instructions ◆ Not covered or valid by Medicare * Carrier discretion

◆ **E2230** Manual wheelchair accessory, manual standing system

∗ **E2231** Manual wheelchair accessory, solid seat support base (replaces sling seat), includes any type mounting hardware

∗ **E2291** Back, planar, for pediatric size wheelchair including fixed attaching hardware

∗ **E2292** Seat, planar, for pediatric size wheelchair including fixed attaching hardware

∗ **E2293** Back, contoured, for pediatric size wheelchair including fixed attaching hardware

∗ **E2294** Seat, contoured, for pediatric size wheelchair including fixed attaching hardware

∗ **E2295** Manual wheelchair accessory, for pediatric size wheelchair, dynamic seating frame, allows coordinated movement of multiple positioning features

∗ **E2300** Power wheelchair accessory, power seat elevation system

∗ **E2301** Power wheelchair accessory, power standing system

∗ **E2310** Power wheelchair accessory, electronic connection between wheelchair controller and one power seating system motor, including all related electronics, indicator feature, mechanical function selection switch, and fixed mounting hardware

∗ **E2311** Power wheelchair accessory, electronic connection between wheelchair controller and two or more power seating system motors, including all related electronics, indicator feature, mechanical function selection switch, and fixed mounting hardware

∗ **E2312** Power wheelchair accessory, hand or chin control interface, mini-proportional remote joystick, proportional, including fixed mounting hardware

∗ **E2313** Power wheelchair accessory, harness for upgrade to expandable controller, including all fasteners, connectors and mounting hardware, each

∗ **E2321** Power wheelchair accessory, hand control interface, remote joystick, nonproportional, including all related electronics, mechanical stop switch, and fixed mounting hardware

∗ **E2322** Power wheelchair accessory, hand control interface, multiple mechanical switches, nonproportional, including all related electronics, mechanical stop switch, and fixed mounting hardware

∗ **E2323** Power wheelchair accessory, specialty joystick handle for hand control interface, prefabricated

∗ **E2324** Power wheelchair accessory, chin cup for chin control interface

∗ **E2325** Power wheelchair accessory, sip and puff interface, nonproportional, including all related electronics, mechanical stop switch, and manual swingaway mounting hardware

∗ **E2326** Power wheelchair accessory, breath tube kit for sip and puff interface

∗ **E2327** Power wheelchair accessory, head control interface, mechanical, proportional, including all related electronics, mechanical direction change switch, and fixed mounting hardware

∗ **E2328** Power wheelchair accessory, head control or extremity control interface, electronic, proportional, including all related electronics and fixed mounting hardware

∗ **E2329** Power wheelchair accessory, head control interface, contact switch mechanism, nonproportional, including all related electronics, mechanical stop switch, mechanical direction change switch, head array, and fixed mounting hardware

∗ **E2330** Power wheelchair accessory, head control interface, proximity switch mechanism, nonproportional, including all related electronics, mechanical stop switch, mechanical direction change switch, head array, and fixed mounting hardware

∗ **E2331** Power wheelchair accessory, attendant control, proportional, including all related electronics and fixed mounting hardware

∗ **E2340** Power wheelchair accessory, nonstandard seat frame width, 20-23 inches

∗ **E2341** Power wheelchair accessory, nonstandard seat frame width, 24-27 inches

▶ New → Revised ✔ Reinstated ~~deleted~~ Deleted
◎ Special coverage instructions ◆ Not covered or valid by Medicare ∗ Carrier discretion

* **E2342** Power wheelchair accessory, nonstandard seat frame depth, 20 or 21 inches

* **E2343** Power wheelchair accessory, nonstandard seat frame depth, 22-25 inches

* **E2351** Power wheelchair accessory, electronic interface to operate speech generating device using power wheelchair control interface

▶ * **E2358** Power wheelchair accessory, Group 34 non-sealed lead acid battery, each

▶ * **E2359** Power wheelchair accessory, Group 34 sealed lead acid battery, each (e.g., gel cell, absorbed glassmat)

* **E2360** Power wheelchair accessory, 22 NF non-sealed lead acid battery, each

* **E2361** Power wheelchair accessory, 22NF sealed lead acid battery, each, (e.g. gel cell, absorbed glassmat)

* **E2362** Power wheelchair accessory, group 24 non-sealed lead acid battery, each

* **E2363** Power wheelchair accessory, group 24 sealed lead acid battery, each (e.g. gel cell, absorbed glassmat)

* **E2364** Power wheelchair accessory, U-1 non-sealed lead acid battery, each

* **E2365** Power wheelchair accessory, U-1 sealed lead acid battery, each (e.g. gel cell, absorbed glassmat)

* **E2366** Power wheelchair accessory, battery charger, single mode, for use with only one battery type, sealed or non-sealed, each

* **E2367** Power wheelchair accessory, battery charger, dual mode, for use with either battery type, sealed or non-sealed, each

* **E2368** Power wheelchair component, motor, replacement only

* **E2369** Power wheelchair component, gear box, replacement only

* **E2370** Power wheelchair component, motor and gear box combination, replacement only

* **E2371** Power wheelchair accessory, group 27 sealed lead acid battery, (e.g. gel cell, absorbed glass mat), each

* **E2372** Power wheelchair accessory, group 27 non-sealed lead acid battery, each

* **E2373** Power wheelchair accessory, hand or chin control interface, compact remote joystick, proportional, including fixed mounting hardware

☺ **E2374** Power wheelchair accessory, hand or chin control interface, standard remote joystick (not including controller), proportional, including all related electronics and fixed mounting hardware, replacement only

☺ **E2375** Power wheelchair accessory, non-expandable controller, including all related electronics and mounting hardware, replacement only

☺ **E2376** Power wheelchair accessory, expandable controller, including all related electronics and mounting hardware, replacement only

☺ **E2377** Power wheelchair accessory, expandable controller, including all related electronics and mounting hardware, upgrade provided at initial issue

☺ **E2381** Power wheelchair accessory, pneumatic drive wheel tire, any size, replacement only, each

☺ **E2382** Power wheelchair accessory, tube for pneumatic drive wheel tire, any size, replacement only, each

☺ **E2383** Power wheelchair accessory, insert for pneumatic drive wheel tire (removable), any type, any size, replacement only, each

☺ **E2384** Power wheelchair accessory, pneumatic caster tire, any size, replacement only, each

☺ **E2385** Power wheelchair accessory, tube for pneumatic caster tire, any size, replacement only, each

☺ **E2386** Power wheelchair accessory, foam filled drive wheel tire, any size, replacement only, each

☺ **E2387** Power wheelchair accessory, foam filled caster tire, any size, replacement only, each

☺ **E2388** Power wheelchair accessory, foam drive wheel tire, any size, replacement only, each

☺ **E2389** Power wheelchair accessory, foam caster tire, any size, replacement only, each

☺ **E2390** Power wheelchair accessory, solid (rubber/plastic) drive wheel tire, any size, replacement only, each

☺ **E2391** Power wheelchair accessory, solid (rubber/plastic) caster tire (removable), any size, replacement only, each

▶ New	→ Revised	✔ Reinstated	~~deleted~~ Deleted
☺ Special coverage instructions		◆ Not covered or valid by Medicare	* Carrier discretion

⊙ **E2392** Power wheelchair accessory, solid (rubber/plastic) caster tire with integrated wheel, any size, replacement only, each

⊙ **E2394** Power wheelchair accessory, drive wheel excludes tire, any size, replacement only, each

⊙ **E2395** Power wheelchair accessory, caster wheel excludes tire, any size, replacement only, each

⊙ **E2396** Power wheelchair accessory, caster fork, any size, replacement only, each

＊ **E2397** Power wheelchair accessory, lithium-based battery, each

Negative Pressure

＊ **E2402** Negative pressure wound therapy electrical pump, stationary or portable

Bill DME/MAC

Document at least every 30 calendar days the quantitative wound characteristics, including wound surface area (length, width and depth)

Medicare coverage up to a maximum of 15 dressing kits (A6550) per wound per month unless documentation states that the wound size requires more than one dressing kit for each dressing change.

Speech Device

E2500-E2599:   Bill DME/MAC

⊙ **E2500** Speech generating device, digitized speech, using pre-recorded messages, less than or equal to 8 minutes recording time

IOM: 100-03, 1, 50.1

⊙ **E2502** Speech generating device, digitized speech, using pre-recorded messages, greater than 8 minutes but less than or equal to 20 minutes recording time

IOM: 100-03, 1, 50.1

⊙ **E2504** Speech generating device, digitized speech, using pre-recorded messages, greater than 20 minutes but less than or equal to 40 minutes recording time

IOM: 100-03, 1, 50.1

⊙ **E2506** Speech generating device, digitized speech, using pre-recorded messages, greater than 40 minutes recording time

IOM: 100-03, 1, 50.1

⊙ **E2508** Speech generating device, synthesized speech, requiring message formulation by spelling and access by physical contact with the device

IOM: 100-03, 1, 50.1

⊙ **E2510** Speech generating device, synthesized speech, permitting multiple methods of message formulation and multiple methods of device access

IOM: 100-03, 1, 50.1

⊙ **E2511** Speech generating software program, for personal computer or personal digital assistant

IOM: 100-03, 1, 50.1

⊙ **E2512** Accessory for speech generating device, mounting system

IOM: 100-03, 1, 50.1

⊙ **E2599** Accessory for speech generating device, not otherwise classified

IOM: 100-03, 1, 50.1

Wheelchair, Cushion and Protection

E2601-E2621:   Bill DME/MAC

＊ **E2601** General use wheelchair seat cushion, width less than 22 inches, any depth

＊ **E2602** General use wheelchair seat cushion, width 22 inches or greater, any depth

＊ **E2603** Skin protection wheelchair seat cushion, width less than 22 inches, any depth

＊ **E2604** Skin protection wheelchair seat cushion, width 22 inches or greater, any depth

＊ **E2605** Positioning wheelchair seat cushion, width less than 22 inches, any depth

＊ **E2606** Positioning wheelchair seat cushion, width 22 inches or greater, any depth

＊ **E2607** Skin protection and positioning wheelchair seat cushion, width less than 22 inches, any depth

＊ **E2608** Skin protection and positioning wheelchair seat cushion, width 22 inches or greater, any depth

＊ **E2609** Custom fabricated wheelchair seat cushion, any size

＊ **E2610** Wheelchair seat cushion, powered

＊ **E2611** General use wheelchair back cushion, width less than 22 inches, any height, including any type mounting hardware

---

▶ New   → Revised   ✔ Reinstated   ~~deleted~~ Deleted

⊙ Special coverage instructions   ◆ Not covered or valid by Medicare   ＊ Carrier discretion

* **E2612** General use wheelchair back cushion, width 22 inches or greater, any height, including any type mounting hardware

* **E2613** Positioning wheelchair back cushion, posterior, width less than 22 inches, any height, including any type mounting hardware

* **E2614** Positioning wheelchair back cushion, posterior, width 22 inches or greater, any height, including any type mounting hardware

* **E2615** Positioning wheelchair back cushion, posterior-lateral, width less than 22 inches, any height, including any type mounting hardware

* **E2616** Positioning wheelchair back cushion, posterior-lateral, width 22 inches or greater, any height, including any type mounting hardware

* **E2617** Custom fabricated wheelchair back cushion, any size, including any type mounting hardware

* **E2619** Replacement cover for wheelchair seat cushion or back cushion, each

* **E2620** Positioning wheelchair back cushion, planar back with lateral supports, width less than 22 inches, any height, including any type mounting hardware

* **E2621** Positioning wheelchair back cushion, planar back with lateral supports, width 22 inches or greater, any height, including any type mounting hardware

SKIN PROTECTION, WHEELCHAIR (E2622-E2625)

▶ * **E2622** Skin protection wheelchair seat cushion, adjustable, width less than 22 inches, any depth

▶ * **E2623** Skin protection wheelchair seat cushion, adjustable, width 22 inches or greater, any depth

▶ * **E2624** Skin protection and positioning wheelchair seat cushion, adjustable, width less than 22 inches, any depth

▶ * **E2625** Skin protection and positioning wheelchair seat cushion, adjustable, width 22 inches or greater, any depth

ARM SUPPORT (E2626-E2633)

▶ * **E2626** Wheelchair accessory, shoulder elbow, mobile arm support attached to wheelchair, balanced, adjustable

▶ * **E2627** Wheelchair accessory, shoulder elbow, mobile arm support attached to wheelchair, balanced, adjustable rancho type

▶ * **E2628** Wheelchair accessory, shoulder elbow, mobile arm support attached to wheelchair, balanced, reclining

▶ * **E2629** Wheelchair accessory, shoulder elbow, mobile arm support attached to wheelchair, balanced, friction arm support (friction dampening to proximal and distal joints)

▶ * **E2630** Wheelchair accessory, shoulder elbow, mobile arm support, monosuspension arm and hand support, overhead elbow forearm hand sling support, yoke type suspension support

▶ * **E2631** Wheelchair accessory, addition to mobile arm support, elevating proximal arm

▶ * **E2632** Wheelchair accessory, addition to mobile arm support, offset or lateral rocker arm with elastic balance control

▶ * **E2633** Wheelchair accessory, addition to mobile arm support, supinator

Gait Trainer

E8000-E8002: Bill DME/MAC

◆ **E8000** Gait trainer, pediatric size, posterior support, includes all accessories and components

◆ **E8001** Gait trainer, pediatric size, upright support, includes all accessories and components

◆ **E8002** Gait trainer, pediatric size, anterior support, includes all accessories and components

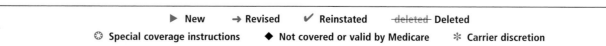

▶ New   → Revised   ✔ Reinstated   ~~deleted~~ Deleted
⊙ Special coverage instructions   ◆ Not covered or valid by Medicare   * Carrier discretion

TEMPORARY PROCEDURES/PROFESSIONAL SERVICES (G0000-G9999)

NOTE: This section contains national codes assigned by CMS on a temporary basis to identify procedures/professional services.

Administration, Vaccine

G0008-G0010: Bill local carrier

✻ **G0008** Administration of influenza virus vaccine

Coinsurance and deductible do not apply. If provided, report significant, separately identifiable E/M for medically necessary services (V04.81)

✻ **G0009** Administration of pneumococcal vaccine

Reported once in a lifetime based on risk; Medicare covers cost of vaccine and administration (V03.82)

Copayment, coinsurance, and deductible waived. (https://www.cms.gov/MLNProducts/downloads/MPS_QuickReferenceChart_1.pdf)

✻ **G0010** Administration of hepatitis B vaccine

Report for other than OPPs. Coinsurance and deductible apply; Medicare covers both cost of vaccine and administration (V05.3)

On or after January 1, 2011 the copayment/coinsurance and deductible are waived.

Semen Analysis

✻ **G0027** Semen analysis; presence and/or motility of sperm excluding Huhner

Bill local carrier

Laboratory Certification: Hematology

Screening, Cervical

✿ **G0101** Cervical or vaginal cancer screening; pelvic and clinical breast examination

Bill local carrier

Covered once every two years and annually if high risk for cervical/vaginal cancer, or if childbearing age patient has had an abnormal Pap smear in preceding three years. High risk diagnosis, V15.89

Screening, Prostate

G0102-G0103: Bill local carrier

✿ **G0102** Prostate cancer screening; digital rectal examination

Covered annually by Medicare (V76.44). Not separately payable with an E/M code (99201-99499).

IOM: 100-02, 6, 10; 100-04, 4, 240
IOM: 100-04, 18, 50.1

✿ **G0103** Prostate cancer screening; prostate specific antigen test (PSA)

Covered annually by Medicare (V76.44)

IOM: 100-02, 6, 10; 100-04, 4, 240
IOM: 100-04, 18, 50
Laboratory Certification: Routine chemistry

Screening, Colorectal

G0104-G0106: Bill local carrier

✿ **G0104** Colorectal cancer screening; flexible sigmoidoscopy

Covered once every 48 months for beneficiaries age 50+

Co-insurance waived under Section 4104.

✿ **G0105** Colorectal cancer screening; colonoscopy on individual at high risk

Screening colonoscopy covered once every 24 months for high risk for developing colorectal cancer. May use modifier 53 if appropriate (physician fee schedule)

Co-insurance waived under Section 4104.

✿ **G0106** Colorectal cancer screening; alternative to G0104, screening sigmoidoscopy, barium enema

Barium enema (not high risk) (alternative to G0104). Covered once every 4 years for beneficiaries age 50+. Use modifier 26 for professional

▶ New　→ Revised　✔ Reinstated　deleted Deleted
✿ Special coverage instructions　◆ Not covered or valid by Medicare　✻ Carrier discretion

component only.

Training Services, Diabetes

G0108-G0109: Bill local carrier

* **G0108** Diabetes outpatient self-management training services, individual, per 30 minutes

  Report for beneficiaries diagnosed with diabetes

* **G0109** Diabetes outpatient self-management training services, group session (2 or more) per 30 minutes

  Report for beneficiaries diagnosed with diabetes

Screening, Glaucoma

G0117-G0118: Bill local carrier

* **G0117** Glaucoma screening for high risk patients furnished by an optometrist or ophthalmologist

  Covered once per year (full 11 months between screenings). Bundled with all other ophthalmic services provided on same day. Diagnosis code V80.1

* **G0118** Glaucoma screening for high risk patient furnished under the direct supervision of an optometrist or ophthalmologist

  Covered once per year (full 11 months between screenings). Diagnosis code V80.1

Screening, Colorectal, Other

G0120-G0122: Bill local carrier

☼ **G0120** Colorectal cancer screening; alternative to G0105, screening colonoscopy, barium enema.

  Barium enema for patients with a high risk of developing colorectal. Covered once every 2 years. Used as an alternative to G0105. Use modifier 26 for professional component only

☼ **G0121** Colorectal cancer screening; colonoscopy on individual not meeting criteria for high risk

  Screening colonoscopy for patients that are not high risk. Covered once every 10 years, but not within 48 months of a G0104. For non-Medicare patients

report 45378.

Co-insurance waived under Section 4104.

◆ **G0122** Colorectal cancer screening; barium enema

  Medicare: this service is denied as noncovered, because it fails to meet the requirements of the benefit. The beneficiary is liable for payment.

Screening, Cytopathology

G0123-G0124: Bill local carrier

☼ **G0123** Screening cytopathology, cervical or vaginal (any reporting system), collected in preservative fluid, automated thin layer preparation, screening by cytotechnologist under physician supervision

  Use G0123 or G0143 or G0144 or G0145 or G0147 or G0148 or P3000 for Pap smears NOT requiring physician interpretation (technical component)

  IOM: 100-03, 3, 190.2; 100-04, 18, 30

  Laboratory Certification: Cytology

☼ **G0124** Screening cytopathology, cervical or vaginal (any reporting system), collected in preservative fluid, automated thin layer preparation, requiring interpretation by physician

  Report professional component for Pap smears requiring physician interpretation

  IOM: 100-03, 3, 190.2; 100-04, 18, 30

  Laboratory Certification: Cytology

Trimming, Nail

☼ **G0127** Trimming of dystrophic nails, any number

  Bill local carrier

  Must be used with a modifier (Q7, Q8, or Q9) to show that the foot care service is needed because the beneficiary has a systemic disease. Limit 1 unit of service

  IOM: 100-02, 15, 290

Service, Nursing and OT

G0128-G0129: Bill local carrier

▶ New	→ Revised	✔ Reinstated	~~deleted~~ Deleted
☼ Special coverage instructions		◆ Not covered or valid by Medicare	* Carrier discretion

⊙ **G0128** Direct (face-to-face with patient) skilled nursing services of a registered nurse provided in a comprehensive outpatient rehabilitation facility, each 10 minutes beyond the first 5 minutes

A separate nursing service that is clearly identifiable in the Plan of Treatment and not part of other services. Documentation must support this service. Examples include: Insertion of a urinary catheter, intramuscular injections, bowel disimpaction, nursing assessment, and education. Restricted coverage by Medicare.

Medicare Statute 1833(a)

* **G0129** Occupational therapy services requiring the skills of a qualified occupational therapist, furnished as a component of a partial hospitalization treatment program, per session (45 minutes or more)

Study, SEXA

⊙ **G0130** Single energy x-ray absorptiometry (SEXA) bone density study, one or more sites; appendicular skeleton (peripheral) (eg, radius, wrist, heel)

Bill local carrier

Covered every 24 months (more frequently if medically necessary). Use modifier 26 for professional component only

IOM: 100-03, 2, 150.3; 100-04, 13, 140.1

Screening, Cytopathology, Other

G0141-G0148: Bill local carrier

* **G0141** Screening cytopathology smears, cervical or vaginal, performed by automated system, with manual rescreening, requiring interpretation by physician

Co-insurance, copay and deductible waived

Report professional component for Pap smears requiring physician interpretation. Refer to diagnosis of V15.89, V76.2, V76.47, or V76.49 to report appropriate risk level

Laboratory Certification: Cytology

* **G0143** Screening cytopathology, cervical or vaginal (any reporting system), collected in preservative fluid, automated thin layer preparation, with manual screening and rescreening by cytotechnologist under physician supervision

Co-insurance, copay and deductible waived

Laboratory Certification: Cytology

* **G0144** Screening cytopathology, cervical or vaginal (any reporting system), collected in preservative fluid, automated thin layer preparation, with screening by automated system, under physician supervision

Co-insurance, copay and deductible waived

Laboratory Certification: Cytology

* **G0145** Screening cytopathology, cervical or vaginal (any reporting system), collected in preservative fluid, automated thin layer preparation, with screening by automated system and manual rescreening under physician supervision

Co-insurance, copay and deductible waived

Laboratory Certification: Cytology

* **G0147** Screening cytopathology smears, cervical or vaginal; performed by automated system under physician supervision

Co-insurance, copay and deductible waived

Laboratory Certification: Cytology

* **G0148** Screening cytopathology smears, cervical or vaginal; performed by automated system with manual rescreening

Co-insurance, copay and deductible waived

Laboratory Certification: Cytology

Services, Allied Health

G0151-G0166: Bill local carrier

→ * **G0151** Services performed by a qualified physical therapist in the home health or hospice setting, each 15 minutes

→ * **G0152** Services performed by a qualified occupational therapist in the home health or hospice setting, each 15 minutes

▶ New   → Revised   ✔ Reinstated   ~~deleted~~ Deleted

⊙ Special coverage instructions   ◆ Not covered or valid by Medicare   * Carrier discretion

→ * **G0153** Services performed by a qualified speech-language pathologist in the home health or hospice setting, each 15 minutes

→ * **G0154** Direct skilled nursing services of a licensed nurse (LPN or RN) in the home health or hospice setting, each 15 minutes

* **G0155** Services of clinical social worker in home health or hospice settings, each 15 minutes

* **G0156** Services of home health/health aide in home health or hospice settings, each 15 minutes

▶ * **G0157** Services performed by a qualified physical therapist assistant in the home health or hospice setting, each 15 minutes

▶ * **G0158** Services performed by a qualified occupational therapist assistant in the home health or hospice setting, each 15 minutes

▶ * **G0159** Services performed by a qualified physical therapist, in the home health setting, in the establishment or delivery of a safe and effective physical therapy maintenance program, each 15 minutes

▶ * **G0160** Services performed by a qualified occupational therapist, in the home health setting, in the establishment or delivery of a safe and effective occupational therapy maintenance program, each 15 minutes

▶ * **G0161** Services performed by a qualified speech-language pathologist, in the home health setting, in the establishment or delivery of a safe and effective speech-language pathology maintenance program, each 15 minutes

▶ * **G0162** Skilled services by a registered nurse (RN) for management and evaluation of the plan of care; each 15 minutes (the patient's underlying condition or complication requires an RN to ensure that essential non-skilled care achieves its purpose in the home health or hospice setting)

Transmittal No. 824 (CR7182)

▶ * **G0163** Skilled services of a licensed nurse (LPN or RN) for the observation and assessment of the patient's condition, each 15 minutes (the change in the patient's condition requires skilled nursing personnel to identify and evaluate the patient's need for possible modification of treatment in the home health or hospice setting)

Transmittal No. 824 (CR7182)

▶ * **G0164** Skilled services of a licensed nurse (LPN or RN), in the training and/or education of a patient or family member, in the home health or hospice setting, each 15 minutes

Transmittal No. 824 (CR7182)

☺ **G0166** External counterpulsation, per treatment session

IOM: 100-03, 1, 20.20

Wound Closure

* **G0168** Wound closure utilizing tissue adhesive(s) only

Bill local carrier

Report for wound closure with only tissue adhesive. If a practitioner utilizes tissue adhesive in addition to staples or sutures to close a wound, HCPCS code G0168 is not separately reportable, but is included in the tissue repair.

The only closure material used for a simple repair, coverage based on payer.

Stereotactic Radiosurgery

☺ **G0173** Linear accelerator based stereotactic radiosurgery, complete course of therapy in one session

Bill local carrier

Do not bill with 77421

Team Conference

* **G0175** Scheduled interdisciplinary team conference (minimum of three exclusive of patient care nursing staff) with patient present

Bill local carrier

▶ New	→ Revised	✔ Reinstated	~~deleted~~ Deleted
☺ Special coverage instructions		◆ Not covered or valid by Medicare	* Carrier discretion

Therapy, Activity

G0176-G0177: Bill local carrier

OPPS not separately payable

✪ **G0176** Activity therapy, such as music, dance, art or play therapies not for recreation, related to the care and treatment of patient's disabling mental health problems, per session (45 minutes or more)

Paid in partial hospitalization

✪ **G0177** Training and educational services related to the care and treatment of patient's disabling mental health problems per session (45 minutes or more)

Paid in partial hospitalization

Physician Services

G0179-G0182: Bill local carrier

✳ **G0179** Physician re-certification for Medicare-covered home health services under a home health plan of care (patient not present), including contacts with home health agency and review of reports of patient status required by physicians to affirm the initial implementation of the plan of care that meets patient's needs, per re-certification period

The recertification code is used after a patient has received services for at least 60 days (or one certification period) when the physician signs the certification after the initial certification period.

✳ **G0180** Physician certification for Medicare-covered home health services under a home health plan of care (patient not present), including contacts with home health agency and review of reports of patient status required by physicians to affirm the initial implementation of the plan of care that meets patient's needs, per certification period

This code can be billed only when the patient has not received Medicare covered home health services for at least 60 days.

✳ **G0181** Physician supervision of a patient receiving Medicare-covered services provided by a participating home health agency (patient not present) requiring complex and multidisciplinary care modalities involving regular physician development and/or revision of care plans, review of subsequent reports of patient status, review of laboratory and other studies, communication (including telephone calls) with other health care professionals involved in the patient's care, integration of new information into the medical treatment plan and/or adjustment of medical therapy, within a calendar month, 30 minutes or more

✳ **G0182** Physician supervision of a patient under a Medicare-approved hospice (patient not present) requiring complex and multidisciplinary care modalities involving regular physician development and/or revision of care plans, review of subsequent reports of patient status, review of laboratory and other studies, communication (including telephone calls) with other health care professionals involved in the patient's care, integration of new information into the medical treatment plan and/or adjustment of medical therapy, within a calendar month, 30 minutes or more

Destruction

✳ **G0186** Destruction of localized lesion of choroid (for example, choroidal neovascularization); photocoagulation, feeder vessel technique (one or more sessions)

Bill local carrier

Mammography

G0202-G0206: Bill local carrier

✳ **G0202** Screening mammography, producing direct digital image, bilateral, all views

Screening mammogram reported based on technique, such as 76082, 76083, 76092, or G0202. Requires coinsurance, but no deductible. Diagnosis codes, V76.11 (high risk) or V76.12 (low risk). Use modifier 26 for professional component only

---

▶ New → Revised ✔ Reinstated ~~deleted~~ Deleted
✪ Special coverage instructions ◆ Not covered or valid by Medicare ✳ Carrier discretion

* **G0204** Diagnostic mammography, producing direct digital image, bilateral, all views

  Use modifier 26 for professional component only

* **G0206** Diagnostic mammography, producing direct digital image, unilateral, all views

  Use modifier 26 for professional component only

Imaging, PET

G0219-G0235: Bill local carrier

◆ **G0219** PET imaging whole body; melanoma for non-covered indications

  Example: Assessing regional lymph nodes in melanoma. Medicare non-covered.

  IOM: 100-03, 4, 220.6

◆ **G0235** PET imaging, any site, not otherwise specified

  Example: Prostate cancer diagnosis and initial staging. Medicare non-covered.

  IOM: 100-03, 4, 220.6

Therapeutic Procedures

G0237-G0239: Bill local carrier

* **G0237** Therapeutic procedures to increase strength or endurance of respiratory muscles, face to face, one on one, each 15 minutes (includes monitoring)

* **G0238** Therapeutic procedures to improve respiratory function, other than described by G0237, one on one, face to face, per 15 minutes (includes monitoring)

* **G0239** Therapeutic procedures to improve respiratory function or increase strength or endurance of respiratory muscles, two or more individuals (includes monitoring)

Physician Service, Diabetic

G0245-G0246: Bill local carrier

⊙ **G0245** Initial physician evaluation and management of a diabetic patient with diabetic sensory neuropathy resulting in a loss of protective sensation (LOPS) which must include (1) the diagnosis of LOPS, (2) a patient history, (3) a physical examination that consist of at least the following elements: (A) visual inspection of the forefoot, hindfoot and toe web spaces, (B) evaluation of a protective sensation, (C) evaluation of foot structure and biomechanics, (D) evaluation of vascular status and skin integrity, and (E) evaluation and recommendation of footwear, and (4) patient education

  Report one of the following diagnosis codes in conjunction with this code: 250.60, 250.61, 250.62, 250.63, or 357.2

  IOM: 100-03, 1, 70.2.1

⊙ **G0246** Follow-up physician evaluation and management of a diabetic patient with diabetic sensory neuropathy resulting in a loss of protective sensation (LOPS) to include at least the following: (1) a patient history, (2) a physical examination that includes: (A) visual inspection of the forefoot, hindfoot and toe web spaces, (B) evaluation of protective sensation, (C) evaluation of foot structure and biomechanics, (D) evaluation of vascular status and skin integrity, and (E) evaluation and recommendation of footwear, and (3) patient education

  IOM: 100-03, 1, 70.2.1; 100-02, 15, 290

Foot Care

⊙ **G0247** Routine foot care by a physician of a diabetic patient with diabetic sensory neuropathy resulting in a loss of protective sensation (LOPS) to include, the local care of superficial wounds (i.e. superficial to muscle and fascia) and at least the following if present: (1) local care of superficial wounds, (2) debridement of corns and calluses, and (3) trimming and debridement of nails

  Bill local carrier

  IOM: 100-03, 1, 70.2.1

▶ New   → Revised   ✔ Reinstated   ~~deleted~~ Deleted
⊙ Special coverage instructions   ◆ Not covered or valid by Medicare   * Carrier discretion

154

Demonstration, INR

G0248-G0250: Bill local carrier

⊛ **G0248** Demonstration, prior to initiation, of home INR monitoring for patient with either mechanical heart valve(s), chronic atrial fibrillation, or venous thromboembolism who meets Medicare coverage criteria, under the direction of a physician; includes: face-to-face demonstration of use and care of the INR monitor, obtaining at least one blood sample, provision of instructions for reporting home INR test results, and documentation of patient's ability to perform testing and report results

⊛ **G0249** Provision of test materials and equipment for home INR monitoring of patient with either mechanical heart valve(s), chronic atrial fibrillation, or venous thromboembolism who meets Medicare coverage criteria; includes provision of materials for use in the home and reporting of test results to physician; testing not occurring more frequently than once a week; testing materials, billing units of service include 4 tests

⊛ **G0250** Physician review, interpretation, and patient management of home INR testing for patient with either mechanical heart valve(s), chronic atrial fibrillation, or venous thromboembolism who meets Medicare coverage criteria; testing not occurring more frequently than once a week; billing units of service include 4 tests

Stereotactic Radiosurgery

⊛ **G0251** Linear accelerator based stereotactic radiosurgery, delivery including collimator changes and custom plugging, fractionated treatment, all lesions, per session, maximum five sessions per course of treatment

Bill local carrier

Cannot bill with 77421. The indicator is "0" and the edit cannot be bypassed with a modifier. (https://www.cms.gov/NationalCorrectCodInitEd/NCCITrans/list.asp)

Imaging, PET

◆ **G0252** PET imaging, full and partial-ring PET scanners only, for initial diagnosis of breast cancer and/or surgical planning for breast cancer (e.g. initial staging of axillary lymph nodes)

Bill local carrier

IOM: 100-03, 4, 220.6

SNCT

◆ **G0255** Current perception threshold/sensory nerve conduction test, (SNCT) per limb, any nerve

Bill local carrier

IOM: 100-03, 2, 160.23

Dialysis, Emergency

⊛ **G0257** Unscheduled or emergency dialysis treatment for an ESRD patient in a hospital outpatient department that is not certified as an ESRD facility

Bill local carrier

Injection, Arthrography

G0259-G0260: Bill local carrier

⊛ **G0259** Injection procedure for sacroiliac joint; arthrography

Used by Part A only (facility), not priced by Part B Medicare.

Replaces 27096 for reporting injections for Medicare beneficiaries

⊛ **G0260** Injection procedure for sacroiliac joint; provision of anesthetic, steroid and/or other therapeutic agent, with or without arthrography

ASCs report when a therapeutic sacroiliac joint injection is administered in ASC

▶ New → Revised ✔ Reinstated ~~deleted~~ Deleted

⊛ Special coverage instructions ◆ Not covered or valid by Medicare ✲ Carrier discretion

Removal, Cerumen

✳ **G0268** Removal of impacted cerumen (one or both ears) by physician on same date of service as audiologic function testing

Bill local carrier

Report only when a physician, not an audiologist, performs the procedure.

Use with DX 380.4 when performed by physician.

Placement, Occlusive Device

✪ **G0269** Placement of occlusive device into either a venous or arterial access site, post surgical or interventional procedure (e.g. angioseal plug, vascular plug)

Bill local carrier

Report for replacement of vasoseal. Hospitals may report the closure device as a supply with C1760. Bundled status on Physician Fee Schedule.

Therapy, Nutrition

G0270-G0271: Bill local carrier

✳ **G0270** Medical nutrition therapy; reassessment and subsequent intervention(s) following second referral in same year for change in diagnosis, medical condition or treatment regimen (including additional hours needed for renal disease), individual, face to face with the patient, each 15 minutes

Requires physician referral for beneficiaries with diabetes or renal disease. Services must be provided by dietitian/nutritionist

✳ **G0271** Medical nutrition therapy, reassessment and subsequent intervention(s) following second referral in same year for change in diagnosis, medical condition, or treatment regimen (including additional hours needed for renal disease), group (2 or more individuals), each 30 minutes

Requires physician referral for beneficiaries with diabetes or renal disease. Services must be provided by dietitian/nutritionist. Co-insurance and deductible waived

Angiography

G0275-G0278: Bill local carrier

✳ **G0275** Renal angiography, non-selective, one or both kidneys, performed at the same time as cardiac catheterization and/or coronary angiography, includes positioning or placement of any catheter in the abdominal aorta at or near the origins (OSTIA) of the renal arteries, injection of dye, flush aortogram, production of permanent images, and radiologic supervision and interpretation (list separately in addition to primary procedure)

Routine "drive-by angiography" at time of cardiac catheterization performed in the absence of accepted clinical indications that support medical necessity will be denied by Medicare

✳ **G0278** Iliac and/or femoral artery angiography, non-selective, bilateral or ipsilateral to catheter insertion, performed at the same time as cardiac catheterization and/or coronary angiography, includes positioning or placement of the catheter in the distal aorta or ipsilateral femoral or iliac artery, injection of dye, production of permanent images, and radiologic supervision and interpretation (list separately in addition to primary procedure)

Medicare specific code not reported for iliac injection used as a guiding shot for a closure device

Stimulation, Electrical

G0281-G0283: Bill local carrier

✳ **G0281** Electrical stimulation, (unattended), to one or more areas, for chronic stage III and stage IV pressure ulcers, arterial ulcers, diabetic ulcers, and venous stasis ulcers not demonstrating measurable signs of healing after 30 days of conventional care, as part of a therapy plan of care

Reported by encounter/areas and not by site. Therapists report G0281 and G0283 rather than 97014

◆ **G0282** Electrical stimulation, (unattended), to one or more areas, for wound care other than described in G0281

IOM: 100-03, 4, 270.1

▶ New → Revised ✔ Reinstated deleted Deleted
✪ Special coverage instructions ◆ Not covered or valid by Medicare ✳ Carrier discretion

* **G0283** Electrical stimulation (unattended), to one or more areas for indication(s) other than wound care, as part of a therapy plan of care

  Reported by encounter/areas and not by site. Therapists report G0281 and G0283 rather than 97014

Angiography, Arthroscopy

G0288-G0289: Bill local carrier

* **G0288** Reconstruction, computed tomographic angiography of aorta for surgical planning for vascular surgery

* **G0289** Arthroscopy, knee, surgical, for removal of loose body, foreign body, debridement/shaving of articular cartilage (chondroplasty) at the time of other surgical knee arthroscopy in a different compartment of the same knee

  Add-on code reported with knee arthroscopy code for major procedure performed—reported once per extra compartment

  "The code may be reported twice (or with a unit of two) if the physician performs these procedures in two compartments, in addition to the compartment where the main procedure was performed." (http://www.ama-assn.org/resources/doc/cpt/orthopaedics.pdf)

Placement, Transcatheter

G0290-G0291: Bill local carrier

  Includes angiography of same vessel.

☺ **G0290** Transcatheter placement of a drug eluting intracoronary stent(s), percutaneous, with or without other therapeutic intervention, any method; single vessel

  Use site specific modifiers -LC, -LD, and -RC to designate artery. Part A claim.

☺ **G0291** Transcatheter placement of a drug eluting intracoronary stent(s), percutaneous, with or without other therapeutic intervention, any method; each additional vessel

  Use site specific modifiers -LC, -LD, and -RC to designate artery. Part A claim.

Procedure, Non-Covered

G0293-G0294: Bill local carrier

☺ **G0293** Noncovered surgical procedure(s) using conscious sedation, regional, general or spinal anesthesia in a Medicare qualifying clinical trial, per day

☺ **G0294** Noncovered procedure(s) using either no anesthesia or local anesthesia only, in a Medicare qualifying clinical trial, per day

Therapy, Electromagnetic

◆ **G0295** Electromagnetic therapy, to one or more areas, for wound care other than described in G0329 or for other uses

  Bill local carrier
  IOM: 100-03, 4, 270.1

Services, Pulmonary Surgery

G0302-G0305: Bill local carrier

* **G0302** Pre-operative pulmonary surgery services for preparation for LVRS, complete course of services, to include a minimum of 16 days of services

* **G0303** Pre-operative pulmonary surgery services for preparation for LVRS, 10 to 15 days of services

* **G0304** Pre-operative pulmonary surgery services for preparation for LVRS, 1 to 9 days of services

* **G0305** Post-discharge pulmonary surgery services after LVRS, minimum of 6 days of services

Laboratory

G0306-G0328: Bill local carrier

→ * **G0306** Complete CBC, automated (HgB, HCT, RBC, WBC, without platelet count) and automated WBC differential count

  Laboratory Certification: Hematology

→ * **G0307** Complete CBC, automated (HgB, HCT, RBC, WBC; without platelet count)

  Laboratory Certification: Hematology

▶ New → Revised ✔ Reinstated ~~deleted~~ Deleted
☺ Special coverage instructions ◆ Not covered or valid by Medicare * Carrier discretion

☺ **G0328** Colorectal cancer screening; fecal occult blood test, immunoassay, 1-3 simultaneous

Co-insurance and deductible waived

Reported for Medicare patients 50+; one FOBT per year, with either G0107 (guaiac-based) or G0328 (immunoassay-based)

Laboratory Certification: Routine Chemistry, Hematology

Therapy, Electromagnetic

✳ **G0329** Electromagnetic therapy, to one or more areas for chronic stage III and stage IV pressure ulcers, arterial ulcers, and diabetic ulcers and venous stasis ulcers not demonstrating measurable signs of healing after 30 days of conventional care as part of a therapy plan of care

Bill local carrier

Fee, Pharmacy

☺ **G0333** Pharmacy dispensing fee for inhalation drug(s); initial 30-day supply as a beneficiary

Bill DME/MAC

Medicare will reimburse an initial dispensing fee to a pharmacy for initial 30-day period of inhalation drugs furnished through DME

Hospice

✳ **G0337** Hospice evaluation and counseling services, pre-election

Bill local carrier

Radiosurgery, Robotic

G0339-G0340: Bill local carrier

→ ✳ **G0339** Image-guided robotic linear accelerator-based stereotactic radiosurgery, complete course of therapy in one session or first session of fractionated treatment

Do not report with 77421

→ ✳ **G0340** Image-guided robotic linear accelerator-based stereotactic radiosurgery, delivery including collimator changes and custom plugging, fractionated treatment, all lesions, per session, second through fifth sessions, maximum five sessions per course of treatment

Do not report with 77421

Islet Cell

G0341-G0343: Bill local carrier

☺ **G0341** Percutaneous islet cell transplant, includes portal vein catheterization and infusion

IOM: 100-03, 4, 260.3; 100-04, 32, 70

☺ **G0342** Laparoscopy for islet cell transplant, includes portal vein catheterization and infusion

IOM: 100-03, 4, 260.3

☺ **G0343** Laparotomy for islet cell transplant, includes portal vein catheterization and infusion

IOM: 100-03, 4, 260.3

Aspiration, Bone Marrow

✳ **G0364** Bone marrow aspiration performed with bone marrow biopsy through the same incision on the same date of service

Bill local carrier

For Medicare patients, reported rather than 38220

Mapping, Vessel

G0365-G0372: Bill local carrier

✳ **G0365** Vessel mapping of vessels for hemodialysis access (services for preoperative vessel mapping prior to creation of hemodialysis access using an autogenous hemodialysis conduit, including arterial inflow and venous outflow)

Includes evaluation of the relevant arterial and venous vessels. Use modifier 26 for professional component only

☺ **G0372** Physician service required to establish and document the need for a power mobility device

Providers should bill the E/M code and G0372 on the same claim.

▶ New → Revised ✔ Reinstated ~~deleted~~ Deleted ☺ Special coverage instructions ◆ Not covered or valid by Medicare ✳ Carrier discretion

Services, Observation and ED

G0378-G0384: Bill local carrier

⊛ **G0378** Hospital observation service, per hour

Report all related services in addition to G0378. Report units of hours spent in observation (rounded to the nearest hour). Hospitals report the ED or clinic visit with a CPT code or, if applicable, G0379 (direct admit to observation) and G0378 (hospital observation services, per hour)

⊛ **G0379** Direct admission of patient for hospital observation care

Report all related services in addition to G0379. Report units of hours spent in observation (rounded to the nearest hour). Hospitals report the ED or clinic visit with a CPT code or, if applicable, G0379 (direct admit to observation) and G0378 (hospital observation services, per hour)

✳ **G0380** Level 1 hospital emergency department visit provided in a type B emergency department; (the ED must meet at least one of the following requirements: (1) it is licensed by the state in which it is located under applicable state law as an emergency room or emergency department; (2) it is held out to the public (by name, posted signs, advertising, or other means) as a place that provides care for emergency medical conditions on an urgent basis without requiring a previously scheduled appointment; or (3) during the calendar year immediately preceding the calendar year in which a determination under 42 CFR 489.24 is being made, based on a representative sample of patient visits that occurred during that calendar year, it provides at least one-third of all of its outpatient visits for the treatment of emergency medical conditions on an urgent basis without requiring a previously scheduled appointment)

✳ **G0381** Level 2 hospital emergency department visit provided in a type B emergency department; (the ED must meet at least one of the following requirements: (1) it is licensed by the state in which it is located under applicable state law as an emergency room or emergency department; (2) it is held out to the public (by name, posted signs, advertising, or other means) as a place that provides care for emergency medical conditions on an urgent basis without requiring a previously scheduled appointment; or (3) during the calendar year immediately preceding the calendar year in which a determination under 42 CFR 489.24 is being made, based on a representative sample of patient visits that occurred during that calendar year, it provides at least one-third of all of its outpatient visits for the treatment of emergency medical conditions on an urgent basis without requiring a previously scheduled appointment)

✳ **G0382** Level 3 hospital emergency department visit provided in a type B emergency department; (the ED must meet at least one of the following requirements: (1) it is licensed by the state in which it is located under applicable state law as an emergency room or emergency department; (2) it is held out to the public (by name, posted signs, advertising, or other means) as a place that provides care for emergency medical conditions on an urgent basis without requiring a previously scheduled appointment; or (3) during the calendar year immediately preceding the calendar year in which a determination under 42 CFR 489.24 is being made, based on a representative sample of patient visits that occurred during that calendar year, it provides at least one-third of all of its outpatient visits for the treatment of emergency medical conditions on an urgent basis without requiring a previously scheduled appointment)

▶ New → Revised ✔ Reinstated deleted Deleted

⊛ Special coverage instructions ◆ Not covered or valid by Medicare ✳ Carrier discretion

* **G0383** Level 4 hospital emergency department visit provided in a type B emergency department; (the ED must meet at least one of the following requirements: (1) it is licensed by the state in which it is located under applicable state law as an emergency room or emergency department; (2) it is held out to the public (by name, posted signs, advertising, or other means) as a place that provides care for emergency medical conditions on an urgent basis without requiring a previously scheduled appointment; or (3) during the calendar year immediately preceding the calendar year in which a determination under 42 CFR 489.24 is being made, based on a representative sample of patient visits that occurred during that calendar year, it provides at least one-third of all of its outpatient visits for the treatment of emergency medical conditions on an urgent basis without requiring a previously scheduled appointment)

* **G0384** Level 5 hospital emergency department visit provided in a type B emergency department; (the ED must meet at least one of the following requirements: (1) it is licensed by the state in which it is located under applicable state law as an emergency room or emergency department; (2) it is held out to the public (by name, posted signs, advertising, or other means) as a place that provides care for emergency medical conditions on an urgent basis without requiring a previously scheduled appointment; or (3) during the calendar year immediately preceding the calendar year in which a determination under 42 CFR § 489.24 is being made, based on a representative sample of patient visits that occurred during that calendar year, it provides at least one-third of all of its outpatient visits for the treatment of emergency medical conditions on an urgent basis without requiring a previously scheduled appointment)

Ultrasound, AAA

☼ **G0389** Ultrasound B-scan and/or real time with image documentation; for abdominal aortic aneurysm (AAA) screening

Bill local carrier

Use modifier 26 for professional component only

Eligible beneficiaries must receive a referral for an AAA ultrasound screening as a result of an IPPE (initial preventative physical examination). This is a once in a lifetime benefit per eligible beneficiary. (http://www.cms.gov/MLNProducts/downloads/MPS_QuickReferenceChart_1.pdf)

Team, Trauma Response

☼ **G0390** Trauma response team associated with hospital critical care service

Bill local carrier

Assessment/Intervention

G0396-G0397: Bill local carrier

* **G0396** Alcohol and/or substance (other than tobacco) abuse structured assessment (e.g., AUDIT, DAST), and brief intervention 15 to 30 minutes

Bill instead of 99408 and 99409

* **G0397** Alcohol and/or substance (other than tobacco) abuse structured assessment (e.g., AUDIT, DAST), and intervention, greater than 30 minutes

Bill instead of 99408 and 99409

Home Sleep Study Test

* **G0398** Home sleep study test (HST) with type II portable monitor, unattended; minimum of 7 channels: EEG, EOG, EMG, ECG/heart rate, airflow, respiratory effort and oxygen saturation

Bill local carrier

* **G0399** Home sleep test (HST) with type III portable monitor, unattended; minimum of 4 channels: 2 respiratory movement/airflow, 1 ECG/heart rate and 1 oxygen saturation

▶ New   → Revised   ✔ Reinstated   deleted Deleted
☼ Special coverage instructions   ◆ Not covered or valid by Medicare   * Carrier discretion

∗ **G0400** Home sleep test (HST) with type IV portable monitor, unattended; minimum of 3 channels

Examination, Initial Medicare

∗ **G0402** Initial preventive physical examination; face-to-face visit, services limited to new beneficiary during the first 12 months of Medicare enrollment

Depending on circumstances, 99201-99215 may be assigned with modifier 25 to report an E/M service as a significant, separately identifiable service in addition to the Initial Preventive Physical Examination (IPPE), G0402.

Copayment and coinsurance waived, deductible waived after 01/01/11. (http://www.cms.gov/MLNProducts/downloads/MPS_QuickReferenceChart_1.pdf)

Electrocardiogram

G0403-G0405: Bill local carrier

∗ **G0403** Electrocardiogram, routine ECG with 12 leads; performed as a screening for the initial preventive physical examination with interpretation and report

Optional service may be ordered or performed at discretion of physician. Once in a life-time screening, stemming from a referral from Initial Preventive Physical Examination (IPPE). Both deductible and co-payment apply.

∗ **G0404** Electrocardiogram, routine ECG with 12 leads; tracing only, without interpretation and report, performed as a screening for the initial preventive physical examination

∗ **G0405** Electrocardiogram, routine ECG with 12 leads; interpretation and report only, performed as a screening for the initial preventive physical examination

Telehealth

G0406-G0408: Bill local carrier

→ ∗ **G0406** Follow-up inpatient consultation, limited, physicians typically spend 15 minutes communicating with the patient via telehealth

These telehealth modifers are required when billing for telehealth services with codes G0406-G0408 and G0425-G0427:
- GT, via interactive audio and video telecommunications system
- GQ, via asynchronous telecommunications system

→ ∗ **G0407** Follow-up inpatient consultation, intermediate, physicians typically spend 25 minutes communicating with the patient via telehealth

→ ∗ **G0408** Follow-up inpatient consultation, complex, physicians typically spend 35 minutes communicating with the patient via telehealth

Services, Social, Psychological

G0409-G0411: Bill local carrier

∗ **G0409** Social work and psychological services, directly relating to and/or furthering the patient's rehabilitation goals, each 15 minutes, face-to-face; individual (services provided by a CORF-qualified social worker or psychologist in a CORF)

∗ **G0410** Group psychotherapy other than of a multiple-family group, in a partial hospitalization setting, approximately 45 to 50 minutes

∗ **G0411** Interactive group psychotherapy, in a partial hospitalization setting, approximately 45 to 50 minutes

Treatment, Bone

G0412-G0415: Bill local carrier

∗ **G0412** Open treatment of iliac spine(s), tuberosity avulsion, or iliac wing fracture(s), unilateral or bilateral for pelvic bone fracture patterns which do not disrupt the pelvic ring includes internal fixation, when performed

▶ New   → Revised   ✔ Reinstated   deleted Deleted
⊙ Special coverage instructions   ◆ Not covered or valid by Medicare   ∗ Carrier discretion

* **G0413** Percutaneous skeletal fixation of posterior pelvic bone fracture and/or dislocation, for fracture patterns which disrupt the pelvic ring, unilateral or bilateral, (includes ilium, sacroiliac joint and/or sacrum)

* **G0414** Open treatment of anterior pelvic bone fracture and/or dislocation for fracture patterns which disrupt the pelvic ring, unilateral or bilateral, includes internal fixation when performed (includes pubic symphysis and/or superior/inferior rami)

* **G0415** Open treatment of posterior pelvic bone fracture and/or dislocation, for fracture patterns which disrupt the pelvic ring, unilateral or bilateral, includes internal fixation, when performed (includes ilium, sacroiliac joint and/or sacrum)

Pathology, Surgical

G0416-G0419: Bill local carrier

* **G0416** Surgical pathology, gross and microscopic examination for prostate needle saturation biopsy sampling, 1-20 specimens

   This testing requires a facility to have either a CLIA certificate of registration (certificate type code 9), a CLIA certificate of compliance (certificate type code 1), or a CLIA certificate of accreditation (certificate type code 3). A facility without a valid, current, CLIA certificate, with a current CLIA certificate of waiver (certificate type code 2) or with a current CLIA certificate for provider-performed microscopy procedures (certificate type code 4) must not be permitted to be paid for these tests. This code has a -TC, -26 (physician), or global component.

   Laboratory Certification: Histopathology

* **G0417** Surgical pathology, gross and microscopic examination for prostate needle saturation biopsy sampling, 21-40 specimens

   Laboratory Certification: Histopathology

* **G0418** Surgical pathology, gross and microscopic examination for prostate needle saturation biopsy sampling, 41-60 specimens

   Use modifier 26 for professional component only

   Laboratory Certification: Histopathology

* **G0419** Surgical pathology, gross and microscopic examination for prostate needle saturation biopsy sampling, greater than 60 specimens

   Use modifier 26 for professional component only

   Laboratory Certification: Histopathology

Educational Services, Rehabilitation, Telehealth, and Drug Screening

G0420-G0441: Bill local carrier

* **G0420** Face-to-face educational services related to the care of chronic kidney disease; individual, per session, per one hour

   CKD is kidney damage of 3 months or longer, regardless of the cause of kidney damage. Sessions billed in increments of one hour (if session is less than 1 hour, it must last at least 31 minutes to be billable. Sessions less than one hour and longer than 31 minutes is billable as one session. No more than 6 sessions of KDE services in a beneficiary's lifetime

* **G0421** Face-to-face educational services related to the care of chronic kidney disease; group, per session, per one hour

   Group setting: 2 to 20, report codes G0420 and G0421 with diagnosis code 585.4.

* **G0422** Intensive cardiac rehabilitation; with or without continuous ECG monitoring with exercise, per session

   Includes the same service as 93798 but at a greater frequency; may be reported with as many as six hourly sessions on a single date of service. Includes medical nutrition services to reduce cardiac disease risk factors.

▶ New   → Revised   ✔ Reinstated   deleted Deleted   ☺ Special coverage instructions   ◆ Not covered or valid by Medicare   * Carrier discretion

* **G0423** Intensive cardiac rehabilitation; with or without continuous ECG monitoring; without exercise, per session

Includes the same service as 93797 but at a greater frequency; may be reported with as many as six hourly sessions on a single date of service. Includes medical nutrition services to reduce cardiac disease risk factors.

* **G0424** Pulmonary rehabilitation, including exercise (includes monitoring), one hour, per session, up to two sessions per day

Includes therapeutic services and all related monitoring services to inprove respiratory function. Do not report with G0237, G0238, or G0239.

→ * **G0425** Telehealth consultation, emergency department or initial inpatient, typically 30 minutes communicating with the patient via telehealth

Problem Focused: Problem focused history and examination, with straightforward medical decision making complexity. Typically 30 minutes communicating with patient via telehealth

→ * **G0426** Telehealth consultation, emergency department or initial inpatient, typically 50 minutes communicating with the patient via telehealth

Detailed: Detailed history and examination, with moderate medical decision making complexity. Typically 50 minutes communicating with patient via telehealth

→ * **G0427** Telehealth consultation, emergency department or initial inpatient, typically 70 minutes or more communicating with the patient via telehealth

Comprehensive: Comprehensive history and examination, with high medical decision making complexity. Typically 70 minutes or more communicating with patient via telehealth.

▶ ◆ **G0428** Collagen meniscus implant procedure for filling meniscal defects (e.g., CMI, collagen scaffold, menaflex)

▶ * **G0429** Dermal filler injection(s) for the treatment of facial lipodystrophy syndrome (LDS) (e.g., as a result of highly active antiretroviral therapy)

Designated for dermal fillers Sculptra® and Radiesse (Medicare). (https://www.cms.gov/ContractorLearningResources/downloads/JA6953.pdf)

→ * **G0431** Drug screen, qualitative; multiple drug classes by high complexity test method (e.g., immunoassay, enzyme assay), per patient encounter

Bill local carrier

http://www.cms.hhs.gov/mlnmattersarticles/downloads/se1001.pdf.

Laboratory Certification: Toxicology

→ * **G0432** Infectious agent antibody detection by enzyme immunoassay (EIA) technique, HIV-1 and/or HIV-2, screening

Bill local carrier

Laboratory Certification: Virology, General immunology

→ * **G0433** Infectious agent antibody detection by enzyme-linked immunosorbent assay (ELISA) technique, HIV-1 and/or HIV-2, screening

Bill local carrier

▶ * **G0434** Drug screen, other than chromatographic; any number of drug classes, by CLIA waived test or moderate complexity test, per patient encounter

Bill local carrier

Laboratory Certification: Virology, General immunology

→ * **G0435** Infectious agent antibody detection by rapid antibody test, HIV-1 and/or HIV-2, screening

Bill local carrier

▶ * **G0436** Smoking and tobacco cessation counseling visit for the asymptomatic patient; intermediate, greater than 3 minutes, up to 10 minutes

Bill local carrier

▶ * **G0437** Smoking and tobacco cessation counseling visit for the asymptomatic patient; intensive, greater than 10 minutes

Bill local carrier

▶ * **G0438** Annual wellness visit; includes a personalized prevention plan of service (PPS), initial visit

Bill local carrier

▶ * **G0439** Annual wellness visit, includes a personalized prevention plan of service (PPS), subsequent visit

Bill local carrier

▶ New	→ Revised	✔ Reinstated	~~deleted~~ Deleted

○ Special coverage instructions   ◆ Not covered or valid by Medicare   * Carrier discretion

~~G0440~~ ~~Application of tissue cultured allogeneic skin substitute or dermal substitute; for use on lower limb, includes the site preparation and debridement if performed; first 25 sq cm or less~~ ✖

~~G0441~~ ~~Application of tissue cultured allogeneic skin substitute or dermal substitute; for use on lower limb, includes the site preparation and debridement if performed; each additional 25 sq cm~~ ✖

▶ ✳ **G0442** Annual alcohol misuse screening, 15 minutes

▶ ✳ **G0443** Brief face-to-face behavioral counseling for alcohol misuse, 15 minutes

▶ ✳ **G0444** Annual depression screening, 15 minutes

▶ ✳ **G0445** High intensity behavioral counseling to prevent sexually transmitted infection; face-to-face, individual, includes: education, skills training and guidance on how to change sexual behavior; performed semi-annually, 30 minutes

▶ ✳ **G0446** Intensive behavioral therapy to reduce cardiovascular disease risk, individual, face-to-face, bi-annual, 15 minutes

▶ ✳ **G0447** Face-to-face behavioral counseling for obesity, 15 minutes

▶ ✳ **G0448** Insertion or replacement of a permanent pacing cardioverter-defibrillator system with transvenous lead(s), single or dual chamber with insertion of pacing electrode, cardiac venous system, for left ventricular pacing

▶ ✳ **G0449** Annual face-to-face obesity screening, 15 minutes

▶ ✳ **G0450** Screening for sexually transmitted infections, includes laboratory tests for chlamydia, gonorrhea, syphilis and hepatitis B

▶ ✳ **G0451** Development testing, with interpretation and report, per standardized instrument form

▶ ✳ **G0908** Most recent hemoglobin (HGB) level >12.0 g/dl

▶ ✳ **G0909** Hemoglobin level measurement not documented, reason not otherwise specified

▶ ✳ **G0910** Most recent hemoglobin level <= 12.0 g/dl

▶ ✳ **G0911** Assessed level of activity and symptoms

▶ ✳ **G0912** Level of activity and symptoms not assessed

▶ ✳ **G0913** Improvement in visual function achieved within 90 days following cataract surgery

▶ ✳ **G0914** Patient care survey was not completed by patient

▶ ✳ **G0915** Improvement in visual function not achieved within 90 days following cataract surgery

▶ ✳ **G0916** Satisfaction with care achieved within 90 days following cataract surgery

▶ ✳ **G0917** Patient satisfaction survey was not completed by patient

▶ ✳ **G0918** Satisfaction with care not achieved within 90 days following cataract surgery

▶ ✳ **G0919** Influenza immunization ordered or recommended (to be given at alternate location or alternate provider); vaccine not available at time of visit

▶ ✳ **G0920** Type, anatomic location, and activity all documented

▶ ✳ **G0921** Documentation of patient reason(s) for not being able to assess

▶ ✳ **G0922** No documentation of disease type, anatomic location, and activity, reason not otherwise specified

Tositumomab

✳ **G3001** Administration and supply of tositumomab, 450 mg

Bill local carrier

The therapeutic regimen consists of a dosimetric step of tositumomab infusion followed 7 – 14 days later by a therapeutic step of iodine I-131 tositumomab infusion.

Documentation

G8126-G9140: Bill local carrier

✳ **G8126** Patient documented as being treated with antidepressant medication during the entire 12 week acute treatment phase

✳ **G8127** Patient not documented as being treated with antidepressant medication during the entire 12 weeks acute treatment phase

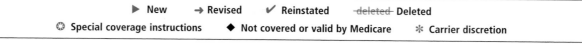

▶ New   → Revised   ✔ Reinstated   ~~deleted~~ Deleted
⊘ Special coverage instructions   ◆ Not covered or valid by Medicare   ✳ Carrier discretion

* **G8128** Clinician documented that patient was not an eligible candidate for antidepressant medication during the entire 12 week acute treatment phase measure

* **G8395** Left ventricular ejection fraction (LVEF) > = 40% or documentation as normal or mildly depressed left ventricular systolic function

* **G8396** Left ventricular ejection fraction (LVEF) not performed or documented

* **G8397** Dilated macular or fundus exam performed, including documentation of the presence or absence of macular edema and level of severity of retinopathy

* **G8398** Dilated macular or fundus exam not performed

* **G8399** Patient with central dual-energy x-ray absorptiometry (DXA) results documented or ordered or pharmacologic therapy (other than minerals/vitamins) for osteoporosis prescribed)

* **G8400** Patient with central dual-energy x-ray absorptiometry (DXA) results not documented or not ordered or pharmacologic therapy (other than minerals/vitamins) for osteoporosis not prescribed

* **G8401** Clinician documented that patient was not an eligible candidate for screening or therapy for osteoporosis for women measure

* **G8404** Lower extremity neurological exam performed and documented

* **G8405** Lower extremity neurological exam not performed

* **G8406** Clinician documented that patient was not an eligible candidate for lower extremity neurological exam measure

* **G8410** Footwear evaluation performed and documented

* **G8415** Footwear evaluation was not performed

* **G8416** Clinician documented that patient was not an eligible candidate for footwear evaluation measure

* **G8417** Calculated BMI above the upper parameter and a follow-up plan was documented in the medical record

* **G8418** Calculated BMI below the lower parameter and a follow-up plan was documented in the medical record

* **G8419** Calculated BMI outside normal parameters, no follow-up plan was documented in the medical record

* **G8420** Calculated BMI within normal parameters and documented

* **G8421** BMI not calculated

* **G8422** Patient not eligible for BMI calculation

→ * **G8427** List of current medications (includes prescription, over-the-counter, herbals, vitamin/mineral/dietary [nutritional] supplements) documented by the provider, including drug name, dosage, frequency and route

→ * **G8428** Current medications (includes prescription, over-the-counter, herbals, vitamin/mineral/dietary [nutritional] supplements) with drug name, dosage, frequency and route not documented by the provider, reason not specified

* **G8430** Provider documentation that patient is not eligible for medication assessment

→ * **G8431** Positive screen for clinical depression using an age-appropriate standardized tool and a follow-up plan documented

→ * **G8432** No documentation of clinical depression screening using an age-appropriate standardized tool

→ * **G8433** Screening for clinical depression using an age-appropriate standardized tool not documented, patient not eligible/ appropriate

~~G8440 Documentation of pain assessment (including location, intensity and description) prior to initiation of therapy or documentation of the absence of pain as a result of assessment through discussion with the patient including the use of a standardized tool and a follow-up plan is documented~~ ✖

~~G8441 No documentation of pain assessment (including location, intensity and description) prior to initiation of therapy~~ ✖

* **G8442** Documentation that patient is not eligible for pain assessment

→ * **G8447** Patient encounter was documented using an EHR system that has been certified by an authorized testing and certification body (ATCB)

→ * **G8448** Patient encounter was documented using a PQRI qualified EHR or other acceptable systems

▶ New → Revised ✔ Reinstated ~~deleted~~ Deleted
⊕ Special coverage instructions ◆ Not covered or valid by Medicare * Carrier discretion

* **G8450** Beta-blocker therapy prescribed for patients with left ventricular ejection fraction (LVEF) <40% or documentation as moderately or severely depressed left ventricular systolic function

* **G8451** Clinician documented patient with left ventricular ejection fraction (LVEF) <40% or documentation as moderately or severely depressed left ventricular systolic function was not eligible candidate for beta-blocker therapy

* **G8452** Beta-blocker therapy not prescribed for patients with left ventricular ejection fraction (LVEF) <40% or documentation as moderately or severely depressed left ventricular systolic function

* **G8458** Clinician documented that patient is not an eligible candidate for genotype testing; patient not receiving antiviral treatment for hepatitis C

* **G8459** Clinician documented that patient is receiving antiviral treatment for hepatitis C

* **G8460** Clinician documented that patient is not an eligible candidate for quantitative RNA testing at week 12; patient not receiving antiviral treatment for hepatitis C

* **G8461** Patient receiving antiviral treatment for hepatitis C

* **G8462** Clinician documented that patient is not an eligible candidate for counseling regarding contraception prior to antiviral treatment; patient not receiving antiviral treatment for hepatitis C

* **G8463** Patient receiving antiviral treatment for hepatitis C documented

* **G8464** Clinician documented that prostate cancer patient is not an eligible candidate for adjuvant hormonal therapy; low or intermediate risk of recurrence or risk of recurrence not determined

* **G8465** High risk of recurrence of prostate cancer

* **G8468** Angiotensin converting enzyme (ACE) inhibitor or angiotensin receptor blocker (ARB) therapy prescribed for patients with a left ventricular ejection fraction (LVEF) <40% or documentation of moderately or severely depressed left ventricular systolic function

* **G8469** Clinician documented that patient with a left ventricular ejection fraction (LVEF) <40% or documentation of moderately or severely depressed left ventricular systolic function was not an eligible candidate for angiotensin converting enzyme (ACE) inhibitor or angiotensin receptor blocker (ARB) therapy

* **G8470** Patient with left ventricular ejection fraction (LVEF) > =40% or documentation as normal or mildly depressed left ventricular systolic function

* **G8471** Left ventricular ejection fraction (LVEF) was not performed or documented

* **G8472** Angiotensin converting enzyme (ACE) inhibitor or angiotensin receptor blocker (ARB) therapy not prescribed for patients with a left ventricular ejection fraction (LVEF) <40% or documentation of moderately or severely depressed left ventricular systolic function, reason not specified

* **G8473** Angiotensin converting enzyme (ACE) inhibitor or angiotensin receptor blocker (ARB) therapy prescribed

* **G8474** Angiotensin converting enzyme (ACE) inhibitor or angiotensin receptor blocker (ARB) therapy not prescribed for reasons documented by the clinician

* **G8475** Angiotensin converting enzyme (ACE) inhibitor or angiotensin receptor blocker (ARB) therapy not prescribed, reason not specified

* **G8476** Most recent blood pressure has a systolic measurement of <130 mm/Hg and a diastolic measurement of <80 mm/Hg

* **G8477** Most recent blood pressure has a systolic measurement of > =130 mm/Hg and/or a diastolic measurement of > =80 mm/Hg

* **G8478** Blood pressure measurement not performed or documented, reason not specified

→ * **G8482** Influenza immunization administered or previously received

* **G8483** Influenza immunization was not ordered or administered for reasons documented by clinician

▶ New	→ Revised	✔ Reinstated	deleted Deleted
⊙ Special coverage instructions		◆ Not covered or valid by Medicare	* Carrier discretion

* **G8484** Influenza immunization was not ordered or administered, reason not specified

* **G8485** I intend to report the diabetes mellitus measures group

* **G8486** I intend to report the preventive care measures group

* **G8487** I intend to report the chronic kidney disease (CKD) measures group

* **G8489** I intend to report the Coronary Artery Disease (CAD) measures group

* **G8490** I intend to report the Rheumatoid Arthritis measures group

* **G8491** I intend to report the HIV/AIDS measures group

* **G8492** I intend to report the Perioperative Care measures group

* **G8493** I intend to report the Back Pain measures group

* **G8494** All quality actions for the applicable measures in the Diabetes Mellitus measures group have been performed for this patient

Composite code, do not report with G8485

* **G8495** All quality actions for the applicable measures in the CKD measures group have been performed for this patient

Composite code, do not report with G8487

* **G8496** All quality actions for the applicable measures in the Preventive Care measures group have been performed for this patient

Composite code, do not report with G8486

* **G8497** All quality actions for the applicable measures in the Coronary Artery Bypass Graft (CABG) measures group have been performed for this patient

Composite code.

* **G8498** All quality actions for the applicable measures in the Coronary Artery Disease (CAD) measures group have been performed for this patient

Composite code.

* **G8499** All quality actions for the applicable measures in the Rheumatoid Arthritis measures group have been performed for this patient

Composite code, do not report with G8490

* **G8500** All quality actions for the applicable measures in the HIV/AIDS measures group have been performed for this patient

Composite code.

* **G8501** All quality actions for the applicable measures in the Perioperative Care measures group have been performed for this patient

Composite code, do not report with G8492

* **G8502** All quality actions for the applicable measures in the Back Pain measures group have been performed for this patient

Composite code, do not report with G8493

* **G8506** Patient receiving angiotensin converting enzyme (ACE) inhibitor or angiotensin receptor blocker (ARB) therapy

G8508 Documentation of pain assessment (including location, intensity and description) prior to initiation of therapy or documentation of the absence of pain as a result of assessment through discussion with the patient including the use of a standardized tool; no documentation of a follow-up plan, patient not eligible ✖

→ * **G8509** Documentation of positive pain assessment; no documentation of a follow-up plan, reason not specified

→ * **G8510** Negative screen for clinical depression using an age-appropriate standardized tool, follow-up not required

→ * **G8511** Positive screen for clinical depression using an age-appropriate standardized tool documented, follow up plan not documented, reason not specified

* **G8524** Patch closure used for patient undergoing conventional CEA

* **G8525** Clinician documented that patient did not receive conventional CEA

* **G8526** Patch closure not used for patient undergoing conventional CEA, reason not specified

▶ New   → Revised   ✔ Reinstated   -deleted- Deleted
🌣 Special coverage instructions   ◆ Not covered or valid by Medicare   * Carrier discretion

* **G8530**   Autogenous AV fistula received

* **G8531**   Clinician documented that patient was not an eligible candidate for autogenous AV fistula

* **G8532**   Clinician documented that patient received vascular access other than autogenous AV fistula, reason not specified

~~G8534~~   ~~Documentation of an elder maltreatment screen and follow-up plan~~   ✖

* **G8535**   No documentation of an elder maltreatment screen, patient not eligible

* **G8536**   No documentation of an elder maltreatment screen, reason not specified

~~G8537~~   ~~Elder maltreatment screen documented, follow up plan not documented, patient not eligible~~   ✖

~~G8538~~   ~~Elder maltreatment screen documented, follow up plan not documented, reason not specified~~   ✖

→ * **G8539**   Documentation of a current functional outcome assessment using a standardized tool and documentation of a care plan based on identified deficiencies

* **G8540**   Documentation that the patient is not eligible for a functional outcome assessment using a standardized tool

* **G8541**   No documentation of a current functional outcome assessment using a standardized tool, reason not specified

→ * **G8542**   Documentation of a current functional outcome assessment using a standardized tool; no functional deficiencies identified, care plan not required

* **G8543**   Documentation of a current functional outcome assessment using a standardized tool; no documentation of a care plan, reason not specified

* **G8544**   I intend to report the coronary artery bypass graft (CABG) measures group

* **G8545**   I intend to report the Hepatitis C measures group

* **G8546**   I intend to report the Community-Acquired Pneumonia (CAP) measures group

* **G8547**   I intend to report the Ischemic Vascular Disease (IVD) measures group

* **G8548**   I intend to report the Heart Failure (HF) measures group

* **G8549**   All quality actions for the applicable measures in the Hepatitis C measures group have been performed for this patient

Composite code, do not report with G8545

* **G8550**   All quality actions for the applicable measures in the Community-Acquired Pneumonia (CAP) measures group have been performed for this patient

Composite code, do not report with G8546

* **G8551**   All quality actions for the applicable measures in the Heart Failure (HF) measures group have been performed for this patient

Composite code.

* **G8552**   All quality actions for the applicable measures in the Ischemic Vascular Disease (IVD) measures group have been performed for this patient

Composite code, do not report with G8547

→ * **G8553**   Prescription generated and transmitted via a qualified ERX system or a certified EHR system

* **G8556**   Referred to a physician (preferably a physician with training in disorders of the ear) for an otologic evaluation

* **G8557**   Patient is not eligible for the referral for otologic evaluation measure

* **G8558**   Not referred to a physician (preferably a physician with training in disorders of the ear) for an otologic evaluation, reason not specified

* **G8559**   Patient referred to a physician (preferably a physician with training in disorders of the ear) for an otologic evaluation

* **G8560**   Patient has a history of active drainage from the ear within the previous 90 days

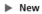

* **G8561** Patient is not eligible for the referral for otologic evaluation for patients with a history of active drainage measure

* **G8562** Patient does not have a history of active drainage from the ear within the previous 90 days

* **G8563** Patient not referred to a physician (preferably a physician with training in disorders of the ear) for an otologic evaluation, reason not specified

* **G8564** Patient was referred to a physician (preferably a physician with training in disorders of the ear) for an otologic evaluation, reason not specified)

* **G8565** Verification and documentation of sudden or rapidly progressive hearing loss

* **G8566** Patient is not eligible for the "referral for otologic evaluation for sudden or rapidly progressive hearing loss" measure

* **G8567** Patient does not have verification and documentation of sudden or rapidly progressive hearing loss

* **G8568** Patient was not referred to a physician (preferably a physician with training in disorders of the ear) for an otologic evaluation, reason not specified

* **G8569** Prolonged intubation (>24 hrs) required

* **G8570** Prolonged intubation (>24 hrs) not required

* **G8571** Development of deep sternal wound infection within 30 days postoperatively

* **G8572** No deep sternal wound infection

→ * **G8573** Stroke following isolated CABG surgery

→ * **G8574** No stroke following isolated CABG surgery

→ * **G8575** Developed postoperative renal failure or required dialysis

→ * **G8576** No postoperative renal failure/dialysis not required

→ * **G8577** Reexploration required due to mediastinal bleeding with or without tamponade, graft occlusion, valve dysfunction, or other cardiac reason

→ * **G8578** Reexploration not required due to mediastinal bleeding with or without tamponade, graft occlusion, valve dysfunction, or other cardiac reason

* **G8579** Antiplatelet medication at discharge

→ * **G8580** Antiplatelet medication contraindicated

* **G8581** No antiplatelet medication at discharge

* **G8582** Beta-blocker at discharge

→ * **G8583** Beta-blocker contraindicated

* **G8584** No beta-blocker at discharge

* **G8585** Anti-lipid treatment at discharge

→ * **G8586** Anti-lipid treatment contraindicated

* **G8587** No anti-lipid treatment at discharge

* **G8588** Most recent systolic blood pressure < 140 mmhg

* **G8589** Most recent systolic blood pressure >= 140 mmhg

* **G8590** Most recent diastolic blood pressure < 90 mmhg

* **G8591** Most recent diastolic blood pressure >= 90 mmhg

* **G8592** No documentation of blood pressure measurement

* **G8593** Lipid profile results documented and reviewed (must include total cholesterol, HDL-C, triglycerides and calculated LDL-C)

* **G8594** Lipid profile not performed, reason not otherwise specified

* **G8595** Most recent LDL-C < 100 mg/dl

* **G8596** LDL-C was not performed

* **G8597** Most recent LDL-C >= 100 mg/dl

* **G8598** Aspirin or another antithrombotic therapy used

* **G8599** Aspirin or another antithrombotic therapy not used, reason not otherwise specified

* **G8600** IV T-PA initiated within three hours (<= 180 minutes) of time last known well

* **G8601** IV T-PA not initiated within three hours (<= 180 minutes) of time last known well for reasons documented by clinician

* **G8602** IV T-PA not initiated within three hours (<= 180 minutes) of time last known well, reason not specified

* **G8603** Score on the spoken language comprehension functional communication measure at discharge was higher than at admission

---

▶ New   → Revised   ✔ Reinstated   ~~deleted~~ Deleted

☺ Special coverage instructions   ◆ Not covered or valid by Medicare   * Carrier discretion

* **G8604** Score on the spoken language comprehension functional communication measure at discharge was not higher than at admission, reason not specified

→ * **G8605** Patient treated for spoken language comprehension but not scored on the spoken language comprehension functional communication measure either at admission or at discharge

* **G8606** Score on the attention functional communication measure at discharge was higher than at admission

* **G8607** Score on the attention functional communication measure at discharge was not higher than at admission, reason not specified

→ * **G8608** Patient treated for attention but not scored on the attention functional communication measure either at admission or at discharge

* **G8609** Score on the memory functional communication measure at discharge was higher than at admission

* **G8610** Score on the memory functional communication measure at discharge was not higher than at admission, reason not specified

→ * **G8611** Patient treated for memory but not scored on the memory functional communication measure either at admission or at discharge

* **G8612** Score on the motor speech functional communication measure at discharge was higher than at admission

* **G8613** Score on the motor speech functional communication measure at discharge was not higher than at admission, reason not specified

→ * **G8614** Patient treated for motor speech but not scored on the motor speech comprehension functional communication measure either at admission or at discharge

* **G8615** Score on the reading functional communication measure at discharge was higher than at admission

* **G8616** Score on the reading functional communication measure at discharge was not higher than at admission, reason not specified

→ * **G8617** Patient treated for reading but not scored on the reading functional communication measure either at admission or at discharge

* **G8618** Score on the spoken language expression functional communication measure at discharge was higher than at admission

* **G8619** Score on the spoken language expression functional communication measure at discharge was not higher than at admission, reason not specified

→ * **G8620** Patient treated for spoken language expression but not scored on the spoken language expression functional communication measure either at admission or at discharge

* **G8621** Score on the writing functional communication measure at discharge was higher than at admission

* **G8622** Score on the writing functional communication measure at discharge was not higher than at admission, reason not specified

→ * **G8623** Patient treated for writing but not scored on the writing functional communication measure either at admission or at discharge

* **G8624** Score on the swallowing functional communication measure at discharge was higher than at admission

* **G8625** Score on the swallowing functional communication measure at discharge was not higher than at admission, reason not specified

→ * **G8626** Patient treated for swallowing but not scored on the swallowing functional communication measure at admission or at discharge

* **G8627** Surgical procedure performed within 30 days following cataract surgery for major complications (e.g. retained nuclear fragments, endophthalmitis, dislocated or wrong power IOL, retinal detachment, or wound dehiscence)

* **G8628** Surgical procedure not performed within 30 days following cataract surgery for major complications (e.g. retained nuclear fragments, endophthalmitis, dislocated or wrong power IOL, retinal detachment, or wound dehiscence)

▶ * **G8629** Documentation of order for prophylactic parenteral antibiotic to be given within one hour (if fluoroquindone or vancomycin, two hours) prior to surgical incision (or start of procedure when no incision is required)

▶ New	→ Revised	✔ Reinstated	~~deleted~~ Deleted
⊙ Special coverage instructions		◆ Not covered or valid by Medicare	* Carrier discretion

▶ ✳ **G8630** Documentation that administration of prophylactic parenteral antibiotics was initiated within one hour (if fluoroquinolone or vancomycin, two hours) prior to surgical incision (or start of procedure when no incision is required), as ordered

▶ ✳ **G8631** Clinician documented that patient was not an eligible candidate for ordering prophylactic parenteral antibiotics to be given within one hour (if fluoroquinolone or vancomycin, two hours) prior to surgical incision (or start of procedure when no incision is required)

▶ ✳ **G8632** Prophylactic parenteral antibiotics were not ordered to be given or given within one hour (if fluoroquinolone or vancomycin, two hours) prior to the surgical incision (or start of procedure when no incision is required), reason not otherwise specified)

▶ ✳ **G8633** Pharmacologic therapy (other than minierals/vitamins) for osteoporosis prescribed

▶ ✳ **G8634** Clinician documented patient not an eligible candidate to receive pharmacologic therapy for osteoporosis

▶ ✳ **G8635** Pharmacologic therapy for osteoporosis was not prescribed, reason not otherwise specified

~~G8636~~ ~~Influenza immunization administered or previously received~~ ✖

~~G8637~~ ~~Clinician documented that patient is not eligible to receive the influenza immunization~~ ✖

~~G8638~~ ~~Influenza immunization not administered or previously received, reason not otherwise specified~~ ✖

~~G8639~~ ~~Influenza immunization was administered or previously received~~ ✖

~~G8640~~ ~~Clinician has documented that patient is not eligible to receive the influenza immunization~~ ✖

~~G8641~~ ~~Influenza immunization was not administered or previously received, reason not otherwise specified~~ ✖

▶ ✳ **G8642** The eligible professional practices in a rural area without sufficient high speed internet access and requests a hardship exemption from the application of the payment adjustment under Section 1848(a)(5)(a) of the Social Security Act

▶ ✳ **G8643** The eligible professional practices in an area without sufficient available pharmacies for electronic prescribing and requests a hardship exemption for the application of the payment adjustment under Section 1848(a)(5)(a) of the Social Security Act

▶ ✳ **G8644** Eligible professional does not have prescribing privileges

▶ ✳ **G8645** I intend to report the asthma measures group

▶ ✳ **G8646** All quality actions for the applicable measures in the asthma measures group have been performed for this patient

▶ ✳ **G8647** Risk-adjusted functional status change residual score for the knee successfully calculated and the score was equal to zero (0) or greater than zero (>0)

▶ ✳ **G8648** Risk-adjusted functional status change residual score for the knee successfully calculated and the score was less than zero (<0)

▶ ✳ **G8649** Risk-adjusted functional status change residual scores for the knee not measured because the patient did not complete FOTO'S functional intake on admission and/or follow up status survey near discharge, patient not eligible/not appropriate

▶ ✳ **G8650** Risk-adjusted functional status change residual scores for the knee not measured because the patient did not complete FOTO'S functional intake on admission and/or follow up status survey near discharge, reason not specified

▶ ✳ **G8651** Risk-adjusted functional status change residual score for the hip successfully calculated and the score was equal to zero (0) or greater than zero (>0)

▶ ✳ **G8652** Risk-adjusted functional status change residual score for the hip successfully calculated and the score was less than zero (<0)

▶ ✳ **G8653** Risk-adjusted functional status change residual scores for the hip not measured because the patient did not complete FOTO'S functional intake on admission and/or follow up status survey near discharge, patient not eligible/not appropriate

---

▶ New   → Revised   ✔ Reinstated   ~~deleted~~ Deleted
☺ Special coverage instructions   ◆ Not covered or valid by Medicare   ✳ Carrier discretion

▶ ✳ **G8654** Risk-adjusted functional status change residual scores for the hip not measured because the patient did not complete FOTO'S functional intake on admission and/or follow up status survey near discharge, reason not specified

▶ ✳ **G8655** Risk-adjusted functional status change residual score for the lower leg, foot or ankle successfully calculated and the score was equal to zero (0) or greater than zero (>0)

▶ ✳ **G8656** Risk-adjusted functional status change residual score for the lower leg, foot or ankle successfully calculated and the score was less than zero (<0)

▶ ✳ **G8657** Risk-adjusted functional status change residual scores for the lower leg, foot or ankle not measured because the patient did not complete FOTO'S functional intake on admission and/or follow up status survey near discharge, patient not eligible/not appropriate

▶ ✳ **G8658** Risk-adjusted functional status change residual scores for the lower leg, foot or ankle not measured because the patient did not complete FOTO'S functional intake on admission and/or follow up status survey near discharge, reason not specified

▶ ✳ **G8659** Risk-adjusted functional status change residual score for the lumbar spine successfully calculated and the score was equal to zero (0) or greater than zero (>0)

▶ ✳ **G8660** Risk-adjusted functional status change residual score for the lumbar spine successfully calculated and the score was less than zero (<0)

▶ ✳ **G8661** Risk-adjusted functional status change residual scores for the lumbar spine not measured because the patient did not complete FOTO'S functional intake on admission and/or follow up status survey near discharge, patient not eligible/not appropriate

▶ ✳ **G8662** Risk-adjusted functional status change residual scores for the lumbar spine not measured because the patient did not complete FOTO'S functional intake on admission and/or follow up status survey near discharge, reason not specified

▶ ✳ **G8663** Risk-adjusted functional status change residual score for the shoulder successfully calculated and the score was equal to zero (0) or greater than zero (>0)

▶ ✳ **G8664** Risk-adjusted functional status change residual score for the shoulder successfully calculated and the score was less than zero (<0)

▶ ✳ **G8665** Risk-adjusted functional status change residual scores for the shoulder not measured because the patient did not complete FOTO'S functional intake on admission and/or follow up status survey near discharge, patient not eligible/not appropriate

▶ ✳ **G8666** Risk-adjusted functional status change residual scores for the shoulder not measured because the patient did not complete FOTO'S functional intake on admission and/or follow up status survey near discharge, reason not specified

▶ ✳ **G8667** Risk-adjusted functional status change residual score for the elbow, wrist or hand successfully calculated and the score was equal to zero (0) or greater than zero (>0)

▶ ✳ **G8668** Risk-adjusted functional status change residual score for the elbow, wrist or hand successfully calculated and the score was less than zero (<0)

▶ ✳ **G8669** Risk-adjusted functional status change residual scores for the elbow, wrist or hand not measured because the patient did not complete FOTO'S functional intake on admission and/or follow up status survey near discharge, patient not eligible/not appropriate

▶ ✳ **G8670** Risk-adjusted functional status change residual scores for the elbow, wrist or hand not measured because the patient did not complete FOTO'S functional intake on admission and/or follow up status survey near discharge, reason not specified

▶ ✳ **G8671** Risk-adjusted functional status change residual score for the neck, cranium, mandible, thoracic spine, ribs, or other general orthopedic impairment successfully calculated and the score was equal to zero (0) or greater than zero (>0)

▶ ✳ **G8672** Risk-adjusted functional status change residual score for the neck, cranium, mandible, thoracic spine, ribs, or other general orthopedic impairment successfully calculated and the score was less than zero (<0)

▶ New   → Revised   ✔ Reinstated   ~~deleted~~ Deleted

⊚ Special coverage instructions   ◆ Not covered or valid by Medicare   ✳ Carrier discretion

▶ ✳ **G8673** Risk-adjusted functional status change residual scores for the neck, cranium, mandible, thoracic spine, ribs, or other general orthopedic impairment not measured because the patient did not complete FOTO'S functional intake on admission and/or follow up status survey near discharge, patient not eligible/not appropriate

▶ ✳ **G8674** Risk-adjusted functional status change residual scores for the neck, cranium, mandible, thoracic spine, ribs, or other general orthopedic impairment not measured because the patient did not complete FOTO'S functional intake on admission and/or follow up status survey near discharge, reason not specified

~~G8675~~ ~~Most recent systolic blood pressure ≥ 140 mm hg~~ ✖

~~G8676~~ ~~Most recent diastolic blood pressure ≥ 90 mm hg~~ ✖

~~G8677~~ ~~Most recent systolic blood pressure < 130 mm hg~~ ✖

~~G8678~~ ~~Most recent systolic blood pressure 130 to 139 mm hg~~ ✖

~~G8679~~ ~~Most recent diastolic blood pressure < 80 mm hg~~ ✖

~~G8680~~ ~~Most recent diastolic blood pressure 80-89 mm hg~~ ✖

~~G8681~~ ~~Patient hospitalized with principal diagnosis of heart failure during the measurement period~~ ✖

▶ ✳ **G8682** Left ventricular function testing performed during the measurement period

▶ ✳ **G8683** Clinician documented that patient is not an eligible candidate for left ventricular function testing during the measurement period

~~G8684~~ ~~Patient not hospitalized with principal diagnosis of heart failure during the measurement period~~ ✖

▶ ✳ **G8685** Left ventricular function testing not performed during the measurement period, reason not specified

~~G8686~~ ~~Currently a tobacco smoker or current exposure to secondhand smoke~~ ✖

~~G8687~~ ~~Currently a tobacco non user and no exposure to secondhand smoke~~ ✖

~~G8688~~ ~~Currently a smokeless tobacco user (eg, chew, snuff) and no exposure to secondhand smoke~~ ✖

~~G8689~~ ~~Tobacco use not assessed, reason not otherwise specified~~ ✖

~~G8690~~ ~~Current tobacco smoker or current exposure to secondhand smoke~~ ✖

~~G8691~~ ~~Current tobacco non-user and no exposure to secondhand smoke~~ ✖

~~G8692~~ ~~Current smokeless tobacco user (eg, chew, snuff) and no exposure to secondhand smoke~~ ✖

~~G8693~~ ~~Tobacco use not assessed, reason not specified~~ ✖

▶ ✳ **G8694** Left ventricular ejection fraction (LVEF) <40%

▶ ✳ **G8695** Left ventricular ejection fraction (LVEF) >= 40% or documentation as mildly depressed left ventricular systolic function or normal

▶ ✳ **G8696** Antithrombotic therapy prescribed at discharge

▶ ✳ **G8697** Antithrombotic therapy not prescribed for documented reasons

▶ ✳ **G8698** Antithrombotic therapy was not prescribed at discharge, reason not otherwise specified

▶ ✳ **G8699** Rehabilitation services (occupational, physical or speech) ordered at or prior to discharge

▶ ✳ **G8700** Rehabilitation services (occupational, physical or speech) not indicated at or prior to discharge

▶ ✳ **G8701** Rehabilitation services were not ordered, reason not otherwise specified

▶ ✳ **G8702** Documentation that prophylactic antibiotics were given within 4 hours prior to surgical incision or intraoperatively

▶ ✳ **G8703** Documentation that prophylactic antibiotics were neither given within 4 hours prior to surgical incision nor intraoperatively

▶ ✳ **G8704** 12-lead electrocardiogram (ECG) performed

▶ ✳ **G8705** Documentation of medical reason(s) for not performing a 12-lead electrocardiogram (ECG)

▶ ✳ **G8706** Documentation of patient reason(s) for not performing a 12-lead electrocardiogram (ECG)

▶ ✳ **G8707** 12-lead electrocardiogram (ECG) not performed, reason not otherwise specified

▶ ✳ **G8708** Patient not prescribed or dispensed antibiotic

▶ **New**   → **Revised**   ✔ **Reinstated**   ~~deleted~~ **Deleted**

◎ **Special coverage instructions**   ◆ **Not covered or valid by Medicare**   ✳ **Carrier discretion**

▶ ✳ **G8709** Patient prescribed or dispensed antibiotic for documented medical reason(s)

▶ ✳ **G8710** Patient prescribed or dispensed antibiotic

▶ ✳ **G8711** Prescribed or dispensed antibiotic

▶ ✳ **G8712** Antibiotic not prescribed or dispensed

▶ ✳ **G8713** SPKT/V greater than or equal to 1.2 (single-pool clearance of urea [KT] / volume [V])

▶ ✳ **G8714** Hemodialysis treatment performed exactly three times per week

▶ ✳ **G8715** Hemodialysis treatment performed less than three times per week or greater than three times per week

▶ ✳ **G8716** Documentation of reason(s) for patient not having greater than or equal to 1.2 (single-pool clearance of urea [KT] / volume [V])

▶ ✳ **G8717** SPKT/V less than 1.2 (single-pool clearance of urea [KT] / volume [V]), reason not specified

▶ ✳ **G8718** Total KT/V greater than or equal to 1.7 per week (total clearance of urea [KT] / volume [V])

▶ ✳ **G8720** Total KT/V less than 1.7 per week (total clearance of urea [KT] / volume [V]), reason not specified

▶ ✳ **G8721** PT category (primary tumor), PN category (regional lymph nodes), and histologic grade were documented in pathology report

▶ ✳ **G8722** Medical reason(s) documented for not including PT category, PN category and histologic grade in the pathology report

▶ ✳ **G8723** Specimen site is other than anatomic location of primary tumor

▶ ✳ **G8724** PT category, PN category and histologic grade were not documented in the pathology report, reason not otherwise specified

▶ ✳ **G8725** Fasting lipid profile performed (triglycerides, LDL-C, HDL-C and total cholesterol)

▶ ✳ **G8726** Clinician has documented reason for not performing fasting lipid profile

▶ ✳ **G8727** Patient receiving hemodialysis, peritoneal dialysis or kidney transplantation

▶ ✳ **G8728** Fasting lipid profile not performed, reason not otherwise specified

▶ ✳ **G8730** Pain assessment documented as positive utilizing a standardized tool and a follow-up plan is documented

▶ ✳ **G8731** Pain assessment documented as negative, no follow-up plan is required

▶ ✳ **G8732** No documentation of pain assessment

▶ ✳ **G8733** Documentation of a positive elder maltreatment screen and documented follow-up plan

▶ ✳ **G8734** Elder maltreatment screen documented as negative, no follow-up required

▶ ✳ **G8735** Elder maltreatment screen documented as positive, follow-up plan not documented, reason not specified

▶ ✳ **G8736** Most current LDL-C <100 mg/dl

▶ ✳ **G8737** Most current LDL-C >=100 mg/dl

▶ ✳ **G8738** Left ventricular ejection fraction (LVEF) <40% or documentation of severely or moderately depressed left ventricular systolic function

▶ ✳ **G8739** Left ventricular ejection fraction (LVEF) >= 40% or documentation as normal or mildly depressed left ventricular systolic function

▶ ✳ **G8740** Left ventricular ejection fraction (LVEF) not performed or assessed, reason not specified

▶ ✳ **G8741** Patient not treated for spoken language comprehension disorder

▶ ✳ **G8742** Patient not treated for attention disorder

▶ ✳ **G8743** Patient not treated for memory disorder

▶ ✳ **G8744** Patient not treated for motor speech disorder

▶ ✳ **G8745** Patient not treated for reading disorder

▶ ✳ **G8746** Patient not treated for spoken language expression disorder

▶ ✳ **G8747** Patient not treated for writing disorder

▶ ✳ **G8748** Patient not treated for swallowing disorder

▶ ✳ **G8749** Absence of signs of melanoma (cough, dyspnea, tenderness, localized neurologic signs such as weakness, jaundice or any other sign suggesting systemic spread) or absence of symptoms of melanoma (pain, paresthesia, or any other symptom suggesting the possibility of systemic spread of melanoma)

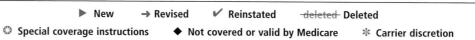

▶ New   → Revised   ✔ Reinstated   ~~deleted~~ Deleted
⊙ Special coverage instructions   ◆ Not covered or valid by Medicare   ✳ Carrier discretion

▶ ✳ **G8750** Presence of signs of melanoma (cough, dyspnea, tenderness, localized neurologic signs such as weakness, jaundice or any other sign suggesting systemic spread) or presence of symptoms of melanoma (pain, paresthesia, or any other symptom suggesting the possibility of systemic spread of melanoma)

▶ ✳ **G8751** Smoking status and exposure to secondhand smoke in the home not assessed, reason not specified

▶ ✳ **G8752** Most recent systolic blood pressure <140 mm hg

▶ ✳ **G8753** Most recent systolic blood pressure >= 140 mm hg

▶ ✳ **G8754** Most recent diastolic blood pressure <90 mm hg

▶ ✳ **G8755** Most recent diastolic blood pressure >= 90 mm hg

▶ ✳ **G8756** No documentation of blood pressure measurement, reason not otherwise specified

▶ ✳ **G8757** All quality actions for the applicable measures in the chronic obstructive pulmonary disease measures group have been performed for this patient

▶ ✳ **G8758** All quality actions for the applicable measures in the inflammatory bowel disease measures group have been performed for this patient

▶ ✳ **G8759** All quality actions for the applicable measures in the obstructive sleep apnea measures group have been performed for this patient

▶ ✳ **G8760** All quality actions for the applicable measures in the epilepsy measures group have been performed for this patient

▶ ✳ **G8761** All quality actions for the applicable measures in the dementia measures group have been performed for this patient

▶ ✳ **G8762** All quality actions for the applicable measures in the Parkinson's disease measures group have been performed for this patient

▶ ✳ **G8763** All quality actions for the applicable measures in the hypertension measures group have been performed for this patient

▶ ✳ **G8764** All quality actions for the applicable measures in the cardiovascular prevention measures group have been performed for this patient

▶ ✳ **G8765** All quality actions for the applicable measures in the cataract measures group have been performed for this patient

▶ ✳ **G8767** Lipid panel results documented and reviewed (must include total cholesterol, HDL-C, triglycerides and calculated LDL-C)

▶ ✳ **G8768** Documentation of medical reason(s) for not performing lipid profile (e.g., patients who have a terminal illness or for whom treatment of hypertension with standard treatment goals is not clinically appropriate)

▶ ✳ **G8769** Lipid profile not performed, reason not otherwise specified

▶ ✳ **G8770** Urine protein test result documented and reviewed

▶ ✳ **G8771** Documentation of diagnosis of chronic kidney disease

▶ ✳ **G8772** Documentation of medical reason(s) for not performing urine protein test (e.g., patients who have a terminal illness or for whom treatment of hypertension with standard treatment goals is not clinically appropriate)

▶ ✳ **G8773** Urine protein test was not performed, reason not otherwise specified

▶ ✳ **G8774** Serum creatinine test result documented and reviewed

▶ ✳ **G8775** Documentation of medical reason(s) for not performing serum creatinine test (e.g., patients who have a terminal illness or for whom treatment of hypertension with standard treatment goals is not clinically appropriate)

▶ ✳ **G8776** Serum creatinine test not performed, reason not otherwise specified

▶ ✳ **G8777** Diabetes screening test performed

▶ ✳ **G8778** Documentation of medical reason(s) for not performing diabetes screening test (e.g., patients who have a terminal illness or for whom treatment of hypertension with standard treatment goals is not clinically appropriate, or patients with a diagnosis of diabetes)

▶ ✳ **G8779** Diabetes screening test not performed, reason not otherwise specified

▶ ✳ **G8780** Counseling for diet and physical activity performed

▶ New   → Revised   ✔ Reinstated   ~~deleted~~ Deleted

⊙ Special coverage instructions   ◆ Not covered or valid by Medicare   ✳ Carrier discretion

▶ * **G8781**   Documentation of medical reason(s) for patient not receiving counseling for diet and physical activity (e.g., patients who have a terminal illness or for whom treatment of hypertension with standard treatment goals is not clinically appropriate)

▶ * **G8782**   Counseling for diet and physical activity not performed, reason not otherwise specified

▶ * **G8783**   Blood pressure screening performed as recommended by the defined screening interval

▶ * **G8784**   Blood pressure not assessed, patient not eligible

▶ * **G8785**   Blood pressure screening not performed as recommended by screening interval, reason not otherwise specified

▶ * **G8786**   Severity of angina assessed according to level of activity

▶ * **G8787**   Angina assessed as present

▶ * **G8788**   Angina assessed as absent

▶ * **G8789**   Severity of angina not assessed according to level of activity

▶ * **G8790**   Most recent office visit systolic blood pressure <130 mm hg

▶ * **G8791**   Most recent office visit systolic blood pressure, 130-139 mm hg

▶ * **G8792**   Most recent office visit systolic blood pressure >=140 mm hg

▶ * **G8793**   Most recent office visit diastolic blood pressure, <80 mm hg

▶ * **G8794**   Most recent office visit diastolic blood pressure, 80-89 mm hg

▶ * **G8795**   Most recent office visit diastolic blood pressure >=90 mm hg

▶ * **G8796**   Blood pressure measurement not documented, reason not otherwise specified

▶ * **G8797**   Specimen site other than anatomic location of esophagus

▶ * **G8798**   Specimen site other than anatomic location of prostate

▶ * **G8799**   Anticoagulation ordered

▶ * **G8800**   Anticoagulation not ordered for reasons documented by clinician

▶ * **G8801**   Anticoagulation was not ordered, reason not specified

▶ * **G8802**   Pregnancy test (urine or serum) ordered

▶ * **G8803**   Pregnancy test (urine or serum) not ordered for reasons documented by clinician

▶ * **G8805**   Pregnancy test (urine or serum) was not ordered, reason not specified

▶ * **G8806**   Performance of trans-abdominal or trans-vaginal ultrasound

▶ * **G8807**   Trans-abdominal or trans-vaginal ultrasound not performed for reasons documented by clinician

▶ * **G8808**   Performance of trans-abdominal or trans-vaginal ultrasound not ordered, reason not specified

▶ * **G8809**   Rh-immunoglobulin (RhoGAM) ordered

▶ * **G8810**   R-immunoglobulin (RhoGAM) not ordered for reasons documented by clinician

▶ * **G8811**   Documentation RH-immunoglobulin (RhoGAM) was not ordered, reason not specified

▶ * **G8812**   Patient is not eligible for follow-up CTA, duplex, or MRA

▶ * **G8813**   Follow-up CTA, duplex, or MRA of the abdomen and pelvis performed

▶ * **G8814**   Follow-up CTA, duplex, or MRA of the abdomen and pelvis not performed

▶ * **G8815**   Statin therapy not prescribed for documented reasons

▶ * **G8816**   Statin medication prescribed at discharge

▶ * **G8817**   Statin therapy not prescribed at discharge, reason not specified

▶ * **G8818**   Patient discharge to home no later than post-operative day #7

▶ * **G8819**   Aneurysm minor diameter <= 5.5 cm

▶ * **G8820**   Aneurysm minor diameter 5.6-6.0 cm

▶ * **G8821**   Abdominal aortic aneurysm is not infareral

▶ * **G8822**   Male patients with aneurysms minor diameter >6 cm

▶ * **G8823**   Female patients with aneurysm minor diameter >6 cm

▶ * **G8824**   Female patients with aneurysm minor diameter 5.6-6.0 cm

▶ * **G8825**   Patient not discharged to home by post-operative day #7

▶ * **G8826**   Patient discharge to home no later than post-operative day #2 following EVAR

▶ * **G8827**   Aneurysm minor diameter <= 5.5 cm for women

▶ New   → Revised   ✔ Reinstated   ~~deleted~~ Deleted

✪ Special coverage instructions   ◆ Not covered or valid by Medicare   * Carrier discretion

176

▶ ✳ **G8828**   Aneurysm minor diameter <= 5.5 cm for men

▶ ✳ **G8829**   Aneurysm minor diameter 5.6-6.0 cm for men

▶ ✳ **G8830**   Aneurysm minor diameter >6 cm for men

▶ ✳ **G8831**   Aneurysm minor diameter >6 cm for women

▶ ✳ **G8832**   Aneurysm minor diameter 5.6-6.0 cm for women

▶ ✳ **G8833**   Patient not discharged to home by post-operative day #2 following EVAR

▶ ✳ **G8834**   Patient discharged to home no later than post-operative day #2 following CEA

▶ ✳ **G8835**   Asymptomatic patient with no history of any transient ischemic attack or stroke in any carotid or vertebrobasilar territory

▶ ✳ **G8836**   Symptomatic patient with ipsilateral stroke or TIA within 120 days prior to CEA

▶ ✳ **G8837**   Other symptomatic patient with ipsilateral carotid territory TIA or stroke >120 days prior to CEA, or contralateral carotid territory TIA or stroke or vertebrobasilar TIA or stroke

▶ ✳ **G8838**   Patient not discharged to home by post-operative day #2

▶ ✳ **G8839**   Sleep apnea symptoms assessed, including presence or absence of snoring and daytime sleepiness

▶ ✳ **G8840**   Documentation of reason(s) for not performing an assessment of sleep symptoms (e.g., patient didn't have initial daytime sleepiness, patient visits between initial testing and initiation of therapy)

▶ ✳ **G8841**   Sleep apnea symptoms not assessed, reason not otherwise specified

▶ ✳ **G8842**   Apnea Hypopnea Index (AHI) or Respiratory Disturbance Index (RDI) measured at the time of initial diagnosis

▶ ✳ **G8843**   Documentation of reason(s) for not measuring an Apnea Hypopnea Index (AHI) or a Respiratory Disturbance Index (RDI) at the time of initial diagnosis

▶ ✳ **G8844**   Apnea Hypopnea Index (AHI) or Respiratory Disturbance Index (RDI) not measured at the time of initial diagnosis, reason not specified

▶ ✳ **G8845**   Positive airway pressure therapy prescribed

▶ ✳ **G8846**   Moderate or severe obstructive sleep apnea (Apnea Hypopnea Index (AHI) or Respiratory Disturbance Index (RDI) of 15 or greater)

▶ ✳ **G8847**   Positive airway pressure therapy not prescribed

▶ ✳ **G8848**   Mild obstructive sleep apnea (Apnea Hypopnea Index (AHI) or Respiratory Disturbance Index (RDI) of less than 15)

▶ ✳ **G8849**   Documentation of reason(s) for not prescribing positive airway pressure therapy

▶ ✳ **G8850**   Positive airway pressure therapy not prescribed, reason not otherwise specified

▶ ✳ **G8851**   Objective measurement of adherence to positive airway pressure therapy, documented

▶ ✳ **G8852**   Positive airway pressure therapy prescribed

▶ ✳ **G8853**   Positive airway pressure therapy not prescribed

▶ ✳ **G8854**   Documentation of reason(s) for not objectively measuring adherence to positive airway pressure therapy

▶ ✳ **G8855**   Objective measurement of adherence to positive airway pressure therapy not performed, reason not otherwise specified

▶ ✳ **G8856**   Referral to a physician for an otologic evaluation performed

▶ ✳ **G8857**   Patient is not eligible for the referral for otologic evaluation measure (e.g., patients who are already under the care of a physician for acute or chronic dizziness)

▶ ✳ **G8858**   Referral to a physician for an otologic evaluation not performed, reason not specified

▶ ✳ **G8859**   Patient receiving corticosteroids greater than or equal to 10 mg/day for 60 or greater consecutive days

▶ ✳ **G8860**   Patients who have received dose of corticosteroids greater than or equal to 10 mg/day for 60 or greater consecutive days

---

▶ New   → Revised   ✔ Reinstated   ~~deleted~~ Deleted

◎ Special coverage instructions   ◆ Not covered or valid by Medicare   ✳ Carrier discretion

▶ ✳ **G8861** Central dual-energy x-ray absorptiometry (DXA) ordered or documented, review of systems and medication history or pharmacologic therapy (other than minerals/vitamins) for osteoporosis prescribed

▶ ✳ **G8862** Patients not receiving corticosteroids greater than or equal to 10 mg/day for 60 or greater consecutive days

▶ ✳ **G8863** Patients not assessed for risk of bone loss, reason not otherwise specified

▶ ✳ **G8864** Pneumococcal vaccine administered or previously received

▶ ✳ **G8865** Documentation of medical reason(s) for not administering or previously receiving pneumococcal vaccine (e.g., patient allergic reaction, potential adverse drug reaction)

▶ ✳ **G8866** Documentation of patient reason(s) for not administering or previously receiving pneumococcal vaccine (e.g., patient refusal)

▶ ✳ **G8867** Pneumococcal vaccine not administered or previously received, reason not otherwise specified

▶ ✳ **G8868** Patients receiving a first course of anti-TNF therapy

▶ ✳ **G8869** Patient has documented immunity to hepatitis B and is receiving a first course of anti-TNF therapy

▶ ✳ **G8870** Hepatitis B vaccine injection administered or previously received and is receiving a first course of anti-TNF therapy

▶ ✳ **G8871** Patient not receiving a first course of anti-TNF therapy

▶ ✳ **G8872** Excised tissue evaluated by imaging intraoperatively to confirm successful inclusion of targeted lesion

▶ ✳ **G8873** Patients with needle localization specimens which are not amenable to intraoperative imaging such as MRI needle wire localization, or targets which are tentatively identified on mammogram or ultrasound which do not contain a biopsy marker but which can be verified on intraoperative inspection or pathology

▶ ✳ **G8874** Excised tissue not evaluated by imaging intraoperatively to confirm successful inclusion of targeted lesion

▶ ✳ **G8875** Clinician diagnosed breast cancer preoperatively by a minimally invasive biopsy method

▶ ✳ **G8876** Documentation of reason(s) for not performing minimally invasive biopsy to diagnose breast cancer properatively

▶ ✳ **G8877** Clinician did not attempt to achieve the diagnosis of breast cancer preoperatively by a minimally invasive biopsy method, reason not otherwise specified

▶ ✳ **G8878** Sentinel lymph node biopsy procedure performed

▶ ✳ **G8879** Clinically node negative (T1N0M0 or T2N0M0) invasive breast cancer

▶ ✳ **G8880** Documentation of reason(s) sentinel lymph node biopsy not performed

▶ ✳ **G8881** Stage of breast cancer is greater than T1N0M0 or T2N0M0

▶ ✳ **G8882** Sentinel lymph node biopsy procedure not performed

▶ ✳ **G8883** Biopsy results reviewed, communicated, tracked and documented

▶ ✳ **G8884** Clinician documented reason that patient's biopsy results were not reviewed

▶ ✳ **G8885** Biopsy results not reviewed, communicated, tracked or documented

▶ ✳ **G8886** Most recent blood pressure under control

▶ ✳ **G8887** Documentation of medical reason(s) for most recent blood pressure not being under control (e.g., patients with comorbid conditions that cause an increase in blood pressure or require treatment with medications that cause an increase in blood pressure, or patients who had a terminal illness or for whom treatment of hypertension with standard treatment goals is not clinically appropriate)

▶ ✳ **G8888** Most recent blood pressure not under control, results documented and reviewed

▶ ✳ **G8889** No documentation of blood pressure measurement, reason not otherwise specified

▶ ✳ **G8890** Most recent LDL-C under control, results documented and reviewed

▶ ✳ **G8891** Documentation of medical reason(s) for most recent LSL-C not under control (e.g., patients who had a terminal illness or for whom treatment of hypertension with standard treatment goals is not clinically appropriate)

▶ New → Revised ✔ Reinstated ~~deleted~~ Deleted ✪ Special coverage instructions ◆ Not covered or valid by Medicare ✳ Carrier discretion

▶ ✳ **G8892** Documentation of medical reason(s) for not performing LDL-C test (e.g., patients who had a terminal illness or for whom treatment of hypertension with standard treatment goals is not clinically appropriate)

▶ ✳ **G8893** Most recent LDL-C not under control, results documented and reviewed

▶ ✳ **G8894** LDL-C not performed, reason not specified

▶ ✳ **G8895** Oral aspirin or other anticoagulant/antiplatelet therapy prescribed

▶ ✳ **G8896** Documentation of medical reason(s) for not prescribing oral aspirin or other anticoagulant/antiplatelet therapy (e.g., under age 30, patient documented to be low risk, patient with terminal illness or treatment of hypertension with standard treatment goals is not clinically appropriate)

▶ ✳ **G8897** Oral aspirin or other anticoagulant/antiplatelet therapy was not prescribed, reason not otherwise specified

▶ ✳ **G8898** I intend to report the chronic obstructive pulmonary disease measures group

▶ ✳ **G8899** I intend to report the inflammatory bowel disease measures group

▶ ✳ **G8900** I intend to report the obstructive sleep apnea measures group

▶ ✳ **G8901** I intend to report the epilepsy measures group

▶ ✳ **G8902** I intend to report the dementia measures group

▶ ✳ **G8903** I intend to report the Parkinson's disease measures group

▶ ✳ **G8904** I intend to report the hypertension measures group

▶ ✳ **G8905** I intend to report the cardiovascular prevention measures group

▶ ✳ **G8906** I intend to report the cataract measures group

⊛ **G9001** Coordinated care fee, initial rate

⊛ **G9002** Coordinated care fee, maintenance rate

⊛ **G9003** Coordinated care fee, risk adjusted high, initial

⊛ **G9004** Coordinated care fee, risk adjusted low, initial

⊛ **G9005** Coordinated care fee, risk adjusted maintenance

⊛ **G9006** Coordinated care fee, home monitoring

⊛ **G9007** Coordinated care fee, scheduled team conference

⊛ **G9008** Coordinated care fee, physician coordinated care oversight services

⊛ **G9009** Coordinated care fee, risk adjusted maintenance, level 3

⊛ **G9010** Coordinated care fee, risk adjusted maintenance, level 4

⊛ **G9011** Coordinated care fee, risk adjusted maintenance, level 5

⊛ **G9012** Other specified case management services not elsewhere classified

◆ **G9013** ESRD demo basic bundle Level I

Medicare non-covered.

◆ **G9014** ESRD demo expanded bundle, including venous access and related services

Medicare non-covered.

◆ **G9016** Smoking cessation counseling, individual, in the absence of or in addition to any other evaluation and management service, per session (6-10 minutes) [demo project code only]

Medicare non-covered.

✳ **G9017** Amantadine hydrochloride, oral, per 100 mg (for use in a Medicare-approved demonstration project)

✳ **G9018** Zanamivir, inhalation powder, administered through inhaler, per 10 mg (for use in a Medicare-approved demonstration project)

✳ **G9019** Oseltamivir phosphate, oral, per 75 mg (for use in a Medicare-approved demonstration project)

✳ **G9020** Rimantadine hydrochloride, oral, per 100 mg (for use in a Medicare-approved demonstration project)

✳ **G9033** Amantadine hydrochloride, oral brand, per 100 mg (for use in a Medicare-approved demonstration project)

✳ **G9034** Zanamivir, inhalation powder, administered through inhaler, brand, per 10 mg (for use in a Medicare-approved demonstration project)

✳ **G9035** Oseltamivir phosphate, oral, brand, per 75 mg (for use in a Medicare-approved demonstration project)

✳ **G9036** Rimantadine hydrochloride, oral, brand, per 100 mg (for use in a Medicare-approved demonstration project)

▶ New　　→ Revised　　✔ Reinstated　　deleted Deleted

⊛ Special coverage instructions　　◆ Not covered or valid by Medicare　　✳ Carrier discretion

G9041   Rehabilitation services for low vision by qualified occupational therapist, direct one on one contact, each 15 minutes ✱

G9042   Rehabilitation services for low vision by certified orientation and mobility specialists, direct one-on-one contact, each 15 minutes ✱

G9043   Rehabilitation services for low vision by certified low vision rehabilitation therapist, direct one-on-one contact, each 15 minutes ✱

G9044   Rehabilitation services for low vision by certified low vision rehabilitation teacher, direct one-on-one contact, each 15 minutes ✱

◆ **G9050**   Oncology; primary focus of visit; work-up, evaluation, or staging at the time of cancer diagnosis or recurrence (for use in a Medicare-approved demonstration project)

◆ **G9051**   Oncology; primary focus of visit; treatment decision-making after disease is staged or restaged, discussion of treatment options, supervising/coordinating active cancer directed therapy or managing consequences of cancer directed therapy (for use in a Medicare-approved demonstration project)

◆ **G9052**   Oncology; primary focus of visit; surveillance for disease recurrence for patient who has completed definitive cancer-directed therapy and currently lacks evidence of recurrent disease; cancer directed therapy might be considered in the future (for use in a Medicare-approved demonstration project)

◆ **G9053**   Oncology; primary focus of visit; expectant management of patient with evidence of cancer for whom no cancer directed therapy is being administered or arranged at present; cancer directed therapy might be considered in the future (for use in a Medicare-approved demonstration project)

◆ **G9054**   Oncology; primary focus of visit; supervising, coordinating or managing care of patient with terminal cancer or for whom other medical illness prevents further cancer treatment; includes symptom management, end-of-life care planning, management of palliative therapies (for use in a Medicare-approved demonstration project)

◆ **G9055**   Oncology; primary focus of visit; other, unspecified service not otherwise listed (for use in a Medicare-approved demonstration project)

◆ **G9056**   Oncology; practice guidelines; management adheres to guidelines (for use in a Medicare-approved demonstration project)

◆ **G9057**   Oncology; practice guidelines; management differs from guidelines as a result of patient enrollment in an institutional review board approved clinical trial (for use in a Medicare-approved demonstration project)

◆ **G9058**   Oncology; practice guidelines; management differs from guidelines because the treating physician disagrees with guideline recommendations (for use in a Medicare-approved demonstration project)

◆ **G9059**   Oncology; practice guidelines; management differs from guidelines because the patient, after being offered treatment consistent with guidelines, has opted for alternative treatment or management, including no treatment (for use in a Medicare-approved demonstration project)

◆ **G9060**   Oncology; practice guidelines; management differs from guidelines for reason(s) associated with patient comorbid illness or performance status not factored into guidelines (for use in a Medicare-approved demonstration project)

▶ New   → Revised   ✔ Reinstated   deleted Deleted
⊙ Special coverage instructions   ◆ Not covered or valid by Medicare   ✱ Carrier discretion

◆ **G9061** Oncology; practice guidelines; patient's condition not addressed by available guidelines (for use in a Medicare-approved demonstration project)

◆ **G9062** Oncology; practice guidelines; management differs from guidelines for other reason(s) not listed (for use in a Medicare-approved demonstration project)

∗ **G9063** Oncology; disease status; limited to non-small cell lung cancer; extent of disease initially established as stage I (prior to neo-adjuvant therapy, if any) with no evidence of disease progression, recurrence, or metastases (for use in a Medicare-approved demonstration project)

∗ **G9064** Oncology; disease status; limited to non-small cell lung cancer; extent of disease initially established as stage II (prior to neo-adjuvant therapy, if any) with no evidence of disease progression, recurrence, or metastases (for use in a Medicare-approved demonstration project)

∗ **G9065** Oncology; disease status; limited to non-small cell lung cancer; extent of disease initially established as stage IIIA (prior to neo-adjuvant therapy, if any) with no evidence of disease progression, recurrence, or metastases (for use in a Medicare-approved demonstration project)

∗ **G9066** Oncology; disease status; limited to non-small cell lung cancer; stage IIIB-IV at diagnosis, metastatic, locally recurrent, or progressive (for use in a Medicare-approved demonstration project)

∗ **G9067** Oncology; disease status; limited to non-small cell lung cancer; extent of disease unknown, staging in progress, or not listed (for use in a Medicare-approved demonstration project)

∗ **G9068** Oncology; disease status; limited to small cell and combined small cell/ non-small cell; extent of disease initially established as limited with no evidence of disease progression, recurrence, or metastases (for use in a Medicare-approved demonstration project)

∗ **G9069** Oncology; disease status; small cell lung cancer, limited to small cell and combined small cell/non-small cell; extensive stage at diagnosis, metastatic, locally recurrent, or progressive (for use in a Medicare-approved demonstration project)

∗ **G9070** Oncology; disease status; small cell lung cancer, limited to small cell and combined small cell/non-small cell; extent of disease unknown, staging in progress, or not listed (for use in a Medicare-approved demonstration project)

∗ **G9071** Oncology; disease status; invasive female breast cancer (does not include ductal carcinoma in situ); adenocarcinoma as predominant cell type; stage I or stage IIA-IIB; or T3, N1, M0; and ER and/or PR positive; with no evidence of disease progression, recurrence, or metastases (for use in a Medicare-approved demonstration project)

∗ **G9072** Oncology; disease status; invasive female breast cancer (does not include ductal carcinoma in situ); adenocarcinoma as predominant cell type; stage I, or stage IIA-IIB; or T3, N1, M0; and ER and PR negative; with no evidence of disease progression, recurrence, or metastases (for use in a Medicare-approved demonstration project)

∗ **G9073** Oncology; disease status; invasive female breast cancer (does not include ductal carcinoma in situ); adenocarcinoma as predominant cell type; stage IIIA-IIIB; and not T3, N1, M0; and ER and/or PR positive; with no evidence of disease progression, recurrence, or metastases (for use in a Medicare-approved demonstration project)

∗ **G9074** Oncology; disease status; invasive female breast cancer (does not include ductal carcinoma in situ); adenocarcinoma as predominant cell type; stage IIIA-IIIB; and not T3, N1, M0; and ER and PR negative; with no evidence of disease progression, recurrence, or metastases (for use in a Medicare-approved demonstration project)

▶ New   → Revised   ✔ Reinstated   ~~deleted~~ Deleted

○ Special coverage instructions   ◆ Not covered or valid by Medicare   ∗ Carrier discretion

TEMPORARY PROCEDURES/PROFESSIONAL SERVICES   G9061 – G9074

✳ **G9075** Oncology; disease status; invasive female breast cancer (does not include ductal carcinoma in situ); adenocarcinoma as predominant cell type; M1 at diagnosis, metastatic, locally recurrent, or progressive (for use in a Medicare-approved demonstration project)

✳ **G9077** Oncology; disease status; prostate cancer, limited to adenocarcinoma as predominant cell type; T1-T2c and Gleason 2-7 and PSA < or equal to 20 at diagnosis with no evidence of disease progression, recurrence, or metastases (for use in a Medicare-approved demonstration project)

✳ **G9078** Oncology; disease status; prostate cancer, limited to adenocarcinoma as predominant cell type; T2 or T3a Gleason 8-10 or PSA > 20 at diagnosis with no evidence of disease progression, recurrence, or metastases (for use in a Medicare-approved demonstration project)

✳ **G9079** Oncology; disease status; prostate cancer, limited to adenocarcinoma as predominant cell type; T3b-T4, any N; any T, N1 at diagnosis with no evidence of disease progression, recurrence, or metastases (for use in a Medicare-approved demonstration project)

✳ **G9080** Oncology; disease status; prostate cancer, limited to adenocarcinoma; after initial treatment with rising PSA or failure of PSA decline (for use in a Medicare-approved demonstration project)

✳ **G9083** Oncology; disease status; prostate cancer, limited to adenocarcinoma; extent of disease unknown, staging in progress, or not listed (for use in a Medicare-approved demonstration project)

✳ **G9084** Oncology; disease status; colon cancer, limited to invasive cancer, adenocarcinoma as predominant cell type; extent of disease initially established as T1-3, N0, M0 with no evidence of disease progression, recurrence, or metastases (for use in a Medicare-approved demonstration project)

✳ **G9085** Oncology; disease status; colon cancer, limited to invasive cancer, adenocarcinoma as predominant cell type; extent of disease initially established as T4, N0, M0 with no evidence of disease progression, recurrence, or metastases (for use in a Medicare-approved demonstration project)

✳ **G9086** Oncology; disease status; colon cancer, limited to invasive cancer, adenocarcinoma as predominant cell type; extent of disease initially established as T1-4, N1-2, M0 with no evidence of disease progression, recurrence, or metastases (for use in a Medicare-approved demonstration project)

✳ **G9087** Oncology; disease status; colon cancer, limited to invasive cancer, adenocarcinoma as predominant cell type; M1 at diagnosis, metastatic, locally recurrent, or progressive with current clinical, radiologic, or biochemical evidence of disease (for use in a Medicare-approved demonstration project)

✳ **G9088** Oncology; disease status; colon cancer, limited to invasive cancer, adenocarcinoma as predominant cell type; M1 at diagnosis, metastatic, locally recurrent, or progressive without current clinical, radiologic, or biochemical evidence of disease (for use in a Medicare-approved demonstration project)

✳ **G9089** Oncology; disease status; colon cancer, limited to invasive cancer, adenocarcinoma as predominant cell type; extent of disease unknown, staging in progress, or not listed (for use in a Medicare-approved demonstration project)

✳ **G9090** Oncology; disease status; rectal cancer, limited to invasive cancer, adenocarcinoma as predominant cell type; extent of disease initially established as T1-2, N0, M0 (prior to neo-adjuvant therapy, if any) with no evidence of disease progression, recurrence, or metastases (for use in a Medicare-approved demonstration project)

▶ New → Revised ✔ Reinstated ~~deleted~~ Deleted

⊘ Special coverage instructions ◆ Not covered or valid by Medicare ✳ Carrier discretion

✳ **G9091** Oncology; disease status; rectal cancer, limited to invasive cancer, adenocarcinoma as predominant cell type; extent of disease initially established as T3, N0, M0 (prior to neo-adjuvant therapy, if any) with no evidence of disease progression, recurrence, or metastases (for use in a Medicare-approved demonstration project)

✳ **G9092** Oncology; disease status; rectal cancer, limited to invasive cancer, adenocarcinoma as predominant cell type; extent of disease initially established as T1-3, N1-2, M0 (prior to neo-adjuvant therapy, if any) with no evidence of disease progression, recurrence or metastases (for use in a Medicare-approved demonstration project)

✳ **G9093** Oncology; disease status; rectal cancer, limited to invasive cancer, adenocarcinoma as predominant cell type; extent of disease initially established as T4, any N, M0 (prior to neo-adjuvant therapy, if any) with no evidence of disease progression, recurrence, or metastases (for use in a Medicare-approved demonstration project)

✳ **G9094** Oncology; disease status; rectal cancer, limited to invasive cancer, adenocarcinoma as predominant cell type; M1 at diagnosis, metastatic, locally recurrent, or progressive (for use in a Medicare-approved demonstration project)

✳ **G9095** Oncology; disease status; rectal cancer, limited to invasive cancer, adenocarcinoma as predominant cell type; extent of disease unknown, staging in progress, or not listed (for use in a Medicare-approved demonstration project)

✳ **G9096** Oncology; disease status; esophageal cancer, limited to adenocarcinoma or squamous cell carcinoma as predominant cell type; extent of disease initially established as T1-T3, N0-N1 or NX (prior to neo-adjuvant therapy, if any) with no evidence of disease progression, recurrence, or metastases (for use in a Medicare-approved demonstration project)

✳ **G9097** Oncology; disease status; esophageal cancer, limited to adenocarcinoma or squamous cell carcinoma as predominant cell type; extent of disease initially established as T4, any N, M0 (prior to neo-adjuvant therapy, if any) with no evidence of disease progression, recurrence, or metastases (for use in a Medicare-approved demonstration project)

✳ **G9098** Oncology; disease status; esophageal cancer, limited to adenocarcinoma or squamous cell carcinoma as predominant cell type; M1 at diagnosis, meta-static, locally recurrent, or progressive (for use in a Medicare-approved demonstration project)

✳ **G9099** Oncology; disease status; esophageal cancer, limited to adenocarcinoma or squamous cell carcinoma as predominant cell type; extent of disease unknown, staging in progress, or not listed (for use in a Medicare-approved demonstration project)

✳ **G9100** Oncology; disease status; gastric cancer, limited to adenocarcinoma as predominant cell type; post R0 resection (with or without neoadjuvant therapy) with no evidence of disease recurrence, progression, or metastases (for use in a Medicare-approved demonstration project)

✳ **G9101** Oncology; disease status; gastric cancer, limited to adenocarcinoma as predominant cell type; post R1 or R2 resection (with or without neoadjuvant therapy) with no evidence of disease progression, or metastases (for use in a Medicare-approved demonstration project)

✳ **G9102** Oncology; disease status; gastric cancer, limited to adenocarcinoma as predominant cell type; clinical or pathologic M0, unresectable with no evidence of disease progression, or metastases (for use in a Medicare-approved demonstration project)

✳ **G9103** Oncology; disease status; gastric cancer, limited to adenocarcinoma as predominant cell type; clinical or pathologic M1 at diagnosis, metastatic, locally recurrent, or progressive (for use in a Medicare-approved demonstration project)

▶ New → Revised ✔ Reinstated deleted Deleted
Special coverage instructions ◆ Not covered or valid by Medicare ✳ Carrier discretion

✳ **G9104** Oncology; disease status; gastric cancer, limited to adenocarcinoma as predominant cell type; extent of disease unknown, staging in progress, or not listed (for use in a Medicare-approved demonstration project)

✳ **G9105** Oncology; disease status; pancreatic cancer, limited to adenocarcinoma as predominant cell type; post R0 resection without evidence of disease progression, recurrence, or metastases (for use in a Medicare-approved demonstration project)

✳ **G9106** Oncology; disease status; pancreatic cancer, limited to adenocarcinoma; post R1 or R2 resection with no evidence of disease progression or metastases (for use in a Medicare-approved demonstration project)

✳ **G9107** Oncology; disease status; pancreatic cancer, limited to adenocarcinoma; unresectable at diagnosis, M1 at diagnosis, metastatic, locally recurrent, or progressive (for use in a Medicare-approved demonstration project)

✳ **G9108** Oncology; disease status; pancreatic cancer, limited to adenocarcinoma; extent of disease unknown, staging in progress, or not listed (for use in a Medicare-approved demonstration project)

✳ **G9109** Oncology; disease status; head and neck cancer, limited to cancers of oral cavity, pharynx and larynx with squamous cell as predominant cell type; extent of disease initially established as T1-T2 and N0, M0 (prior to neo-adjuvant therapy, if any) with no evidence of disease progression, recurrence, or metastases (for use in a Medicare-approved demonstration project)

✳ **G9110** Oncology; disease status; head and neck cancer, limited to cancers of oral cavity, pharynx, and larynx with squamous cell as predominant cell type; extent of disease initially established as T3-4 and/ or N1-3, M0 (prior to neo-adjuvant therapy, if any) with no evidence of disease progression, recurrence, or metastases (for use in a Medicare-approved demonstration project)

✳ **G9111** Oncology; disease status; head and neck cancer, limited to cancers of oral cavity, pharynx and larynx with squamous cell as predominant cell type; M1 at diagnosis, metastatic, locally recurrent, or progressive (for use in a Medicare-approved demonstration project)

✳ **G9112** Oncology; disease status; head and neck cancer, limited to cancers of oral cavity, pharynx and larynx with squamous cell as predominant cell type; extent of disease unknown, staging in progress, or not listed (for use in a Medicare-approved demonstration project)

✳ **G9113** Oncology; disease status; ovarian cancer, limited to epithelial cancer; pathologic stage IA-B (grade 1) without evidence of disease progression, recurrence, or metastases (for use in a Medicare-approved demonstration project)

✳ **G9114** Oncology; disease status; ovarian cancer, limited to epithelial cancer; pathologic stage IA-B (grade 2-3); or stage IC (all grades); or stage II; without evidence of disease progression, recurrence, or metastases (for use in a Medicare-approved demonstration project)

✳ **G9115** Oncology; disease status; ovarian cancer, limited to epithelial cancer; pathologic stage III-IV; without evidence of progression, recurrence, or metastases (for use in a Medicare-approved demonstration project)

✳ **G9116** Oncology; disease status; ovarian cancer, limited to epithelial cancer; evidence of disease progression, or recurrence and/or platinum resistance (for use in a Medicare-approved demonstration project)

✳ **G9117** Oncology; disease status; ovarian cancer, limited to epithelial cancer; extent of disease unknown, staging in progress, or not listed (for use in a Medicare-approved demonstration project)

✳ **G9123** Oncology; disease status; chronic myelogenous leukemia, limited to Philadelphia chromosome positive and/ or BCR-ABL positive; chronic phase not in hematologic, cytogenetic, or molecular remission (for use in a Medicare-approved demonstration project)

▶ New   → Revised   ✔ Reinstated   ~~deleted~~ Deleted

⊙ Special coverage instructions   ◆ Not covered or valid by Medicare   ✳ Carrier discretion

✳ **G9124** Oncology; disease status; chronic myelogenous leukemia, limited to Philadelphia chromosome positive and/or BCR-ABL positive; accelerated phase not in hematologic cytogenetic, or molecular remission (for use in a Medicare-approved demonstration project)

✳ **G9125** Oncology; disease status; chronic myelogenous leukemia, limited to Philadelphia chromosome positive and/or BCR-ABL positive; blast phase not in hematologic, cytogenetic, or molecular remission (for use in a Medicare-approved demonstration project)

✳ **G9126** Oncology; disease status; chronic myelogenous leukemia, limited to Philadelphia chromosome positive and/or BCR-ABL positive; in hematologic, cytogenetic, or molecular remission (for use in a Medicare-approved demonstration project)

G9128 Oncology: disease status; limited to multiple myeloma, systemic disease; smouldering, stage I (for use in a Medicare-approved demonstration project)

✳ **G9129** Oncology; disease status; limited to multiple myeloma, systemic disease; stage II or higher (for use in a Medicare-approved demonstration project)

✳ **G9130** Oncology; disease status; limited to multiple myeloma, systemic disease; extent of disease unknown, staging in progress, or not listed (for use in a Medicare-approved demonstration project)

✳ **G9131** Oncology; disease status; invasive female breast cancer (does not include ductal carcinoma in situ); adenocarcinoma as predominant cell type; extent of disease unknown, staging in progress, or not listed (for use in a Medicare-approved demonstration project)

✳ **G9132** Oncology; disease status; prostate cancer, limited to adenocarcinoma; hormone-refractory/androgen-independent (e.g., rising PSA on anti-androgen therapy or post-orchiectomy); clinical metastases (for use in a Medicare-approved demonstration project)

✳ **G9133** Oncology; disease status; prostate cancer, limited to adenocarcinoma; hormone-responsive; clinical metastases or M1 at diagnosis (for use in a Medicare-approved demonstration project)

✳ **G9134** Oncology; disease status; non-Hodgkin's lymphoma, any cellular classification; stage I, II at diagnosis, not relapsed, not refractory (for use in a Medicare-approved demonstration project)

✳ **G9135** Oncology; disease status; non-Hodgkin's lymphoma, any cellular classification; stage III, IV, not relapsed, not refractory (for use in a Medicare-approved demonstration project)

✳ **G9136** Oncology; disease status; non-Hodgkin's lymphoma, transformed from original cellular diagnosis to a second cellular classification (for use in a Medicare-approved demonstration project)

✳ **G9137** Oncology; disease status; non-Hodgkin's lymphoma, any cellular classification; relapsed/refractory (for use in a Medicare-approved demonstration project)

✳ **G9138** Oncology; disease status; non-Hodgkin's lymphoma, any cellular classification; diagnostic evaluation, stage not determined, evaluation of possible relapse or non-response to therapy, or not listed (for use in a Medicare-approved demonstration project)

✳ **G9139** Oncology; disease status; chronic myelogenous leukemia, limited to Philadelphia chromosome positive and/or BCR-ABL positive; extent of disease unknown, staging in progress, not listed (for use in a Medicare-approved demonstration project)

▶ New   → Revised   ✔ Reinstated   ~~deleted~~ Deleted

○ Special coverage instructions   ◆ Not covered or valid by Medicare   ✳ Carrier discretion

* **G9140** Frontier extended stay clinic demonstration; for a patient stay in a clinic approved for the CMS demonstration project; the following measures should be present: the stay must be equal to or greater than 4 hours; weather or other conditions must prevent transfer or the case falls into a category of monitoring and observation cases that are permitted by the rules of the demonstration; there is a maximum frontier extended stay clinic (FESC) visit of 48 hours, except in the case when weather or other conditions prevent transfer; payment is made on each period up to 4 hours, after the first 4 hours

Influenza A (H1N1) and Warfarin Responsiveness Testing

* **G9141** Influenza A (H1N1) immunization administration (includes the physician counseling the patient/family)

Payment for G9141 will be the same as that for G0008 and G0009, which is currently based on 90471. Beneficiary copayment and deductible do not apply. Bill the H1N1 flu administration with V04.81

* **G9142** Influenza A (H1N1) vaccine, any route of administration

Under OPPS, G9142 will be assigned status indicator "E," indicating that payment will not be made by Medicare when this code is submitted for an outpatient service. (Transmittal 1803, October 1, 2009)

http://www.cdc.gov/h1n1flu/

* **G9143** Warfarin responsiveness testing by genetic technique using any method, any number of specimen(s)

This would be a once-in-a-lifetime test unless there is a reason to believe that the patient's personal genetic characteristics would change over time. (https://www.cms.gov/ContractorLearningResources/downloads/JA6715.pdf)

▶ ◆ **G9147** Outpatient intravenous insulin treatment (OIVIT) either pulsatile or continuous, by any means, guided by the results of measurements for: respiratory quotient; and/or, urine urea nitrogen (UUN); and/or, arterial, venous or capillary glucose; and/or potassium concentration

On December 23, 2009, CMS issued a national non-coverage decision on the use of OIVIT. CR 6775.

Not covered on Physician Fee Schedule.

▶ * **G9156** Evaluation for wheelchair requiring face to face visit with physician

BEHAVIORAL HEALTH AND/OR SUBSTANCE ABUSE TREATMENT SERVICES (H0001-H9999)

Used by Medicaid state agencies because no national code exists to meet the reporting needs of these agencies.

◆ **H0001** Alcohol and/or drug assessment

◆ **H0002** Behavioral health screening to determine eligibility for admission to treatment program

◆ **H0003** Alcohol and/or drug screening; laboratory analysis of specimens for presence of alcohol and/or drugs

◆ **H0004** Behavioral health counseling and therapy, per 15 minutes

◆ **H0005** Alcohol and/or drug services; group counseling by a clinician

◆ **H0006** Alcohol and/or drug services; case management

◆ **H0007** Alcohol and/or drug services; crisis intervention (outpatient)

◆ **H0008** Alcohol and/or drug services; sub-acute detoxification (hospital inpatient)

◆ **H0009** Alcohol and/or drug services; acute detoxification (hospital inpatient)

◆ **H0010** Alcohol and/or drug services; sub-acute detoxification (residential addiction program inpatient)

◆ **H0011** Alcohol and/or drug services; acute detoxification (residential addiction program inpatient)

◆ **H0012** Alcohol and/or drug services; sub-acute detoxification (residential addiction program outpatient)

◆ **H0013** Alcohol and/or drug services; acute detoxification (residential addiction program outpatient)

◆ **H0014** Alcohol and/or drug services; ambulatory detoxification

◆ **H0015** Alcohol and/or drug services; intensive outpatient (treatment program that operates at least 3 hours/day and at least 3 days/week and is based on an individualized treatment plan), including assessment, counseling; crisis intervention, and activity therapies or education

◆ **H0016** Alcohol and/or drug services; medical/somatic (medical intervention in ambulatory setting)

◆ **H0017** Behavioral health; residential (hospital residential treatment program), without room and board, per diem

◆ **H0018** Behavioral health; short-term residential (non-hospital residential treatment program), without room and board, per diem

◆ **H0019** Behavioral health; long-term residential (non-medical, non-acute care in a residential treatment program where stay is typically longer than 30 days), without room and board, per diem

◆ **H0020** Alcohol and/or drug services; methadone administration and/or service (provision of the drug by a licensed program)

◆ **H0021** Alcohol and/or drug training service (for staff and personnel not employed by providers)

◆ **H0022** Alcohol and/or drug intervention service (planned facilitation)

◆ **H0023** Behavioral health outreach service (planned approach to reach a targeted population)

◆ **H0024** Behavioral health prevention information dissemination service (one-way direct or non-direct contact with service audiences to affect knowledge and attitude)

◆ **H0025** Behavioral health prevention education service (delivery of services with target population to affect knowledge, attitude and/or behavior)

◆ **H0026** Alcohol and/or drug prevention process service, community-based (delivery of services to develop skills of impactors)

◆ **H0027** Alcohol and/or drug prevention environmental service (broad range of external activities geared toward modifying systems in order to mainstream prevention through policy and law)

◆ **H0028** Alcohol and/or drug prevention problem identification and referral service (e.g. student assistance and employee assistance programs), does not include assessment

◆ **H0029** Alcohol and/or drug prevention alternatives service (services for populations that exclude alcohol and other drug use e.g. alcohol-free social events)

◆ **H0030** Behavioral health hotline service

◆ **H0031** Mental health assessment, by non-physician

◆ **H0032** Mental health service plan development by non-physician

◆ **H0033** Oral medication administration, direct observation

▶ New → Revised ✔ Reinstated ~~deleted~~ Deleted
☼ Special coverage instructions ◆ Not covered or valid by Medicare ✳ Carrier discretion

◆ **H0034** Medication training and support, per 15 minutes

◆ **H0035** Mental health partial hospitalization, treatment, less than 24 hours

◆ **H0036** Community psychiatric supportive treatment, face-to-face, per 15 minutes

◆ **H0037** Community psychiatric supportive treatment program, per diem

◆ **H0038** Self-help/peer services, per 15 minutes

◆ **H0039** Assertive community treatment, face-to-face, per 15 minutes

◆ **H0040** Assertive community treatment program, per diem

◆ **H0041** Foster care, child, non-therapeutic, per diem

◆ **H0042** Foster care, child, non-therapeutic, per month

◆ **H0043** Supported housing, per diem

◆ **H0044** Supported housing, per month

◆ **H0045** Respite care services, not in the home, per diem

◆ **H0046** Mental health services, not otherwise specified

◆ **H0047** Alcohol and/or other drug abuse services, not otherwise specified

◆ **H0048** Alcohol and/or other drug testing: collection and handling only, specimens other than blood

◆ **H0049** Alcohol and/or drug screening

◆ **H0050** Alcohol and/or drug services, brief intervention, per 15 minutes

◆ **H1000** Prenatal care, at-risk assessment

◆ **H1001** Prenatal care, at-risk enhanced service; antepartum management

◆ **H1002** Prenatal care, at-risk enhanced service; care coordination

◆ **H1003** Prenatal care, at-risk enhanced service; education

◆ **H1004** Prenatal care, at-risk enhanced service; follow-up home visit

◆ **H1005** Prenatal care, at-risk enhanced service package (includes H1001-H1004)

◆ **H1010** Non-medical family planning education, per session

◆ **H1011** Family assessment by licensed behavioral health professional for state defined purposes

◆ **H2000** Comprehensive multidisciplinary evaluation

◆ **H2001** Rehabilitation program, per 1/2 day

◆ **H2010** Comprehensive medication services, per 15 minutes

◆ **H2011** Crisis intervention service, per 15 minutes

◆ **H2012** Behavioral health day treatment, per hour

◆ **H2013** Psychiatric health facility service, per diem

◆ **H2014** Skills training and development, per 15 minutes

◆ **H2015** Comprehensive community support services, per 15 minutes

◆ **H2016** Comprehensive community support services, per diem

◆ **H2017** Psychosocial rehabilitation services, per 15 minutes

◆ **H2018** Psychosocial rehabilitation services, per diem

◆ **H2019** Therapeutic behavioral services, per 15 minutes

◆ **H2020** Therapeutic behavioral services, per diem

◆ **H2021** Community-based wrap-around services, per 15 minutes

◆ **H2022** Community-based wrap-around services, per diem

◆ **H2023** Supported employment, per 15 minutes

◆ **H2024** Supported employment, per diem

◆ **H2025** Ongoing support to maintain employment, per 15 minutes

◆ **H2026** Ongoing support to maintain employment, per diem

◆ **H2027** Psychoeducational service, per 15 minutes

◆ **H2028** Sexual offender treatment service, per 15 minutes

◆ **H2029** Sexual offender treatment service, per diem

◆ **H2030** Mental health clubhouse services, per 15 minutes

◆ **H2031** Mental health clubhouse services, per diem

◆ **H2032** Activity therapy, per 15 minutes

◆ **H2033** Multisystemic therapy for juveniles, per 15 minutes

◆ **H2034** Alcohol and/or drug abuse halfway house services, per diem

◆ **H2035** Alcohol and/or other drug treatment program, per hour

◆ **H2036** Alcohol and/or other drug treatment program, per diem

◆ **H2037** Developmental delay prevention activities, dependent child of client, per 15 minutes

---

▶ **New**   → **Revised**   ✔ **Reinstated**   ~~deleted~~ **Deleted**

⊙ **Special coverage instructions**   ◆ **Not covered or valid by Medicare**   ✳ **Carrier discretion**

DRUGS OTHER THAN CHEMOTHERAPY (J0100-J9999)

J0120-J3570:   Bill local carrier if incident to a physician's service or used in an implanted infusion pump. If other, bill DME/MAC

✪ **J0120**   Injection, tetracycline, **up to 250 mg**

Other: Achromycin

IOM: 100-02, 15, 50

→ ✳ **J0129**   Injection, abatacept, **10 mg** (code may be used for Medicare when drug administered under the direct supervision of a physician; not for use when drug is self-administered)

Other: Orencia

✪ **J0130**   Injection, abciximab, **10 mg**

NDC: ReoPro

IOM: 100-02, 15, 50

▶ ✳ **J0131**   Injection, acetaminophen, **10 mg**

✳ **J0132**   Injection, acetylcysteine, **100 mg**

✳ **J0133**   Injection, acyclovir, **5 mg**

✳ **J0135**   Injection, adalimumab, **20 mg**

NDC: Humira

IOM: 100-02, 15, 50

✪ **J0150**   Injection, adenosine, for therapeutic use, **6 mg** (not to be used to report any adenosine phosphate compounds, instead use A9270)

NDC: Adenocard

IOM: 100-02, 15, 50

✳ **J0152**   Injection, adenosine, for diagnostic use, **30 mg** (not to be used to report any adenosine phosphate compounds; instead use A9270)

NDC: Adenoscan

▶ ✪ **J0171**   Injection, adrenalin, epinephrine, **0.1 mg**

IOM: 100-02, 15, 50

✳ **J0180**   Injection, agalsidase beta, **1 mg**

NDC: Fabrazyme

IOM: 100-02, 15, 50

✪ **J0190**   Injection, biperiden lactate, **per 5 mg**

Other: Akineton

IOM: 100-02, 15, 50

✪ **J0200**   Injection, alatrofloxacin mesylate, **100 mg**

Other: Trovan

IOM: 100-02, 15, 50

✪ **J0205**   Injection, alglucerase, **per 10 units**

NDC: Ceredase

IOM: 100-02, 15, 50

✪ **J0207**   Injection, amifostine, **500 mg**

NDC: Ethyol

IOM: 100-02, 15, 50

✪ **J0210**   Injection, methyldopate HCL, **up to 250 mg**

Other: Aldomet

IOM: 100-02, 15, 50

✳ **J0215**   Injection, alefacept, **0.5 mg**

NDC: Amevive

→ ✳ **J0220**   Injection, alglucosidase alfa, not otherwise specified, **10 mg**

NDC: Myozyme

▶ ✳ **J0221**   Injection, alglucosidase alfa, (lumizyme), **10 mg**

→ ✪ **J0256**   Injection, alpha 1 - proteinase inhibitor (human), not otherwise specified, **10 mg**

NDC: Aralast, Aralast NP, Prolastin, Prolastin-C, Zemaira

IOM: 100-02, 15, 50

▶ ✪ **J0257**   Injection, alpha 1 proteinase inhibitor (human), (glassia), **10 mg**

IOM: 100-02, 15, 50

✪ **J0270**   Injection, alprostadil, **per 1.25 mcg** (Code may be used for Medicare when drug administered under the direct supervision of a physician, not for use when drug is self administered)

NDC: Caverject, Caverject Impulse, Edex, Prostin VR

Other: Prostaglandin E1

IOM: 100-02, 15, 50

✪ **J0275**   Alprostadil urethral suppository (Code may be used for Medicare when drug administered under the direct supervision of a physician, not for use when drug is self administered)

Other: Muse

IOM: 100-02, 15, 50

✳ **J0278**   Injection, amikacin sulfate, **100 mg**

Other: Amikin

▶ New   → Revised   ✔ Reinstated   ~~deleted~~ Deleted

✪ Special coverage instructions   ◆ Not covered or valid by Medicare   ✳ Carrier discretion

⊛ **J0280** Injection, aminophylline, **up to 250 mg**

IOM: 100-02, 15, 50

⊛ **J0282** Injection, amiodarone hydrochloride, **30 mg**

Other: Cordarone

IOM: 100-02, 15, 50

⊛ **J0285** Injection, amphotericin B, **50 mg**

Other: ABLC, Amphocin, Fungizone

IOM: 100-02, 15, 50

⊛ **J0287** Injection, amphotericin B lipid complex, **10 mg**

NDC: Abelcet

IOM: 100-02, 15, 50

⊛ **J0288** Injection, amphotericin B cholesteryl sulfate complex, **10 mg**

NDC: Amphotec

Other: Abelcet

IOM: 100-02, 15, 50

⊛ **J0289** Injection, amphotericin B liposome, **10 mg**

NDC: AmBisome

Other: Abelcet

IOM: 100-02, 15, 50

⊛ **J0290** Injection, ampicillin sodium, **500 mg**

Other: Omnipen-N, Polycillin-N, Totacillin-N

IOM: 100-02, 15, 50

⊛ **J0295** Injection, ampicillin sodium/sulbactam sodium, **per 1.5 gm**

NDC: Unasyn

Other: Omnipen-N, Polycillin-N, Totacillin-N

IOM: 100-02, 15, 50

⊛ **J0300** Injection, amobarbital, **up to 125 mg**

Other: Amytal

IOM: 100-02, 15, 50

⊛ **J0330** Injection, succinylcholine chloride, **up to 20 mg**

Other: Anectine, Quelicin

IOM: 100-02, 15, 50

✳ **J0348** Injection, anidulafungin, **1 mg**

NDC: Eraxis

⊛ **J0350** Injection, anistreplase, **per 30 units**

Other: Eminase

IOM: 100-02, 15, 50

⊛ **J0360** Injection, hydralazine hydrochloride, **up to 20 mg**

Other: Apresoline

IOM: 100-02, 15, 50

✳ **J0364** Injection, apomorphine hydrochloride, **1 mg**

NDC: Apokyn

⊛ **J0365** Injection, aprotinin, **10,000 KIU**

NDC: Trasylol

IOM: 100-02, 15, 50

⊛ **J0380** Injection, metaraminol bitartrate, **per 10 mg**

Other: Aramine

IOM: 100-02, 15, 50

⊛ **J0390** Injection, chloroquine hydrochloride, **up to 250 mg**
Benefit only for diagnosed malaria or amebiasis

Other: Aralen

IOM: 100-02, 15, 50

⊛ **J0395** Injection, arbutamine HCL, **1 mg**

IOM: 100-02, 15, 50

✳ **J0400** Injection, aripiprazole, intramuscular, **0.25 mg**

Other: Abilify

⊛ **J0456** Injection, azithromycin, **500 mg**

NDC: Zithromax

IOM: 100-02, 15, 50

⊛ **J0461** Injection, atropine sulfate, **0.01 mg**

IOM: 100-02, 15, 50

⊛ **J0470** Injection, dimercaprol, per 100 mg

NDC: BAL In Oil

IOM: 100-02, 15, 50

⊛ **J0475** Injection, baclofen, **10 mg**

NDC: Gablofen, Lioresal

IOM: 100-02, 15, 50

⊛ **J0476** Injection, baclofen **50 mcg** for intrathecal trial

NDC: Gablofen, Lioresal

IOM: 100-02, 15, 50

⊛ **J0480** Injection, basiliximab, **20 mg**

NDC: Simulect

IOM: 100-02, 15, 50

▶ ✳ **J0490** Injection, belimumab, **10 mg**

⊛ **J0500** Injection, dicyclomine HCL, **up to 20 mg**

NDC: Bentyl

Other: Antispas, Dibent, Dicyclocot, Dilomine, Di-Spa, Neoquess, Or-Tyl, Spasmoject

IOM: 100-02, 15, 50

▶ New   → Revised   ✔ Reinstated   ~~deleted~~ Deleted

⊛ Special coverage instructions   ◆ Not covered or valid by Medicare   ✳ Carrier discretion

❂ **J0515** Injection, benztropine mesylate, **per 1 mg**

NDC: Cogentin

IOM: 100-02, 15, 50

❂ **J0520** Injection, bethanechol chloride, myotonachol or urecholine, **up to 5 mg**

IOM: 100-02, 15, 50

▶ ✳ **J0558** Injection, penicillin G benzathine and penicillin G procaine, **100,000 units**

NDC: Bicillin C-R

▶ ❂ **J0561** Injection, penicillin G benzathine, **100,000 units**

NDC: Bicillin L-A

IOM: 100-02, 15, 50

✳ **J0583** Injection, bivalirudin, **1 mg**

NDC: Angiomax

✳ **J0585** Injection, onabotulinumtoxinaA, **1 unit**

NDC: Botox, Botox Cosmetic

Other: Oculinum

IOM: 100-02, 15, 50

✳ **J0586** Injection, abobotulinumtoxinA, **5 units**

NDC: Dysport

✳ **J0587** Injection, rimabotulinumtoxinB, **100 units**

NDC: Myobloc

IOM: 100-02, 15, 50

▶ ✳ **J0588** Injection, incobotulinumtoxin A, **1 unit**

❂ **J0592** Injection, buprenorphine hydrochloride, **0.1 mg**

NDC: Buprenex

IOM: 100-02, 15, 50

✳ **J0594** Injection, busulfan, **1 mg**

✳ **J0595** Injection, butorphanol tartrate, **1 mg**

NDC: Stadol

▶ ✳ **J0597** Injection, C-1 esterase inhibitor (human), Berinet, **10 units**

→ ✳ **J0598** Injection, C1 esterase inhibitor (human), cinryze, **10 units**

❂ **J0600** Injection, edetate calcium disodium, **up to 1000 mg**

NDC: Calcium Disodium Versenate

IOM: 100-02, 15, 50

❂ **J0610** Injection, calcium gluconate, **per 10 ml**

Other: Kaleinate

IOM: 100-02, 15, 50

❂ **J0620** Injection, calcium glycerophosphate and calcium lactate, **per 10 ml**

Other: Calphosan

MCM 2049

IOM: 100-02, 15, 50

❂ **J0630** Injection, calcitonin (salmon), **up to 400 units**

NDC: Miacalcin

Other: Calcimar, Calcitonin-salmon

IOM: 100-02, 15, 50

❂ **J0636** Injection, calcitriol, **0.1 mcg**

Non-dialysis use

NDC: Calcijex

Other: Calcitriol in almond oil

IOM: 100-02, 15, 50

✳ **J0637** Injection, caspofungin acetate, **5 mg**

NDC: Cancidas

▶ ✳ **J0638** Injection, canakinumab, **1 mg**

NDC: Ilaris

❂ **J0640** Injection, leucovorin calcium, **per 50 mg**

Other: Wellcovorin

IOM: 100-02, 15, 50

❂ **J0641** Injection, levoleucovorin calcium, **0.5 mg**

Part of treatment regimen for osteosarcoma

❂ **J0670** Injection, mepivacaine HCL, **per 10 ml**

NDC: Carbocaine, Polocaine, Polocaine-MPF

Other: Isocaine HCl

IOM: 100-02, 15, 50

❂ **J0690** Injection, cefezolin sodium, **500 mg**

NDC: Ancef, Kefzol

IOM: 100-02, 15, 50

✳ **J0692** Injection, cefepime HCL, **500 mg**

NDC: Maxipime

❂ **J0694** Injection, cefoxitin sodium, **1 gm**

NDC: Mefoxin

IOM: 100-02, 15, 50,

Cross Reference Q0090

▶ New	→ Revised	✔ Reinstated	~~deleted~~ Deleted

❂ Special coverage instructions ◆ Not covered or valid by Medicare ✳ Carrier discretion

⊛ **J0696** Injection, ceftriaxone sodium, **per 250 mg**

NDC: Rocephin

IOM: 100-02, 15, 50

⊛ **J0697** Injection, sterile cefuroxime sodium, **per 750 mg**

NDC: Zinacef

Other: Kefurox

IOM: 100-02, 15, 50

⊛ **J0698** Injection, cefotaxime sodium, **per g**

NDC: Claforan

IOM: 100-02, 15, 50

⊛ **J0702** Injection, betamethasone acetate **3 mg** and betamethasone sodium phosphate **3 mg**

NDC: Celestone Soluspan

IOM: 100-02, 15, 50

⁎ **J0706** Injection, caffeine citrate, **5 mg**

Other: Cafcit, Cipro IV, Ciprofloxacin

⊛ **J0710** Injection, cephapirin sodium, **up to 1 gm**

Other: Cefadyl

IOM: 100-02, 15, 50

▶ ⁎ **J0712** Injection, ceftaroline fosamil, **10 mg**

⊛ **J0713** Injection, ceftazidime, **per 500 mg**

NDC: Fortaz, Tazicef

IOM: 100-02, 15, 50

⊛ **J0715** Injection, ceftizoxime sodium, **per 500 mg**

Other: Cefizox

IOM: 100-02, 15, 50

⁎ **J0718** Injection, certolizumab pegol, **1 mg**

NDC: Cimzia

⊛ **J0720** Injection, chloramphenicol sodium succinate, **up to 1 gm**

IOM: 100-02, 15, 50

⊛ **J0725** Injection, chorionic gonadotropin, **per 1,000 USP units**

NDC: Pregnyl, Novarel

Other: A.P.L., Chorex-5, Chorex-10, Chorignon, Choron-10, Corgonject-5, Follutein, Glukor, Gonic, Profasi HP

IOM: 100-02, 15, 50

⊛ **J0735** Injection, clonidine hydrochloride (HCL), **1 mg**

NDC: Duraclon

IOM: 100-02, 15, 50

⊛ **J0740** Injection, cidofovir, **375 mg**

NDC: Vistide

IOM: 100-02, 15, 50

⊛ **J0743** Injection, cilastatin sodium; imipenem, **per 250 mg**

NDC: Primaxin

IOM: 100-02, 15, 50

⁎ **J0744** Injection, ciprofloxacin for intravenous infusion, **200 mg**

Other: Cipro IV

⊛ **J0745** Injection, codeine phosphate, **per 30 mg**

IOM: 100-02, 15, 50

⊛ **J0760** Injection, colchicine, **per 1 mg**

IOM: 100-02, 15, 50

⊛ **J0770** Injection, colistimethate sodium, **up to 150 mg**

NDC: Coly-Mycin M

IOM: 100-02, 15, 50

▶ ⁎ **J0775** Injection, collagenase, clostridium histolyticum, **0.01 mg**

NDC: Xiaflex

⊛ **J0780** Injection, prochlorperazine, **up to 10 mg**

Other: Compa-Z, Compazine, Cotranzine, Ultrazine-10

IOM: 100-02, 15, 50

⊛ **J0795** Injection, corticorelin ovine triflutate, **1 microgram**

NDC: Acthrel

IOM: 100-02, 15, 50

⊛ **J0800** Injection, corticotropin, **up to 40 units**

NDC: Acthar H.P.

Other: H.P. Acthar, ACTH

IOM: 100-02, 15, 50

⁎ **J0833** Injection, cosyntropin, not otherwise specified, **0.25 mg**

⁎ **J0834** Injection, cosyntropin (Cortrosyn), **0.25 mg**

▶ ⁎ **J0840** Injection, crotalidae polyvalent immune fab (ovine), **up to 1 gram**

⊛ **J0850** Injection, cytomegalovirus immune globulin intravenous (human), **per vial**

Prophylaxis to prevent cytomegalovirus disease associated with transplantation of kidney, lung, liver, pancreas, and heart.

NDC: CytoGam

IOM: 100-02, 15, 50

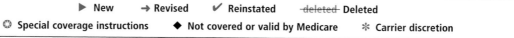

▶ New	→ Revised	✔ Reinstated	~~deleted~~ Deleted
⊛ Special coverage instructions	◆ Not covered or valid by Medicare		⁎ Carrier discretion

✳ **J0878**   Injection, daptomycin, **1 mg**

   NDC: Cubicin

☻ **J0881**   Injection, darbepoetin alfa, **1 microgram** (non-ESRD use)

   NDC: Aranesp

☻ **J0882**   Injection, darbepoetin alfa, **1 microgram** (for ESRD on dialysis)

   NDC: Aranesp

   IOM: 100-02, 6, 10; 100-04, 4, 240

☻ **J0885**   Injection, epoetin alfa, (for non-ESRD use), **1000 units**

   NDC: Epogen, Procrit

   IOM: 100-02, 15, 50

☻ **J0886**   Injection, epoetin alfa, **1000 units** (for ESRD on dialysis)

   NDC: Epogen, Procrit

   IOM: 100-02, 6, 10; 100-04, 4, 240

✳ **J0894**   Injection, decitabine, **1 mg**

   Indicated for treatment of myelodysplastic syndromes (MDS)

☻ **J0895**   Injection, deferoxamine mesylate, **500 mg**

   NDC: Desferal

   Other: Desferal mesylate

   IOM: 100-02, 15, 50,

   Cross Reference Q0087

▶ ✳ **J0897**   Injection, denosumab, **1 mg**

☻ **J0900**   Injection, testosterone enanthate and estradiol valerate, **up to 1 cc**

   Other: Andrest 90-4, Andro-Estro 90-4, Androgyn L.A., Deladumone, Deladumone OB, Delatest, Delatestadiol, Ditate-DS, Dua-Gen LA, Duoval PA, Estra-Testrin, TEEV, Testadiate, Testradiol 90/4, Valertest

   IOM: 100-02, 15, 50

☻ **J0945**   Injection, brompheniramine maleate, **per 10 mg**

   Other: Codimal-A, Cophene-B, Dehist, Histaject, Nasahist B, ND Stat, Oraminic II, Sinusol-B

   IOM: 100-02, 15, 50

☻ **J1000**   Injection, depo-estradiol cypionate, **up to 5 mg**

   Other: Depogen, DepGynogen, Dura-Estrin, Estra-D, Estro-Cyp, Estroject LA, Estronol-LA

   IOM: 100-02, 15, 50

☻ **J1020**   Injection, methylprednisolone acetate, **20 mg**

   NDC: Depo-Medrol, Methylpred

   Other: DepMedalone, Depoject, Depopred, D-Med 80, Duralone, Medralone, M-Prednisol, Rep-Pred

   IOM: 100-02, 15, 50

☻ **J1030**   Injection, methylprednisolone acetate, **40 mg**

   NDC: Depo-Medrol

   Other: DepMedalone, Depoject, Depopred, D-Med 80, Duralone, Medralone, M-Prednisol, Rep-Pred

   IOM: 100-02, 15, 50

☻ **J1040**   Injection, methylprednisolone acetate, **80 mg**

   NDC: Depo-Medrol

   Other: DepMedalone, Depoject, Depopred, D-Med 80, Duralone, Medralone, M-Prednisol, Rep-Pred

   IOM: 100-02, 15, 50

☻ **J1051**   Injection, medroxyprogesterone acetate, **50 mg**

   NDC: Depo-Provera

   IOM: 100-02, 15, 50

◆ **J1055**   Injection, medroxyprogesterone acetate for contraceptive use, **150 mg**

   Other: Depo Provera

   Medicare Statute 1862a1

✳ **J1056**   Injection, medroxyprogesterone acetate/ estradiol cypionate, **5 mg/25 mg**

   Other: Lunelle

☻ **J1060**   Injection, testosterone cypionate and estradiol cypionate, **up to 1 ml**

   Other: Andro/Fem, De-Comberol, DepAndrogyn, Depo-Testadiol, Depotestogen, Duratestrin, Estradiol cypionate, Test-Estro-C, Test-Estro Cypionates, Valertest No. 1

   IOM: 100-02, 15, 50

☻ **J1070**   Injection, testosterone cypionate, **up to 100 mg**

   NDC: Depo-Testosterone

   Other: Andro-Cyp, Andronaq-LA, Andronate, DepAndro, Depotest, Duratest, Testa-C, Testadiate-Depo, Testaject-LA, Testoject-LA,

   IOM: 100-02, 15, 50

▶ **New**   → **Revised**   ✔ **Reinstated**   ~~deleted~~ **Deleted**

☻ **Special coverage instructions**   ◆ **Not covered or valid by Medicare**   ✳ **Carrier discretion**

⊛ **J1080** Injection, testosterone cypionate, **1 cc, 200 mg**

NDC: Depo-Testosterone

Other: Andro-Cyp, Andronaq-LA, Andronate, DepAndro, Depotest, Duratest, Testa-C, Testadiate-Depo, Testaject-LA, Testoject-LA

IOM: 100-02, 15, 50

⊛ **J1094** Injection, dexamethasone acetate, **1 mg**

Other: Cortastat LA, Dalalone LA, Decadrone LA, Decaject LA, Dexacen-LA-8, Dexamethasone Micronized, Dexasone L.A., Dexone-LA

IOM: 100-02, 15, 50

⊛ **J1100** Injection, dexamethasone sodium phosphate, **1 mg**

Other: Cortastat 10, Dalalone, Decadron Phosphate, Decaject, Dexacen-4, Dexone, Hexadrol Phosphate, Solurex

IOM: 100-02, 15, 50

⊛ **J1110** Injection, dihydroergotamine mesylate, **per 1 mg**

NDC: D.H.E. 45

IOM: 100-02, 15, 50

⊛ **J1120** Injection, acetazolamide sodium, **up to 500 mg**

Other: Diamox

IOM: 100-02, 15, 50

⊛ **J1160** Injection, digoxin, **up to 0.5 mg**

NDC: Lanoxin

IOM: 100-02, 15, 50

⊛ **J1162** Injection, digoxin immune Fab (ovine), **per vial**

NDC: Digibind, DigiFab

IOM: 100-02, 15, 50

⊛ **J1165** Injection, phenytoin sodium, **per 50 mg**

Other: Dilantin

IOM: 100-02, 15, 50

⊛ **J1170** Injection, hydromorphone, **up to 4 mg**

NDC: Dilaudid, Dilaudid-HP

IOM: 100-02, 15, 50

⊛ **J1180** Injection, dyphylline, **up to 500 mg**

Other: Dilor, Lufyllin

IOM: 100-02, 15, 50

⊛ **J1190** Injection, dexrazoxane hydrochloride, **per 250 mg**

NDC: Totect, Zinecard

IOM: 100-02, 15, 50

⊛ **J1200** Injection, diphenhydramine HCL, **up to 50 mg**

NDC: Benadryl

Other: Bena-D, Truxadryl

IOM: 100-02, 15, 50

⊛ **J1205** Injection, chlorothiazide sodium, **per 500 mg**

NDC: Diuril

IOM: 100-02, 15, 50

⊛ **J1212** Injection, DMSO, dimethyl sulfoxide, 50%, **50 ml**

NDC: Rimso-50

IOM: 100-02, 15, 50; 100-03, 4, 230.12

⊛ **J1230** Injection, methadone HCL, **up to 10 mg**

MCM 2049

IOM: 100-02, 15, 50

⊛ **J1240** Injection, dimenhydrinate, **up to 50 mg**

Other: Dinate, Dommanate, Dramamine, Dramanate, Dramilin, Dramocen, Dramoject, Dymenate, Hydrate, Marmine, Wehamine

IOM: 100-02, 15, 50

⊛ **J1245** Injection, dipyridamole, **per 10 mg**

Other: Persantine

IOM: 100-04, 15, 50; 100-04, 12, 30.6

⊛ **J1250** Injection, dobutamine HCL, **per 250 mg**

Other: Dobutrex

IOM: 100-02, 15, 50

⊛ **J1260** Injection, dolasetron mesylate, **10 mg**

NDC: Anzemet

IOM: 100-02, 15, 50

✳ **J1265** Injection, dopamine HCL, **40 mg**

✳ **J1267** Injection, doripenem, **10 mg**

NDC: Doribax

✳ **J1270** Injection, doxercalciferol, **1 mcg**

NDC: Hectorol

▶ ✳ **J1290** Injection, ecallantide, **1 mg**

NDC: Ralbitor

✳ **J1300** Injection, eculizumab, **10 mg**

NDC: Soliris

⊛ **J1320** Injection, amitriptyline HCL, **up to 20 mg**

Other: Elavil, Enovil

IOM: 100-02, 15, 50

▶ New   → Revised   ✔ Reinstated   ~~deleted~~ Deleted

⊛ Special coverage instructions   ◆ Not covered or valid by Medicare   ✳ Carrier discretion

✳ **J1324**   Injection, enfuvirtide, **1 mg**
Other: Fuzeon

✪ **J1325**   Injection, epoprostenol, **0.5 mg**
NDC: Flolan
IOM: 100-02, 15, 50

✪ **J1327**   Injection, eptifibatide, **5 mg**
NDC: Integrilin
IOM: 100-02, 15, 50

✪ **J1330**   Injection, ergonovine maleate, **up to 0.2 mg**
Benefit limited to obstetrical diagnosis
IOM: 100-02, 15, 50

✳ **J1335**   Injection, ertapenem sodium, **500 mg**
NDC: Invanz

✪ **J1364**   Injection, erythromycin lactobionate, **per 500 mg**
IOM: 100-02, 15, 50

✪ **J1380**   Injection, estradiol valerate, **up to 10 mg**
NDC: Delestrogen
Other: Dioval, Duragen, Estra-L, Gynogen L.A. L.A.E. 20, Valergen
IOM: 100-02, 15, 50

✪ **J1410**   Injection, estrogen conjugated, **per 25 mg**
NDC: Premarin
IOM: 100-02, 15, 50

✪ **J1430**   Injection, ethanolamine oleate, **100 mg**
Other: Ethamolin
IOM: 100-02, 15, 50

✪ **J1435**   Injection, estrone, **per 1 mg**
Other: Estragyn, Estronol, Kestrone 5, Theelin Aqueous
IOM: 100-02, 15, 50

✪ **J1436**   Injection, etidronate disodium, **per 300 mg**
Other: Didronel
IOM: 100-02, 15, 50

✪ **J1438**   Injection, etanercept, **25 mg** (Code may be used for Medicare when drug administered under the direct supervision of a physician, not for use when drug is self-administered.)
NDC: Enbrel
IOM: 100-02, 15, 50

✪ **J1440**   Injection, filgrastim (G-CSF), **300 mcg**
NDC: Neupogen
IOM: 100-02, 15, 50

✪ **J1441**   Injection, filgrastim (G-CSF), **480 mcg**
Other: Neupogen
IOM: 100-02, 15, 50

✪ **J1450**   Injection, fluconazole, **200 mg**
NDC: Diflucan
IOM: 100-02, 15, 50

✪ **J1451**   Injection, fomepizole, **15 mg**
NDC: Antizol
IOM: 100-02, 15, 50

✪ **J1452**   Injection, fomivirsen sodium, intraocular, **1.65 mg**
IOM: 100-02, 15, 50

✳ **J1453**   Injection, fosaprepitant, **1 mg**
Prevents chemotherapy-induced nausea and vomiting
NDC: Emend

✪ **J1455**   Injection, foscarnet sodium, **per 1000 mg**
NDC: Foscavir
IOM: 100-02, 15, 50

✳ **J1457**   Injection, gallium nitrate, **1 mg**
NDC: Ganite

✳ **J1458**   Injection, galsulfase, **1 mg**
NDC: Naglazyme

✳ **J1459**   Injection, immune globulin (Privigen), intravenous, non-lyophilized (e.g., liquid), **500 mg**

✪ **J1460**   Injection, gamma globulin, intramuscular, **1 cc**
NDC: GamaSTAN, Immune Globulin (Human)
Other: Gammar
IOM: 100-02, 15, 50

▶ ✳ **J1557**   Injection, immune globulin, (gammaplex), intravenous, non-lyophilized (e.g., liquid), **500 mg**

▶ ✳ **J1559**   Injection, immune globulin, (hizentra), **100 mg**

✪ **J1560**   Injection, gamma globulin, intramuscular, **over 10 cc**
NDC: GamaSTAN, Immune Globin (Human)
Other: Gammar
IOM: 100-02, 15, 50

▶ New   → Revised   ✔ Reinstated   ~~deleted~~ Deleted
✪ Special coverage instructions   ◆ Not covered or valid by Medicare   ✳ Carrier discretion

→ ☼ **J1561** Injection, immune globulin, (Gamunex/Gamunex-C/Gammaked), non-lyophilized (e.g. liquid), **500 mg**

NDC: Gamunex

IOM: 100-02, 15, 50

✳ **J1562** Injection, immune globulin (Vivaglobin), **100 mg**

☼ **J1566** Injection, immune globulin, intravenous, lyophilized (e.g., powder), not otherwise specified, **500 mg**

NDC: Carimune Gammagard S/D, Panglobulin NF

Other: Polygam

IOM: 100-02, 15, 50

✳ **J1568** Injection, immune globulin, (Octagam), intravenous, non-lyophilized (e.g., liquid), **500 mg**

☼ **J1569** Injection, immune globulin, (Gammagard Liquid), intravenous, non-lyophilized, (e.g. liquid), **500 mg**

IOM: 100-02, 15, 50

☼ **J1570** Injection, ganciclovir sodium, **500 mg**

NDC: Cytovene

IOM: 100-02, 15, 50

☼ **J1571** Injection, hepatitis B immune globulin (HepaGam B), intramuscular, **0.5 ml**

IOM: 100-02, 15, 50

☼ **J1572** Injection, immune globulin, (flebogamma/flebogamma DIF) intravenous, non-lyophilized (e.g. liquid), **500 mg**

IOM: 100-02, 15, 50

✳ **J1573** Injection, hepatitis B immune globulin (HepaGam B), intravenous, **0.5 ml**

☼ **J1580** Injection, Garamycin, gentamicin, **up to 80 mg**

NDC: Gentamicin Sulfate

Other: Jenamicin

IOM: 100-02, 15, 50

✳ **J1590** Injection, gatifloxacin, **10 mg**

Other: Tequin

☼ **J1595** Injection, glatiramer acetate, **20 mg**

Other: Copaxone

IOM: 100-02, 15, 50

▶ ✳ **J1599** Injection, immune globulin, intravenous, non-lyophilized (e.g., liquid), not otherwise specified, **500 mg**

☼ **J1600** Injection, gold sodium thiomalate, **up to 50 mg**

NDC: Myochrysine

IOM: 100-02, 15, 50

☼ **J1610** Injection, glucagon hydrochloride, **per 1 mg**

NDC: GlucaGen, Glucagon Emergency

IOM: 100-02, 15, 50

☼ **J1620** Injection, gonadorelin hydrochloride, **per 100 mcg**

Other: Factrel

IOM: 100-02, 15, 50

☼ **J1626** Injection, granisetron hydrochloride, **100 mcg**

NDC: Kytril

IOM: 100-02, 15, 50

☼ **J1630** Injection, haloperidol, **up to 5 mg**

NDC: Haldol, Haloperidol Lactate

IOM: 100-02, 15, 50

☼ **J1631** Injection, haloperidol decanoate, **per 50 mg**

NDC: Haldol Decanoate

IOM: 100-02, 15, 50

☼ **J1640** Injection, hemin, **1 mg**

NDC: Panhematin

IOM: 100-02, 15, 50

☼ **J1642** Injection, heparin sodium, (heparin lock flush), **per 10 units**

NDC: Heparine Combination, Heparine (Porcine) In Nacl, Heparin (Porcine) Lock Flush, Heparin Sodium Flush, Heparin Sodium Lock Flush, Hep Flush-10, Hep-Lock, Hep-Lock Flush, Vasceze

Other: Hep-Lock U/P

IOM: 100-02, 15, 50

☼ **J1644** Injection, heparin sodium, **per 1000 units**

NDC: Heparin (Porcine), Heparin Sodium (Porcine)

Other: Liquaemin Sodium

IOM: 100-02, 15, 50

☼ **J1645** Injection, dalteparin sodium, **per 2500 IU**

NDC: Fragmin

IOM: 100-02, 15, 50

✳ **J1650** Injection, enoxaparin sodium, **10 mg**

NDC: Lovenox

▶ New   → Revised   ✔ Reinstated   ~~deleted~~ Deleted
☼ Special coverage instructions   ◆ Not covered or valid by Medicare   ✳ Carrier discretion

⚙ **J1652** Injection, fondaparinux sodium, **0.5 mg**

NDC: Arixtra

IOM: 100-02, 15, 50

✳ **J1655** Injection, tinzaparin sodium, **1000 IU**

NDC: Innohep

⚙ **J1670** Injection, tetanus immune globulin, human, **up to 250 units**

Indicated for transient protection against tetanus post-exposure to tetanus (V03.7).

NDC: Hypertet S/D

Other: Hyper-tet

IOM: 100-02, 15, 50

⚙ **J1675** Injection, histrelin acetate, **10 micrograms**

IOM: 100-02, 15, 50

✳ **J1680** Injection, human fibrinogen concentrate, **100 mg**

⚙ **J1700** Injection, hydrocortisone acetate, **up to 25 mg**

Other: Hydrocortone Acetate

IOM: 100-02, 15, 50

⚙ **J1710** Injection, hydrocortisone sodium phosphate, **up to 50 mg**

Other: A-hydroCort, Hydrocortone phosphate, Solu-Cortef

IOM: 100-02, 15, 50

▶ ✳ **J1725** Injection, hydroxyprogesterone caproate, **1 mg**

⚙ **J1720** Injection, hydrocortisone sodium succinate, **up to 100 mg**

NDC: A-Hydrocort, Solu-Cortef

IOM: 100-02, 15, 50

⚙ **J1730** Injection, diazoxide, **up to 300 mg**

Other: Hyperstat

IOM: 100-02, 15, 50

✳ **J1740** Injection, ibandronate sodium, **1 mg**

Other: Boniva

⚙ **J1742** Injection, ibutilide fumarate, **1 mg**

NDC: Corvert

IOM: 100-02, 15, 50

✳ **J1743** Injection, idursulfase, **1 mg**

Other: Elaprase

⚙ **J1745** Injection, infliximab, **10 mg**

Report total number of 10 mg increments administered; medical record must document failed or incomplete control of arthritis with use of other antirheumatic modalities

NDC: Remicade

IOM: 100-02, 15, 50

⚙ **J1750** Injection, iron dextran, **50 mg**

IOM: 100-02, 15, 50

NDC: Dexferrum, Infed

✳ **J1756** Injection, iron sucrose, **1 mg**

NDC: Venofer

▶ ⚙ **J1786** Injection, imiglucerase, **10 units**

NDC: Cerezyme

IOM: 100-02, 15, 50

⚙ **J1790** Injection, droperidol, **up to 5 mg**

NDC: Inapsine

IOM: 100-02, 15, 50

⚙ **J1800** Injection, propranolol HCL, **up to 1 mg**

NDC: Inderal

IOM: 100-02, 15, 50

⚙ **J1810** Injection, droperidol and fentanyl citrate, **up to 2 ml ampule**

Other: Innovar

IOM: 100-02, 15, 50

⚙ **J1815** Injection, insulin, **per 5 units**

NDC: Apidra, Humalog, Iletin-I, Lantus, Novolin, Novolog, Relion

Other: Lispro-PFC

IOM: 100-02, 15, 50; 100-03, 4, 280.14

✳ **J1817** Insulin for administration through DME (i.e., insulin pump) **per 50 units**

NDC: Apidra, Humalog, Humulin, Iletin, Lantus, Novolin, Novolog, Relion

▶ ◆ **J1826** Injection, interferon beta-1a, **30 mcg**

⚙ **J1830** Injection interferon beta-1b, **0.25 mg** (Code may be used for Medicare when drug administered under the direct supervision of a physician, not for use when drug is self administered)

Other: Betaseron

IOM: 100-02, 15, 50

▶ New → Revised ✔ Reinstated deleted Deleted

⚙ Special coverage instructions ◆ Not covered or valid by Medicare ✳ Carrier discretion

* **J1835** Injection, itraconazole, **50 mg**
  Other: Sporanox

⊛ **J1840** Injection, kanamycin sulfate, **up to 500 mg**
  Other: Kantrex, Klebcil
  IOM: 100-02, 15, 50

⊛ **J1850** Injection, kanamycin sulfate, **up to 75 mg**
  Other: Kantrex, Klebcil
  IOM: 100-02, 15, 50

⊛ **J1885** Injection, ketorolac tromethamine, **per 15 mg**
  Other: Toradol
  Other: 100-02, 15, 50

⊛ **J1890** Injection, cephalothin sodium, **up to 1 gram**
  Other: Keflin
  IOM: 100-02, 15, 50

* **J1930** Injection, lanreotide, **1 mg**
  Treats acromegaly and symptoms caused by neuroendocrine tumors
  NDC: Somatuline Depot

* **J1931** Injection, laronidase, **0.1 mg**
  NDC: Aldurazyme

⊛ **J1940** Injection, furosemide, **up to 20 mg**
  Other: Lasix
  MCM 2049
  IOM: 100-02, 15, 50

⊛ **J1945** Injection, lepirudin, **50 mg**
  NDC: Refludan
  IOM: 100-02, 15, 50

⊛ **J1950** Injection, leuprolide acetate (for depot suspension), **per 3.75 mg**
  NDC: Lupron Depot, Lupron Depot-Ped
  IOM: 100-02, 15, 50

* **J1953** Injection, levetiracetam, **10 mg**

⊛ **J1955** Injection, levocarnitine, **per 1 gm**
  NDC: Carnitor
  Other: L-Carnitine
  IOM: 100-02, 15, 50

⊛ **J1956** Injection, levofloxacin, **250 mg**
  NDC: Levaquin
  IOM: 100-02, 15, 50

⊛ **J1960** Injection, levorphanol tartrate, **up to 2 mg**
  Other: Levo-Dromoran
  MCM 2049
  IOM: 100-02, 15, 50

⊛ **J1980** Injection, hyoscyamine sulfate, **up to 0.25 mg**
  NDC: Levsin
  IOM: 100-02, 15, 50

⊛ **J1990** Injection, chlordiazepoxide HCL, **up to 100 mg**
  Other: Librium
  IOM: 100-02, 15, 50

⊛ **J2001** Injection, lidocaine HCL for intravenous infusion, **10 mg**
  NDC: Lidocaine in D5W, Xylocaine (Cardiac)
  Other: Anestacaine, Caine-1, Dilocaine, L-Caine, Lidoject, Nervocaine, Nulicaine, Xylocaine
  IOM: 100-02, 15, 50

⊛ **J2010** Injection, lincomycin HCL, **up to 300 mg**
  NDC: Lincocin
  IOM: 100-02, 15, 50

* **J2020** Injection, linezolid, **200 mg**
  NDC: Zyvox

⊛ **J2060** Injection, lorazepam, **2 mg**
  NDC: Ativan
  IOM: 100-02, 15, 50

⊛ **J2150** Injection, mannitol, **25% in 50 ml**
  MCM 2049
  IOM: 100-02, 15, 50

* **J2170** Injection, mecasermin, **1 mg**
  Other: Increlex

⊛ **J2175** Injection, meperidine hydrochloride, **per 100 mg**
  NDC: Demerol
  IOM: 100-02, 15, 50

⊛ **J2180** Injection, meperidine and promethazine HCL, **up to 50 mg**
  Other: Mepergan
  IOM: 100-02, 15, 50

* **J2185** Injection, meropenem, **100 mg**
  NDC: Merrem

⊛ **J2210** Injection, methylergonovine maleate, **up to 0.2 mg**
  Benefit limited to obstetrical diagnoses for prevention and control of post-partum hemorrhage
  NDC: Methergine
  IOM: 100-02, 15, 50

▶ New → Revised ✔ Reinstated ~~deleted~~ Deleted ⊛ Special coverage instructions ◆ Not covered or valid by Medicare * Carrier discretion

✳ **J2248** Injection, micafungin sodium, **1 mg**

Other: Mycamine

☺ **J2250** Injection, midazolam hydrochloride, **per 1 mg**

Other: Versed

IOM: 100-02, 15, 50

☺ **J2260** Injection, milrinone lactate, **5 mg**

NDC: Primacor

IOM: 100-02, 15, 50

▶ ✳ **J2265** Injection, minocycline hydrochloride, **1 mg**

☺ **J2270** Injection, morphine sulfate, **up to 10 mg**

Other: Astromorph PF, Duramorph

IOM: 100-02, 15, 50

☺ **J2271** Injection, morphine sulfate, **100 mg**

Other: Astramorph PF, Duramorph

IOM: 100-02, 15, 50; 100-03, 4, 280.1

☺ **J2275** Injection, morphine sulfate (preservative-free sterile solution), **per 10 mg**

NDC: Astramorph, Duramorph, Infumorph

IOM: 100-02, 15, 50; 100-03, 4, 280.1

☺ **J2278** Injection, ziconotide, **1 microgram**

NDC: Prialt

✳ **J2280** Injection, moxifloxacin, **100 mg**

NDC: Avelox

☺ **J2300** Injection, nalbuphine hydrochloride, **per 10 mg**

NDC: Nubain

IOM: 100-02, 15, 50

☺ **J2310** Injection, naloxone hydrochloride, **per 1 mg**

Other: Narcan

IOM: 100-02, 15, 50

✳ **J2315** Injection, naltrexone, depot form, **1 mg**

NDC: Vivitrol

☺ **J2320** Injection, nandrolone decanoate, **up to 50 mg**

Other: Anabolin LA 100, Androlone, Deca-Durabolin, Decolone, Hybolin Decanoate, Nandrobolic LA, Neo-Durabolic

IOM: 100-02, 15, 50

✳ **J2323** Injection, natalizumab, **1 mg**

Other: Tysabri

☺ **J2325** Injection, nesiritide, **0.1 mg**

NDC: Natrecor

IOM: 100-02, 15, 50

✳ **J2353** Injection, octreotide, depot form for intramuscular injection, **1 mg**

NDC: Sandostatin LAR Depot

✳ **J2354** Injection, octreotide, non-depot form for subcutaneous or intravenous injection, **25 mcg**

Other: Sandostatin LAR Depot

☺ **J2355** Injection, oprelvekin, **5 mg**

NDC: Neumega

IOM: 100-02, 15, 50

✳ **J2357** Injection, omalizumab, **5 mg**

NDC: Xolair

▶ ✳ **J2358** Injection, olanzapine, long-acting, **1 mg**

NDC: Zyprexa Relprevv

☺ **J2360** Injection, orphenadrine citrate, **up to 60 mg**

NDC: Norflex

Other: Antiflex, Banflex, Flexoject, Flexon, K-Flex, Mio-Rel, Neocyten, O-Flex, Orfro, Orphenate

IOM: 100-02, 15, 50

☺ **J2370** Injection, phenylephrine HCL, **up to 1 ml**

NDC: Neo-Synephrine

IOM: 100-02, 15, 50

☺ **J2400** Injection, chloroprocaine hydrochloride, **per 30 ml**

NDC: Nesacaine, Nesacaine-MPF

IOM: 100-02, 15, 50

☺ **J2405** Injection, ondansetron hydrochloride, **per 1 mg**

NDC: Zofran

IOM: 100-02, 15, 50

☺ **J2410** Injection, oxymorphone HCL, **up to 1 mg**

NDC: Numorphan, Opana

IOM: 100-02, 15, 50

✳ **J2425** Injection, palifermin, **50 micrograms**

NDC: Kepivance

▶ ✳ **J2426** Injection, paliperidone palmitate extended release, **1 mg**

NDC: Invega Sustenna

▶ New   → Revised   ✔ Reinstated   ~~deleted~~ Deleted

☺ Special coverage instructions   ◆ Not covered or valid by Medicare   ✳ Carrier discretion

⚙ **J2430** Injection, pamidronate disodium, **per 30 mg**

NDC: Aredia

IOM: 100-02, 15, 50

⚙ **J2440** Injection, papaverine HCL, **up to 60 mg**

IOM: 100-02, 15, 50

⚙ **J2460** Injection, oxytetracycline HCL, **up to 50 mg**

Other: Terramycin IM

IOM: 100-02, 15, 50

✳ **J2469** Injection, palonosetron HCL, **25 mcg**

Example: 0.25 mgm dose = 10 units. Example of use is acute, delayed, nausea and vomiting due to chemotherpy.

NDC: Aloxi

⚙ **J2501** Injection, paricalcitol, **1 mcg**

NDC: Zemplar

IOM: 100-02, 15, 50

✳ **J2503** Injection, pegaptanib sodium, **0.3 mg**

NDC: Macugen

⚙ **J2504** Injection, pegademase bovine, **25 IU**

NDC: Adagen

IOM: 100-02, 15, 50

✳ **J2505** Injection, pegfilgrastim, **6 mg**

Report 1 unit per 6 mg.

NDC: Neulasta

▶ ✳ **J2507** Injection, pegloticase, **1 mg**

⚙ **J2510** Injection, penicillin G procaine, aqueous, **up to 600,000 units**

NDC: Wycillin

Other: Crysticillin, Duracillin AS, Penicillin G procaine aqueous, Pfizerpen AS

IOM: 100-02, 15, 50

⚙ **J2513** Injection, pentastarch, 10% solution, **100 ml**

IOM: 100-02, 15, 50

⚙ **J2515** Injection, pentobarbital sodium, **per 50 mg**

NDC: Nembutal

IOM: 100-02, 15, 50

⚙ **J2540** Injection, penicillin G potassium, **up to 600,000 units**

NDC: Pfizerpen-G

IOM: 100-02, 15, 50

⚙ **J2543** Injection, piperacillin sodium/ tazobactam sodium, **1 gram/ 0.125 grams (1.125 grams)**

NDC: Zosyn

IOM: 100-02, 15, 50

⚙ **J2545** Pentamidine isethionate, inhalation solution, FDA-approved final product, non-compounded, administered through DME, unit dose form, **per 300 mg**

NDC: Nebupent

⚙ **J2550** Injection, promethazine HCL, **up to 50 mg**

Administration of phenergan suppository considered part of E/M encounter

NDC: Phenergan

Other: Anergan, Phenazine, Prorex, Prothazine

IOM: 100-02, 15, 50

⚙ **J2560** Injection, phenobarbital sodium, **up to 120 mg**

NDC: Luminal

IOM: 100-02, 15, 50

✳ **J2562** Injection, plerixafor, **1 mg**

FDA approved for non-Hodgkin lymphoma and multiple myeloma in 2008.

NDC: Mozobil

⚙ **J2590** Injection, oxytocin, **up to 10 units**

NDC: Pitocin

Other: Syntocinon

IOM: 100-02, 15, 50

⚙ **J2597** Injection, desmopressin acetate, **per 1 mcg**

NDC: DDAVP

IOM: 100-02, 15, 50

⚙ **J2650** Injection, prednisolone acetate, **up to 1 ml**

Other: Cotolone, Key-Pred, Predalone, Predcor, Predicort

IOM: 100-02, 15, 50

⚙ **J2670** Injection, tolazoline HCL, **up to 25 mg**

Other: Priscoline Hydrochloride

IOM: 100-02, 15, 50

⚙ **J2675** Injection, progesterone, **per 50 mg**

Other: Gesterol 50, Progestaject

IOM: 100-02, 15, 50

▶ New → Revised ✔ Reinstated deleted Deleted ⚙ Special coverage instructions ◆ Not covered or valid by Medicare ✳ Carrier discretion

⊛ **J2680** Injection, fluphenazine decanoate, **up to 25 mg**

Other: Prolixin Decanoate

MCM 2049

IOM: 100-02, 15, 50

⊛ **J2690** Injection, procainamide HCL, **up to 1 gm**

Benefit limited to obstetrical diagnoses

Other: Pronestyl, Prostaphlin

IOM: 100-02, 15, 50

⊛ **J2700** Injection, oxacillin sodium, **up to 250 mg**

NDC: Bactocill

IOM: 100-02, 15, 50

⊛ **J2710** Injection, neostigmine methylsulfate, **up to 0.5 mg**

Other: Prostigmin

IOM: 100-02, 15, 50

⊛ **J2720** Injection, protamine sulfate, **per 10 mg**

IOM: 100-02, 15, 50

✳ **J2724** Injection, protein C concentrate, intravenous, human, **10 IU**

NDC: Ceprotin

⊛ **J2725** Injection, protirelin, **per 250 mcg**

Other: Relefact TRH, Thypinone

IOM: 100-02, 15, 50

⊛ **J2730** Injection, pralidoxime chloride, **up to 1 gm**

NDC: Protopam Chloride

IOM: 100-02, 15, 50

⊛ **J2760** Injection, phentolamine mesylate, **up to 5 mg**

Other: Regitine

IOM: 100-02, 15, 50

⊛ **J2765** Injection, metoclopramide HCL, **up to 10 mg**

NDC: Reglan

IOM: 100-02, 15, 50

⊛ **J2770** Injection, quinupristin/dalfopristin, **500 mg (150/350)**

NDC: Synercid

IOM: 100-02, 15, 50

✳ **J2778** Injection, ranibizumab, **0.1 mg**

May be reported for exudative senile macular degeneration (wet AMD) with 67028 (RT or LT)

Other: Lucentis

⊛ **J2780** Injection, ranitidine hydrochloride, **25 mg**

NDC: Zantac

IOM: 100-02, 15, 50

✳ **J2783** Injection, rasburicase, **0.5 mg**

NDC: Elitek

✳ **J2785** Injection, regadenoson, **0.1 mg**

One billing unit equal to 0.1 mg of regadenoson

⊛ **J2788** Injection, Rho D immune globulin, human, minidose, **50 mcg (250 IU)**

NDC: Bay Rho-D, MicRhoGAM

Other: HypRho-D, RhoGam

IOM: 100-02, 15, 50

⊛ **J2790** Injection, Rho D immune globulin, human, full dose, **300 mcg (1500 IU)**

Administered to pregnant female to prevent hemolistic disease of newborn. Report 90384 to private payer

NDC: Hyperrho S/D, RhoGAM

Other: Gamulin Rh, HypRho-D, Rhesonativ

IOM: 100-02, 15, 50

⊛ **J2791** Injection, Rho(D) immune globulin (human), (Rhophylac), intramuscular or intravenous, **100 IU**

Agent must be billed per 100 IU in both physician office and hospital outpatient settings

IOM: 100-02, 15, 50

⊛ **J2792** Injection, Rho D immune globulin intravenous, human, solvent detergent, **100 IU**

NDC: WinRHo-SDF

Other: Gamulin RH, Hyperrho S/D

IOM: 100-02, 15, 50

⊛ **J2793** Injection, rilonacept, **1 mg**

IOM: 100-02, 15, 50

✳ **J2794** Injection, risperidone, long acting, **0.5 mg**

NDC: Risperdal Costa

✳ **J2795** Injection, ropivacaine hydrochloride, **1 mg**

NDC: Naropin

✳ **J2796** Injection, romiplostim, **10 micrograms**

Stimulates bone marrow megakarocytes to produce platelets (i.e., ITP).

NDC: Nplate

▶ New → Revised ✔ Reinstated ~~deleted~~ Deleted

⊛ Special coverage instructions ◆ Not covered or valid by Medicare ✳ Carrier discretion

⊛ **J2800** Injection, methocarbamol, **up to 10 ml**
NDC: Robaxin
IOM: 100-02, 15, 50

✳ **J2805** Injection, sincalide, **5 micrograms**

⊛ **J2810** Injection, theophylline, **per 40 mg**
IOM: 100-02, 15, 50

⊛ **J2820** Injection, sargramostim (GM-CSF), **50 mcg**
NDC: Leukine
Other: Prokine
IOM: 100-02, 15, 50

⊛ **J2850** Injection, secretin, synthetic, human, **1 microgram**
NDC: Chirhostim
IOM: 100-02, 15, 50

⊛ **J2910** Injection, aurothioglucose, **up to 50 mg**
Other: Solganal
IOM: 100-02, 15, 50

⊛ **J2916** Injection, sodium ferric gluconate complex in sucrose injection, **12.5 mg**
NDC: Ferrlecit
IOM: 100-02, 15, 50

⊛ **J2920** Injection, methylprednisolone sodium succinate, **up to 40 mg**
NDC: A-MethaPred, Solu-Medrol
IOM: 100-02, 15, 50

⊛ **J2930** Injection, methylprednisolone sodium succinate, **up to 125 mg**
NDC: A-MethaPred, Solu-Medrol
IOM: 100-02, 15, 50

⊛ **J2940** Injection, somatrem, **1 mg**
IOM: 100-02, 15, 50,
Medicare Statute 1861s2b

⊛ **J2941** Injection, somatropin, **1 mg**
Other: Genotropin, Humatrope, Nutropin, Omnitrope, Saizen, Serostim, Zorbtive
IOM: 100-02, 15, 50,
Medicare Statute 1861s2b

⊛ **J2950** Injection, promazine HCL, **up to 25 mg**
Other: Prozine-50, Sparine
IOM: 100-02, 15, 50

⊛ **J2993** Injection, reteplase, **18.1 mg**
NDC: Retavase
IOM: 100-02, 15, 50

⊛ **J2995** Injection, streptokinase, **per 250,000 IU**
Bill 1 unit for each 250,000 IU
Other: Kabikinase, Streptase
IOM: 100-02, 15, 50

⊛ **J2997** Injection, alteplase recombinant, **1 mg**
Thrombolytic agent, treatment of occluded catheters. Bill units of 1 mg administered
NDC: Activase, Cathflo Activase
IOM: 100-02, 15, 50

⊛ **J3000** Injection, streptomycin, **up to 1 gm**
IOM: 100-02, 15, 50

⊛ **J3010** Injection, fentanyl citrate, **0.1 mg**
NDC: Sublimaze
IOM: 100-02, 15, 50

⊛ **J3030** Injection, sumatriptan succinate, **6 mg (Code may be used for Medicare when drug administered under the direct supervision of a physician, not for use when drug is self administered)**
NDC: Imitrex, Sumavel Dosepro
IOM: 100-02, 15, 150

⊛ **J3070** Injection, pentazocine, **30 mg**
NDC: Talwin
IOM: 100-02, 15, 50

▶ ✳ **J3095** Injection, televancin, **10 mg**
Prescribed for the treatment of adults with complicated skin and skin structure infections (cSSSI) of the following Gram-positive microorganisms: Staphylococcus aureus ; Streptococcus pyogenes, Streptococcus agalactiae, Streptococcus anginosus group. Separately payable under the ASC payment system.
NDC: Vibativ

✳ **J3101** Injection, tenecteplase, **1 mg**
NDC: TNKase

⊛ **J3105** Injection, terbutaline sulfate, **up to 1 mg**
Other: Brethine
IOM: 100-02, 15, 50

⊛ **J3110** Injection, teriparatide, **10 mcg**
Other: Forteo

▶ New   → Revised   ✔ Reinstated   ~~deleted~~ Deleted

⊛ Special coverage instructions   ◆ Not covered or valid by Medicare   ✳ Carrier discretion

⊕ **J3120** Injection, testosterone enanthate, **up to 100 mg**

NDC: Delatestryl

Other: Andro LA 200, Andropository 100, Andryl 200, Delatest, Durathate-200, Everone, Testone LA, Testrin PA

IOM: 100-02, 15, 50

⊕ **J3130** Injection, testosterone enanthate, **up to 200 mg**

NDC: Delatestryl

Other: Andro LA 200, Andropository 100, Andryl 200, Delatest, Durathate-200, Everone, Testone LA, Testrin PA

IOM: 100-02, 15, 50

⊕ **J3140** Injection, testosterone suspension, **up to 50 mg**

Other: Adronaq-50, Histerone, Testaqua, Testro AQ, Testoject-50

IOM: 100-02, 15, 50

⊕ **J3150** Injection, testosterone propionate, **up to 100 mg**

Other: DepAndro 100, Testex

IOM: 100-02, 15, 50

⊕ **J3230** Injection, chlorpromazine HCL, **up to 50 mg**

Other: Ormazine, Thorazine

IOM: 100-02, 15, 50

⊕ **J3240** Injection, thyrotropin alfa, **0.9 mg provided in 1.1 mg vial**

NDC: Thyrogen

IOM: 100-02, 15, 50

✻ **J3243** Injection, tigecycline, **1 mg**

✻ **J3246** Injection, tirofiban HCL, **0.25 mg**

NDC: Aggrastat

⊕ **J3250** Injection, trimethobenzamide HCL, **up to 200 mg**

NDC: Benzacot, Tigan

Other: Arrestin, Tiject 20

IOM: 100-02, 15, 50

⊕ **J3260** Injection, tobramycin sulfate, **up to 80 mg**

Other: Nebcin

IOM: 100-02, 15, 50

▶ ✻ **J3262** Injection, tocilizumab, **1 mg**

Indicated for the treatment of adult patients with moderately to severely active rheumatoid arthritis (RA) who have had an inadequate response to one or more tumor necrosis factor (TNF) antagonist therapies.

NDC: Actemra

⊕ **J3265** Injection, torsemide, **10 mg/ml**

Other: Demadex

IOM: 100-02, 15, 50

⊕ **J3280** Injection, thiethylperazine maleate, **up to 10 mg**

Other: Norzine, Torecan

IOM: 100-02, 15, 50

✻ **J3285** Injection, treprostinil, **1 mg**

NDC: Remodulin

⊕ **J3300** Injection, triamcinolone acetonide, preservative free, **1 mg**

⊕ **J3301** Injection, triamcinolone acetonide, not otherwise specified, **10 mg**

NDC: Kenalog

Other: Cenacort A-40, Kenaject-40, Triam A, Triesence, Tri-Kort, Trilog

IOM: 100-02, 15, 50

⊕ **J3302** Injection, triamcinolone diacetate, **per 5 mg**

NDC: Clincacort

Other: Amcort, Aristocort, Cenacort Forte, Triamcot, Trilone

IOM: 100-02, 15, 50

⊕ **J3303** Injection, triamcinolone hexacetonide, **per 5 mg**

NDC: Aristospan

IOM: 100-02, 15, 50

⊕ **J3305** Injection, trimetrexate glucuronate, **per 25 mg**

Other: NeuTrexin

IOM: 100-02, 15, 50

⊕ **J3310** Injection, perphenazine, **up to 5 mg**

Other: Trilafon

IOM: 100-02, 15, 50

⊕ **J3315** Injection, triptorelin pamoate, **3.75 mg**

NDC: Trelstar

IOM: 100-02, 15, 50

▶ New → Revised ✔ Reinstated ~~deleted~~ Deleted

⊕ Special coverage instructions ◆ Not covered or valid by Medicare ✻ Carrier discretion

⊛ **J3320** Injection, spectinomycin dihydrochloride, **up to 2 gm**

Other: Trobicin

IOM: 100-02, 15, 50

⊛ **J3350** Injection, urea, **up to 40 gm**

Other: Ureaphil

IOM: 100-02, 15, 50

⊛ **J3355** Injection, urofollitropin, **75 IU**

NDC: Bravelle

Other: Metrodin

IOM: 100-02, 15, 50

▶ ✻ **J3357** Injection, ustekinumab, **1 mg**

NDC: Stelara

⊛ **J3360** Injection, diazepam, **up to 5 mg**

Other: Valium, Zetran

IOM: 100-02, 15, 50

⊛ **J3364** Injection, urokinase, **5000 IU vial**

NDC: Abbokinase

IOM: 100-02, 15, 50

⊛ **J3365** Injection, IV, urokinase, **250,000 IU vial**

Other: Kinlytic

IOM: 100-02, 15, 50,

Cross Reference Q0089

⊛ **J3370** Injection, vancomycin HCL, **500 mg**

NDC: Vancocin

Other: Vancoled

IOM: 100-02, 15, 50; 100-03, 4, 280.14

▶ ✻ **J3385** Injection, velaglucerase alfa, **100 units**

Enzyme replacement therapy in Gaucher Disease that results from a specific enzyme deficiency in the body, caused by a genetic mutation received from both parents. Type 1 is the most prevalent Ashkenazi Jewish genetic disease, occurring in one in every 1,000.

NDC: VPRIV

⊛ **J3396** Injection, verteporfin, **0.1 mg**

NDC: Visudyne

IOM: 100-03, 1, 80.2; 100-03, 1, 80.3

⊛ **J3400** Injection, triflupromazine HCL, **up to 20 mg**

Other: Vesprin

IOM: 100-02, 15, 50

⊛ **J3410** Injection, hydroxyzine HCL, **up to 25 mg**

NDC: Restall

Other: Hyzine-50, Vistacot, Vistaject 25

IOM: 100-02, 15, 50

✻ **J3411** Injection, thiamine HCL, **100 mg**

✻ **J3415** Injection, pyridoxine HCL, **100 mg**

Other: Rodex

⊛ **J3420** Injection, vitamin B-12 cyanocobalamin, **up to 1000 mcg**

Medicare carriers may have local coverage decisions regarding vitamin B_{12} injections that provide reimbursement only for patients with certain types of anemia and other conditions

NDC: Cobal-1000, Nervidox-6 S

Other: Cobolin-M, Hydroxocobalamin, Neuroforte-R, Redisol, Rubramin PC, Sytobex, Vita #12

IOM: 100-02, 15, 50; 100-03, 2, 150.6

⊛ **J3430** Injection, phytonadione (vitamin K), **per 1 mg**

NDC: Vitamin K1

Other: Aqua-Mephyton, Konakion, Menadione, Synkavite

IOM: 100-02, 15, 50

⊛ **J3465** Injection, voriconazole, **10 mg**

NDC: VFEND

IOM: 100-02, 15, 50

⊛ **J3470** Injection, hyaluronidase, **up to 150 units**

NDC: Amphadase

Other: Vitrase, Wydase

IOM: 100-02, 15, 50

⊛ **J3471** Injection, hyaluronidase, ovine, preservative free, **per 1 USP unit (up to 999 USP units)**

NDC: Vitrase

⊛ **J3472** Injection, hyaluronidase, ovine, preservative free, **per 1000 USP units**

NDC: Vitrase

⊛ **J3473** Injection, hyaluronidase, recombinant, **1 USP unit**

Other: Hylenex

IOM: 100-02, 15, 50

▶ New	→ Revised	✔ Reinstated	~~deleted~~ Deleted
⊛ Special coverage instructions		◆ Not covered or valid by Medicare	✻ Carrier discretion

⊕ **J3475**   Injection, magnesium sulfate, **per 500 mg**

IOM: 100-02, 15, 50

⊕ **J3480**   Injection, potassium chloride, **per 2 meq**

IOM: 100-02, 15, 50

⊕ **J3485**   Injection, zidovudine, **10 mg**

NDC: Retrovir

IOM: 100-02, 15, 50

✳ **J3486**   Injection, ziprasidone mesylate, **10 mg**

NDC: Geodon

✳ **J3487**   Injection, zoledronic acid (Zometa), **1 mg**

NDC: Zometa

⊕ **J3488**   Injection, zoledronic acid (Reclast), **1 mg**

Physician to specify 5 units for approved 5 mg dosing of Reclast

NDC: Reclast

⊕ **J3490**   Unclassified drugs

Bill on paper. Bill one unit. Identify drug and total dosage in "Remarks" field.

Other: Acthib, Aminocaproic Acid, Baciim, Bacitracin, Benzocaine, Betamethasone Acetate, Brevital Sodium, Bumetanide, Bupivacaine, Cefotetan, Cimetidine, Ciprofloxacin, Cleocin Phosphate, Clindamycin, Cortisone Acetate, Definity, Diprivan, Engerix-B, Ethanolamine, Famotidine, Ganirelix, Gonal-F, Gonal-F RFF, Hyaluronic Acid, Kineret, Marcaine, Metronidazole, Nafcillin, Naltrexone, Ovidrel, Pegasys, Peg-Intron, Penicillin G Sodium, Prodrox, Propofol, Protonix, Recombivax, Rifadin, Rifampin, Sensorcaine-MPF, Smz-TMP, Sodium Hyaluronate, Sufenta, Sufentanil Citrate, Timentin, Treanda, Twinrix, Valcyte, Veritas Collagen Matrix

IOM: 100-02, 15, 50

◆ **J3520**   Edetate disodium, **per 150 mg**

Other: Chealamide, Disotate, Endrate ethylenediamine-tetra-acetic

IOM: 100-03, 1, 20.21; 100-03, 1, 20.22

⊕ **J3530**   Nasal vaccine inhalation

IOM: 100-02, 15, 50

◆ **J3535**   Drug administered through a metered dose inhaler

Other: Ipratropium bromide

IOM: 100-02, 15, 50

◆ **J3570**   Laetrile, amygdalin, vitamin B-17

IOM: 100-03, 1, 30.7

✳ **J3590**   Unclassified biologics

Bill local carrier

Bill on paper. Bill one unit. Identify drug and total dosage in "Remarks" field.

Other: Bayhep B, Hyperhep-B, NABI-HB

Miscellaneous Drugs and Solutions

⊕ **J7030**   Infusion, normal saline solution, **1000 cc**

NDC: Sodium Chloride

IOM: 100-02, 15, 50

⊕ **J7040**   Infusion, normal saline solution, sterile **(500 ml=1 unit)**

Bill local carrier if incident to a physician's service or used in an implanted infusion pump. If other, bill DME/MAC.

NDC: Sodium Chloride

IOM: 100-02, 15, 50

⊕ **J7042**   5% dextrose/normal saline **(500 ml = 1 unit)**

Bill local carrier if incident to a physician's service or used in an implanted infusion pump. If other, bill DME/MAC.

NDC: Dextrose-Nacl

IOM: 100-02, 15, 50

⊕ **J7050**   Infusion, normal saline solution, **250 cc**

Bill local carrier if incident to a physician's service or used in an implanted infusion pump. If other, bill DME/MAC.

NDC: Sodium Chloride

IOM: 100-02, 15, 50

⊕ **J7060**   5% dextrose/water **(500 ml = 1 unit)**

Bill local carrier if incident to a physician's service or used in an implanted infusion pump. If other, bill DME/MAC.

IOM: 100-02, 15, 50

⊕ **J7070**   Infusion, D 5 W, **1000 cc**

Bill local carrier if incident to a physician's service or used in an implanted infusion pump. If other, bill DME/MAC.

NDC: Dextrose

IOM: 100-02, 15, 50

▶ New   → Revised   ✔ Reinstated   ~~deleted~~ Deleted

⊕ Special coverage instructions   ◆ Not covered or valid by Medicare   ✳ Carrier discretion

⊙ **J7100** Infusion, dextran 40, **500 ml**

Bill local carrier if incident to a physician's service or used in an implanted infusion pump. If other, bill DME/MAC.

Other: Gentran, LMD, LMD in Dextrose, Rheomacrodex

IOM: 100-02, 15, 50

⊙ **J7110** Infusion, dextran 75, **500 ml**

Bill local carrier if incident to a physician's service or used in an implanted infusion pump. If other, bill DME/MAC.

NDC: Dextran 70 w/NACL, Dextran 75 in D5W

Other: Gentran

IOM: 100-02, 15, 50

⊙ **J7120** Ringer's lactate infusion, **up to 1000 cc**

Bill local carrier if incident to a physician's service or used in an implanted infusion pump. If other, bill DME/MAC.

Replacement fluid or electrolytes.

NDC: Lactated Ringers

IOM: 100-02, 15, 50

J7130   Hypertonic saline solution, 50 or 100 meq, 20 cc vial   ✖

▶ ⊙ **J7131** Hypertonic saline solution, **1 ml**

IOM: 100-02, 15, 50

▶ ✳ **J7180** Injection, factor XIII (antihemophilic factor, human), 1 i.u.

▶ ⊙ **J7183** Injection, von Willebrand factor complex (human), wilate, **1 i.u. vwf:rco**

J7184   Injection, von Willebrand factor complex (human), Wilate, per 100 IU VWF:RCO   ✖

✳ **J7185** Injection, Factor VIII (antihemophilic factor, recombinant) (Xyntha), **per IU**

Reported in place of temporary code Q2023.

⊙ **J7186** Injection, anti-hemophilic factor VIII/von Willebrand factor complex (human), **per factor VIII IU**

Bill local carrier

NDC: Alphanate

IOM: 100-02, 15, 50

⊙ **J7187** Injection, von Willebrand factor complex (HUMATE-P), **per IU VWF: RCO**

Bill local carrier

NDC: Humate-P Low Dilutent

Other: Wilate

IOM: 100-02, 15, 50

⊙ **J7189** Factor VIIa (anti-hemophilic factor, recombinant), **per 1 microgram**

Bill local carrier

NDC: NovoSeven

IOM: 100-02, 15, 50

⊙ **J7190** Factor VIII anti-hemophilic factor, human, **per IU**

Bill local carrier

NDC: Alphanate, Alphanate/von Willebrand factor complex, Hemofil M, Koate DVI, Monarc-M, Monoclate-P

Other: Koate-HP, Kogenate, Recombinate

IOM: 100-02, 15, 50

⊙ **J7191** Factor VIII, anti-hemophilic factor (porcine), **per IU**

Bill local carrier

Other: Hyate C, Koate-HP, Recombinate

IOM: 100-02, 15, 50

✳ **J7192** Factor VIII (anti-hemophilic factor, recombinant) **per IU,** not otherwise specified

Bill local carrier

NDC: Advate, Helixate FS, Kogenate FS, Poly Bio-Set, Recombinate

Other: Refracto

IOM: 100-02, 15, 50

⊙ **J7193** Factor IX (anti-hemophilic factor, purified, non-recombinant) **per IU**

Bill local carrier

NDC: AlphaNine SD, Mononine

IOM: 100-02, 15, 50

⊙ **J7194** Factor IX, complex, **per IU**

Bill local carrier

NDC: Bebulin VH, Profilnine SD

Other: Konyne-80, Profilnine Heat-treated, Proplex SX-T, Proplex T

IOM: 100-02, 15, 50

⊙ **J7195** Factor IX (anti-hemophilic factor, recombinant) **per IU**

Bill local carrier

NDC: Benefix

Other: Konyne 80, Proplex T

IOM: 100-02, 15, 50

▶ **New**   → **Revised**   ✔ **Reinstated**   deleted **Deleted**

⊙ **Special coverage instructions**   ◆ **Not covered or valid by Medicare**   ✳ **Carrier discretion**

▶ ✳ **J7196** Injection, antithrombin recombinant, **50 IU**

Other: ATryn

☺ **J7197** Anti-thrombin III (human), **per IU**

Bill local carrier

NDC: Thrombate III

IOM: 100-02, 15, 50

☺ **J7198** Anti-inhibitor, **per IU**

Bill local carrier

Diagnosis examples: 286.0 Congenital Factor VIII disorder; 286.1 Congenital Factor IX disorder; 286.4 VonWillebrand's disease

NDC: Feiba VH Immuno

Other: Autoplex T, Hemophilia clotting factors

IOM: 100-02, 15, 50; 100-03, 2, 110.3

☺ **J7199** Hemophilia clotting factor, not otherwise classified

Bill local carrier

Other: Autoplex T

IOM: 100-02, 15, 50; 100-03, 2, 110.3

◆ **J7300** Intrauterine copper contraceptive

Bill local carrier

Report IVD insertion with 58300. Bill usual and customary charge.

Other: Paragard T 380 A

Medicare Statute 1862a1

◆ **J7302** Levonorgestrel-releasing intrauterine contraceptive system, **52 mg**

Bill local carrier

Other: Mirena

Medicare Statute 1862a1

◆ **J7303** Contraceptive supply, hormone containing vaginal ring, each

Bill local carrier

Medicare Statute 1862.1

◆ **J7304** Contraceptive supply, hormone containing patch, each

Bill local carrier

Only billed by Family Planning Clinics

Medicare Statute 1862.1

◆ **J7306** Levonorgestrel (contraceptive) implant system, including implants and supplies

Bill local carrier

◆ **J7307** Etonogestrel (contraceptive) implant system, including implant and supplies

✳ **J7308** Aminolevulinic acid HCL for topical administration, 20%, single unit dosage form **(354 mg)**

NDC: Levulan Kerastick

▶ ☺ **J7309** Methyl aminolevulinate (MAL) for topical administration, 16.8%, **1 gram**

☺ **J7310** Ganciclovir, **4.5 mg,** long-acting implant

Bill local carrier

NDC: Vitrasert

IOM: 100-02, 15, 50

✳ **J7311** Fluocinolone acetonide, intravitreal implant

Bill local carrier

Treatment of chronic noninfectious posterior segment uveitis

Other: Retisert

▶ ✳ **J7312** Injection, dexamethasone, intravitreal implant, **0.1 mg**

To bill for Ozurdex services submit the following codes: J7312 and 67028 with the modifier -22 (for the increased work difficulty and increased risk). Indicated for the treatment of macular edema occurring after branch retinal vein occlusion (BRVO) or central retinal vein occlusion (CRVO) and non-infectious uveitis affecting the posterior segment of the eye.

NDC: Ozurdex

✳ **J7321** Hyaluronan or derivative, Hyalgan or Supartz, for intra-articular injection, **per dose**

Bill local carrier

Therapeutic goal is to restore visco-elasticity of synovial hyaluronan, thereby decreasing pain, improving mobility and restoring natural protective functions of hyaluronan in joint

✳ **J7323** Hyaluronan or derivative, Euflexxa, for intra-articular injection, **per dose**

Bill local carrier

✳ **J7324** Hyaluronan or derivative, Orthovisc, for intra-articular injection, **per dose**

Bill local carrier

▶ New → Revised ✔ Reinstated ~~deleted~~ Deleted
☺ Special coverage instructions ◆ Not covered or valid by Medicare ✳ Carrier discretion

▶ ✳ **J7325** Hyaluronan or derivative, Synvisc or Synvisc-One, for intra-articular injection, **1 mg**

▶ ✳ **J7326** Hyaluronan or derivative, Gel-One, for intra-articular injection, **per dose**

✳ **J7330** Autologous cultured chondrocytes, **implant**

Bill local carrier

NDC: Carticel

▶ ✳ **J7335** Capsaicin 8% patch, **per 10 square centimeters**

NDC: Qutenza

Immunosuppressive Drugs (Includes Non-injectibles)

J7500-J7599: Bill local carrier if incident to a physician's service or used in an implanted infusion pump. If other, bill DME/MAC.

✪ **J7500** Azathioprine, oral, **50 mg**

NDC: Azasan, Imuran

IOM: 100-02, 15, 50

✪ **J7501** Azathioprine, parenteral, **100 mg**

Other: Imuran

IOM: 100-02, 15, 50

✪ **J7502** Cyclosporine, oral, **100 mg**

NDC: Gengraf, Neoral, Sandimmune

IOM: 100-02, 15, 50

✪ **J7504** Lymphocyte immune globulin, antithymocyte globulin, equine, parenteral, **250 mg**

NDC: Atgam

IOM: 100-02, 15, 50; 100-03, 2, 110.3

✪ **J7505** Muromonab-CD3, parenteral, **5 mg**

NDC: Orthoclone OKT3

Other: Monoclonal antibodies (parenteral)

IOM: 100-02, 15, 50

✪ **J7506** Prednisone, oral, **per 5 mg**

Unit billing example, fifty 10 mg prednisone tablets dispensed, report J7506, 100 units (1 unit of J7506 = 5 mg)

NDC: Deltasone, Liquid Pred, Sterapred

Other: Prednicot

IOM: 100-02, 15, 50

✪ **J7507** Tacrolimus, oral, **per 1 mg**

NDC: Prograf

IOM: 100-02, 15, 50

✪ **J7509** Methylprednisolone oral, **per 4 mg**

NDC: Medrol

Other: Methylpred DP

IOM: 100-02, 15, 50

✪ **J7510** Prednisolone oral, **per 5 mg**

Other: Cotolone, Delta-Cortef Prelone

IOM: 100-02, 15, 50

✳ **J7511** Lymphocyte immune globulin, antithymocyte globulin, rabbit, parenteral, **25 mg**

NDC: Thymoglobulin

✪ **J7513** Daclizumab, parenteral, **25 mg**

NDC: Zenapax

IOM: 100-02, 15, 50

✳ **J7515** Cyclosporine, oral, **25 mg**

NDC: Gengraf, Neoral, Sandimmune

✳ **J7516** Cyclosporin, parenteral, **250 mg**

NDC: Sandimmune

✳ **J7517** Mycophenolate mofetil, oral, **250 mg**

NDC: CellCept

✪ **J7518** Mycophenolic acid, oral, **180 mg**

NDC: Myfortic

IOM: 100-04, 4, 240; 100-4, 17, 80.3.1

✪ **J7520** Sirolimus, oral, **1 mg**

NDC: Rapamune

IOM: 100-02, 15, 50

✪ **J7525** Tacrolimus, parenteral, **5 mg**

NDC: Prograf

IOM: 100-02, 15, 50

✪ **J7599** Immunosuppressive drug, not otherwise classified

Bill on paper. Bill one unit. Identify drug and total dosage in "Remarks" field.

IOM: 100-02, 15, 50

Inhalation Solutions

J7604-J7799: If "incident to" a physician's service, do not bill; otherwise, bill DME/MAC.

✳ **J7604** Acetylcysteine, inhalation solution, compounded product, administered through DME, unit dose form, **per gram**

Other: Mucomyst (unit dose form), N-acetyl-L-cysteine

▶ New → Revised ✔ Reinstated deleted Deleted
✪ Special coverage instructions ◆ Not covered or valid by Medicare ✳ Carrier discretion

✳ **J7605** Arformoterol, inhalation solution, FDA approved final product, non-compounded, administered through DME, unit dose form, **15 micrograms**

Maintenance treatment of bronchoconstriction in patients with chronic obstructive pulmonary disease (COPD)

Other: Brovana

✳ **J7606** Formoterol fumarate, inhalation solution, FDA approved final product, non-compounded, administered through DME, unit dose form, **20 micrograms**

NDC: Perforomist

✳ **J7607** Levalbuterol, inhalation solution, compounded product, administered through DME, concentrated form, **0.5 mg**

☼ **J7608** Acetylcysteine, inhalation solution, FDA-approved final product, non-compounded, administered through DME, unit dose form, **per gram**

Other: Mucomyst

✳ **J7609** Albuterol, inhalation solution, compounded product, administered through DME, unit dose, **1 mg**

Patient's home, medications—such as albuterol when administered through a nebulizer—are considered DME and are payable under Part B.

Other: Xopenex

✳ **J7610** Albuterol, inhalation solution, compounded product, administered through DME, concentrated form, **1 mg**

Other: Xopenex

☼ **J7611** Albuterol, inhalation solution, FDA-approved final product, non-compounded, administered through DME, concentrated form, **1 mg**

Report once for each milligram administered. For example, 2 mg of concentrated albuterol (usually diluted with saline), reported with J7611×2

NDC: Albuteral Sulfate, Proventil, Ventolin

Other: Xopenet

☼ **J7612** Levalbuterol, inhalation solution, FDA-approved final product, non-compounded, administered through DME, concentrated form, **0.5 mg**

NDC: Xopenex

☼ **J7613** Albuterol, inhalation solution, FDA-approved final product, non-compounded, administered through DME, unit dose, **1 mg**

NDC: Accuneb

☼ **J7614** Levalbuterol, inhalation solution, FDA-approved final product, non-compounded, administered through DME, unit dose, **0.5 mg**

NDC: Xopenex

✳ **J7615** Levalbuterol, inhalation solution, compounded product, administered through DME, unit dose, **0.5 mg**

☼ **J7620** Albuterol, **up to 2.5 mg** and ipratropium bromide, **up to 0.5 mg,** FDA-approved final product, non-compounded, administered through DME

NDC: DuoNeb

✳ **J7622** Beclomethasone, inhalation solution, compounded product, administered through DME, unit dose form, **per milligram**

✳ **J7624** Betamethasone, inhalation solution, compounded product, administered through DME, unit dose form, **per mg**

Other: Celestone, Soluspan

✳ **J7626** Budesonide inhalation solution, FDA-approved final product, non-compounded, administered through DME, unit dose form, **up to 0.5 mg**

NDC: Pulmicort

✳ **J7627** Budesonide, inhalation solution, compounded product, administered through DME, unit dose form, **up to 0.5 mg**

Other: Pulmicort Respulses

☼ **J7628** Bitolterol mesylate, inhalation solution, compounded product, administered through DME, concentrated form, **per milligram**

Other: Tornalate

☼ **J7629** Bitolterol mesylate, inhalation solution, compounded product, administered through DME, unit dose form, **per milligram**

Other: Tornalate

▶ New   → Revised   ✔ Reinstated   ~~deleted~~ Deleted

☼ Special coverage instructions   ◆ Not covered or valid by Medicare   ✳ Carrier discretion

✪ **J7631** Cromolyn sodium, inhalation solution, FDA-approved final product, non-compounded, administered through DME, unit dose form, **per 10 milligrams**

NDC: Intal

✳ **J7632** Cromolyn sodium, inhalation solution, compounded product, administered through DME, unit dose form, **per 10 milligrams**

✳ **J7633** Budesonide, inhalation solution, FDA-approved final product, non-compounded, administered through DME, concentrated form, **per 0.25 milligram**

Other: Pulmicort Respules

✳ **J7634** Budesonide, inhalation solution, compounded product, administered through DME, concentrated form, **per 0.25 milligram**

✪ **J7635** Atropine, inhalation solution, compounded product, administered through DME, concentrated form, **per milligram**

✪ **J7636** Atropine, inhalation solution, compounded product, administered through DME, unit dose form, **per milligram**

✪ **J7637** Dexamethasone, inhalation solution, compounded product, administered through DME, concentrated form, **per milligram**

✪ **J7638** Dexamethasone, inhalation solution, compounded product, administered through DME, unit dose form, **per milligram**

✪ **J7639** Dornase alfa, inhalation solution, FDA-approved final product, non-compounded, administered through DME, unit dose form, **per milligram**

NDC: Pulmozyme

✳ **J7640** Formoterol, inhalation solution, compounded product, administered through DME, unit dose form, **12 micrograms**

✳ **J7641** Flunisolide, inhalation solution, compounded product, administered through DME, unit dose, **per milligram**

✪ **J7642** Glycopyrrolate, inhalation solution, compounded product, administered through DME, concentrated form, **per milligram**

✪ **J7643** Glycopyrrolate, inhalation solution, compounded product, administered through DME, unit dose form, **per milligram**

Other: Robinul

✪ **J7644** Ipratropium bromide, inhalation solution, FDA-approved final product, non-compounded, administered through DME, unit dose form, **per milligram**

NDC: Atrovent

✳ **J7645** Ipratropium bromide, inhalation solution, compounded product, administered through DME, unit dose form, **per milligram**

✳ **J7647** Isoetharine HCL, inhalation solution, compounded product, administered through DME, concentrated form, **per milligram**

Other: Bronkosol

✪ **J7648** Isoetharine HCL, inhalation solution, FDA-approved final product, non-compounded, administered through DME, concentrated form, **per milligram**

Other: Bronkosol

✪ **J7649** Isoetharine HCL, inhalation solution, FDA-approved final product, non-compounded, administered through DME, unit dose form, **per milligram**

Other: Bronkosol

✳ **J7650** Isoetharine HCL, inhalation solution, compounded product, administered through DME, unit dose form, **per milligram**

Other: Bronkosol

✳ **J7657** Isoproterenol HCL, inhalation solution, compounded product, administered through DME, concentrated form, **per milligram**

Other: Isuprel

✪ **J7658** Isoproterenol HCL inhalation solution, FDA-approved final product, non-compounded, administered through DME, concentrated form, **per milligram**

Other: Isuprel

✪ **J7659** Isoproterenol HCL, inhalation solution, FDA-approved final product, non-compounded, administered through DME, unit dose form, **per milligram**

Other: Isuprel

✳ **J7660** Isoproterenol HCL, inhalation solution, compounded product, administered through DME, unit dose form, **per milligram**

Other: Isuprel

▶ ✳ **J7665** Mannitol, administered through an inhaler, **5 mg**

▶ New   → Revised   ✔ Reinstated   ~~deleted~~ Deleted

✪ Special coverage instructions   ◆ Not covered or valid by Medicare   ✳ Carrier discretion

210

✳ **J7667** Metaproterenol sulfate, inhalation solution, compounded product, concentrated form, **per 10 milligrams**

Other: Metaprel

✪ **J7668** Metaproterenol sulfate, inhalation solution, FDA-approved final product, non-compounded, administered through DME, concentrated form, **per 10 milligrams**

Other: Metaprel

✪ **J7669** Metaproterenol sulfate, inhalation solution, FDA-approved final product, non-compounded, administered through DME, unit dose form, **per 10 milligrams**

NDC: Alupent

Other: Metaprel

✳ **J7670** Metaproterenol sulfate, inhalation solution, compounded product, administered through DME, unit dose form, **per 10 milligrams**

Other: Metaprel

✳ **J7674** Methacholine chloride administered as inhalation solution through a nebulizer, **per 1 mg**

NDC: Provocholine

✳ **J7676** Pentamidine isethionate, inhalation solution, compounded product, administered through DME, unit dose form, **per 300 mg**

Other: Pentam

✪ **J7680** Terbutaline sulfate, inhalation solution, compounded product, administered through DME, concentrated form, **per milligram**

Other: Brethine

✪ **J7681** Terbutaline sulfate, inhalation solution, compounded product, administered through DME, unit dose form, **per milligram**

Other: Brethine

✪ **J7682** Tobramycin, inhalation solution, FDA-approved final product, non-compounded unit dose form, administered through DME, **per 300 milligrams**

NDC: Tobi

Other: Nebcin

✪ **J7683** Triamcinolone, inhalation solution, compounded product, administered through DME, concentrated form, **per milligram**

✪ **J7684** Triamcinolone, inhalation solution, compounded product, administered through DME, unit dose form, **per milligram**

Other: Triamcinolone acetonide

✳ **J7685** Tobramycin, inhalation solution, compounded product, administered through DME, unit dose form, **per 300 milligrams**

Other: Tobramycin sulfate

▶ ✳ **J7686** Treprostinil, inhalation solution, FDA-approved final product, non-compounded, administered through DME, unit dose form, **1.74 mg**

NDC: Tyvasco

✪ **J7699** NOC drugs, inhalation solution administered through DME

Other: Gentamicin Sulfate, Sodium chloride, Tyvasco

✪ **J7799** NOC drugs, other than inhalation drugs, administered through DME

Bill on paper. Bill one unit and identify drug and total dosage in the "Remark" field.

Other: Dextrose, Epinephrine, Mannitol, Osmitrol, Phenylephrine, Resectisol, Sodium chloride

IOM: 100-02, 15, 110.3

Other

✪ **J8498** Antiemetic drug, rectal/suppository, not otherwise specified

Bill DME/MAC

Other: Compazine, Compro, Phenadoz, Phenergan, Prochlorperazine, Promethazine, Promethegan, Thorazine

Medicare Statute 1861(s)2t

◆ **J8499** Prescription drug, oral, non chemotherapeutic, NOS

If "incident to" a physician's service, do not bill; otherwise, bill DME/MAC

Other: Acyclovir, Millipred, Zovirax

IOM: 100-02, 15, 50

✪ **J8501** Aprepitant, oral, **5 mg**

Bill DME/MAC

NDC: Emend

✪ **J8510** Busulfan; oral, **2 mg**

Bill DME/MAC

NDC: Myleran

IOM 100-02, 15, 50; 100-04, 4, 240; 100-04, 17, 80.1.1

▶ New → Revised ✔ Reinstated ~~deleted~~ Deleted
✪ Special coverage instructions ◆ Not covered or valid by Medicare ✳ Carrier discretion

◆ **J8515** Cabergoline, oral, **0.25 mg**

Bill DME/MAC

IOM: 100-02, 15, 50; 100-04, 4, 240

✪ **J8520** Capecitabine, oral, **150 mg**

Bill DME/MAC

NDC: Xeloda

IOM: 100-02, 15, 50; 100-04, 4, 240; 100-04, 17, 80.1.1

✪ **J8521** Capecitabine, oral, **500 mg**

Bill DME/MAC

NDC: Xeloda

IOM: 100-02, 15, 50; 100-04, 4, 240; 100-04, 17, 80.1.1

✪ **J8530** Cyclophosphamide; oral, **25 mg**

Bill DME/MAC

NDC: Cytoxan

IOM: 100-02, 15, 50; 100-04, 4, 240; 100-04, 17, 80.1.1

✪ **J8540** Dexamethasone, oral, **0.25 mg**

Bill DME/MAC

Other: Decadron, Dexone, Dexpak

Medicare Statute 1861(s)2t

✪ **J8560** Etoposide; oral, **50 mg**

Bill DME/MAC

NDC: VePesid

IOM: 100-02, 15, 50; 100-04, 4, 230.1; 100-04, 4, 240; 100-04, 17, 80.1.1

▶ ✪ **J8561** Everolimus, oral, **0.25 mg**

IOM: 100-02, 15, 50

▶ ✳ **J8562** Fludarabine phosphate, oral, **10 mg**

Bill DME/MAC

Other: Oforta

◆ **J8565** Gefitinib, oral, **250 mg**

Bill DME/MAC

Other: Iressa

✪ **J8597** Antiemetic drug, oral, not otherwise specified

Bill DME/MAC

Medicare Statute 1861(s)2t

✪ **J8600** Melphalan; oral, **2 mg**

Bill DME/MAC

NDC: Alkeran

IOM: 100-02, 15, 50; 100-04, 4, 240; 100-04, 17, 80.1.1

✪ **J8610** Methotrexate; oral, **2.5 mg**

Bill DME/MAC

NDC: Rheumatrex, Trexall

IOM: 100-02, 15, 50; 100-04, 4, 240; 100-04, 17, 80.1.1

✳ **J8650** Nabilone, oral, **1 mg**

Bill DME/MAC

✪ **J8700** Temozolomide, oral, **5 mg**

Bill DME/MAC

NDC: Temodar

IOM: 100-02, 15, 50; 100-04, 4, 240

✳ **J8705** Topotecan, oral, **0.25 mg**

Bill DME/MAC

Treatment for ovarian and lung cancers, etc. Report J9350 (Topotecan, 4 mg) for intravenous version

✪ **J8999** Prescription drug, oral, chemotherapeutic, NOS

Bill DME/MAC

Other: Arimidex, Aromasin, Ceenu, Droxia, Flutamide, Hydrea, Hydroxyurea, Leukeran, Malulane, Megace, Megestrol Acetate, Mercaptopurine, Nolvadex, Purinethol, Tamoxifen Citrate

IOM: 100-02, 15, 50; 100-04, 4, 250; 100-04, 17, 80.1.1; 100-04, 17, 80.1.2

CHEMOTHERAPY DRUGS (J9000-J9999)

NOTE: These codes cover the cost of the chemotherapy drug only, not to include the administration

J9000-J9999: Bill local carrier if incident to a physician's service or used in an implanted infusion pump. If other, bill DME/MAC.

✪ **J9000** Injection, doxorubicin hydrochloride, **10 mg**

NDC: Adriamycin

Other: Rubex

IOM: 100-02, 15, 50

✪ **J9001** Injection, doxorubicin hydrochloride, all lipid formulations, **10 mg**

NDC: Doxil

IOM: 100-02, 15, 50

✪ **J9010** Injection, alemtuzumab, **10 mg**

NDC: Campath

Medicare Statute 1833(t)

▶ New	→ Revised	✔ Reinstated	~~deleted~~ Deleted
✪ Special coverage instructions		◆ Not covered or valid by Medicare	✳ Carrier discretion

⊙ **J9015** Injection, aldesleukin, **per single use vial**

NDC: Proleukin

IOM: 100-02, 15, 50

✳ **J9017** Injection, arsenic trioxide, **1 mg**

NDC: Trisenox

⊙ **J9020** Injection, asparaginase, **10,000 units**

NDC: Elspar

IOM: 100-02, 15, 50

✳ **J9025** Injection, azacitidine, **1 mg**

NDC: Vidaza

✳ **J9027** Injection, clofarabine, **1 mg**

NDC: Clolar

⊙ **J9031** BCG (intravesical), **per instillation**

NDC: TheraCys, Tice BCG

IOM: 100-02, 15, 50

✳ **J9033** Injection, bendamustine HCL, **1 mg**

Treatment for form of non-Hodgkin's lymphoma; standard administration time is as an intravenous infusion over 30 minutes

NDC: Treanda

✳ **J9035** Injection, bevacizumab, **10 mg**

For malignant neoplasm of breast, considered J9207.

NDC: Avastin

⊙ **J9040** Injection, bleomycin sulfate, **15 units**

NDC: Blenoxane

IOM: 100-02, 15, 50

✳ **J9041** Injection, bortezomib, **0.1 mg**

NDC: Velcade

▶ ✳ **J9043** Injection, cabazitaxel, **1 mg**

⊙ **J9045** Injection, carboplatin, **50 mg**

NDC: Paraplatin

IOM: 100-02, 15, 50

⊙ **J9050** Injection, carmustine, **100 mg**

NDC: BiCNU

IOM: 100-02, 15, 50

✳ **J9055** Injection, cetuximab, **10 mg**

NDC: Erbitux

→ ⊙ **J9060** Injection, cisplatin, powder or solution, **10 mg**

Bill local carrier if incident to a physician's service or used in an implanted infusion pump. If other, bill DME/MAC.

NDC: Plantinol AQ

IOM: 100-02, 15, 50

⊙ **J9065** Injection, cladribine, **per 1 mg**

NDC: Leustatin

IOM: 100-02, 15, 50

⊙ **J9070** Cyclophosphamide, **100 mg**

NDC: Cytoxan

Other: Neosar

IOM: 100-02, 15, 50

✳ **J9098** Injection, cytarabine liposome, **10 mg**

NDC: DepoCyt

⊙ **J9100** Injection, cytarabine, **100 mg**

Other: Cytosar-U

IOM: 100-02, 15, 50

⊙ **J9120** Injection, dactinomycin, **0.5 mg**

NDC: Cosmegen

IOM: 100-02, 15, 50

⊙ **J9130** Dacarbazine, **100 mg**

Other: DTIC-Dome

IOM: 100-02, 15, 50

⊙ **J9150** Injection, daunorubicin, **10 mg**

NDC: Cerubidine

IOM: 100-02, 15, 50

⊙ **J9151** Injection, daunorubicin citrate, liposomal formulation, **10 mg**

NDC: Daunoxome

IOM: 100-02, 15, 50

✳ **J9155** Injection, degarelix, **1 mg**

Report 1 unit for every 1 mg.

NDC: Firmagon

✳ **J9160** Injection, denileukin diftitox, **300 micrograms**

NDC: Ontak

⊙ **J9165** Injection, diethylstilbestrol diphosphate, **250 mg**

Other: Stilphostrol

IOM: 100-02, 15, 50

⊙ **J9171** Injection, docetaxel, **1 mg**

Report 1 unit for every 1 mg.

NDC: Taxotere

IOM: 100-02, 15, 50

⊙ **J9175** Injection, Elliott's B solution, **1 ml**

NDC: Elliott's b

IOM: 100-02, 15, 50

▶ New   → Revised   ✔ Reinstated   ~~deleted~~ Deleted

⊙ Special coverage instructions   ◆ Not covered or valid by Medicare   ✳ Carrier discretion

✳ **J9178** Injection, epirubicin HCL, **2 mg**
NDC: Ellence

▶ ✳ **J9179** Injection, eribulin mesylate, **0.1 mg**

◎ **J9181** Injection, etoposide, **10 mg**
NDC: Etopophos, VePesid
IOM: 100-02, 15, 50

◎ **J9185** Injection, fludarabine phosphate, **50 mg**
NDC: Fludara
IOM: 100-02, 15, 50

◎ **J9190** Injection, fluorouracil, **500 mg**
NDC: Adrucil
IOM: 100-02, 15, 50

◎ **J9200** Injection, floxuridine, **500 mg**
Other: FUDR
IOM: 100-02, 15, 50

◎ **J9201** Injection, gemcitabine hydrochloride, **200 mg**
NDC: Gemzar
IOM: 100-02, 15, 50

◎ **J9202** Goserelin acetate implant, **per 3.6 mg**
NDC: Zoladex
IOM: 100-02, 15, 50

◎ **J9206** Injection, irinotecan, **20 mg**
NDC: Camptosar
IOM: 100-02, 15, 50

✳ **J9207** Injection, ixabepilone, **1 mg**

→ ◎ **J9208** Injection, ifosfamide, **1 gm**
NDC: Ifex
IOM: 100-02, 15, 50

◎ **J9209** Injection, mesna, **200 mg**
NDC: Mesnex
IOM: 100-02, 15, 50

◎ **J9211** Injection, idarubicin hydrochloride, **5 mg**
NDC: Idamycin PFS
IOM: 100-02, 15, 50

◎ **J9212** Injection, interferon alfacon-1, recombinant, **1 mcg**
Other: Infergen
IOM: 100-02, 15, 50

◎ **J9213** Injection, interferon, alfa-2a, recombinant, **3 million units**
IOM: 100-02, 15, 50

◎ **J9214** Injection, interferon, alfa-2b, recombinant, **1 million units**
NDC: Intron-A
IOM: 100-02, 15, 50

◎ **J9215** Injection, interferon, alfa-n3 (human leukocyte derived), **250,000 IU**
Other: Alferon N
IOM: 100-02, 15, 50

◎ **J9216** Injection, interferon, gamma-1B, **3 million units**
Other: Actimmune
IOM: 100-02, 15, 50

◎ **J9217** Leuprolide acetate (for depot suspension), **7.5 mg**
NDC: Eligard, Lupron Depot
IOM: 100-02, 15, 50

◎ **J9218** Leuprolide acetate, **per 1 mg**
NDC: Lupron
IOM: 100-02, 15, 50

◎ **J9219** Leuprolide acetate implant, **65 mg**
NDC: Viadur
IOM: 100-02, 15, 50

◎ **J9225** Histrelin implant (Vantas), **50 mg**
IOM: 100-02, 15, 50

◎ **J9226** Histrelin implant (Supprelin LA), **50 mg**
Other: Vantas
IOM: 100-02, 15, 50

▶ ✳ **J9228** Injection, ipilimumab, **1 mg**

◎ **J9230** Injection, mechlorethamine hydrochloride, (nitrogen mustard), **10 mg**
NDC: Mustargen
IOM: 100-02, 15, 50

◎ **J9245** Injection, melphalan hydrochloride, **50 mg**
NDC: Alkeran
IOM: 100-02, 15, 50

◎ **J9250** Methotrexate sodium, **5 mg**
Other: Folex
IOM: 100-02, 15, 50

◎ **J9260** Methotrexate sodium, **50 mg**
Other: Folex
IOM: 100-02, 15, 50

✳ **J9261** Injection, nelarabine, **50 mg**
NDC: Arranon

✳ **J9263** Injection, oxaliplatin, **0.5 mg**
Eloxatin, platinum-based anticancer drug that destroys cancer cells
NDC: Eloxatin

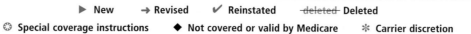

▶ New   → Revised   ✔ Reinstated   ~~deleted~~ Deleted

◎ Special coverage instructions   ◆ Not covered or valid by Medicare   ✳ Carrier discretion

✳ **J9264** Injection, paclitaxel protein-bound particles, **1 mg**
NDC: Abraxane

☙ **J9265** Injection, paclitaxel, **30 mg**
NDC: Onxol, Taxol
IOM: 100-02, 15, 50

☙ **J9266** Injection, pegaspargase, **per single dose vial**
NDC: Oncaspar
IOM: 100-02, 15, 50

☙ **J9268** Injection, pentostatin, **10 mg**
NDC: Nipent
IOM: 100-02, 15, 50

☙ **J9270** Injection, plicamycin, **2.5 mg**
Other: Mithracin
IOM: 100-02, 15, 50

☙ **J9280** Mitomycin, **5 mg**
NDC: Mutamycin
IOM: 100-02, 15, 50

☙ **J9293** Injection, mitoxantrone hydrochloride, **per 5 mg**
Other: Novantrone
IOM: 100-02, 15, 50

✳ **J9300** Injection, gemtuzumab ozogamicin, **5 mg**
NDC: Mylotarg

▶ ✳ **J9302** Injection, ofatumumab, **10 mg**
NDC: Arzerra
Other: Doulinum

✳ **J9303** Injection, panitumumab, **10 mg**
Other: Vectibix

✳ **J9305** Injection, pemetrexed, **10 mg**
NDC: Alimta

▶ ✳ **J9307** Injection, pralatrexate, **1 mg**
NDC: Folotyn

☙ **J9310** Injection, rituximab, **100 mg**
NDC: RituXan
IOM: 100-02, 15, 50

▶ ✳ **J9315** Injection, romidepsin, **1 mg**
NDC: Istodax

☙ **J9320** Injection, streptozocin, **1 gram**
NDC: Zanosar
IOM: 100-02, 15, 50

✳ **J9328** Injection, temozolomide, **1 mg**
Intravenous formulation, not for oral administration
NDC: Temodar

✳ **J9330** Injection, temsirolimus, **1 mg**
Treatment for advanced renal cell carcinoma; standard administration is intravenous infusion greater than 30-60 minutes
Other: Torisel

☙ **J9340** Injection, thiotepa, **15 mg**
Other: Thiethylenethiophosphoramide/T
IOM: 100-02, 15, 50

▶ ✳ **J9351** Injection, topotecan, **0.1 mg**
NDC: Hycamtin

✳ **J9355** Injection, trastuzumab, **10 mg**
NDC: Herceptin

☙ **J9357** Injection, valrubicin, intravesical, **200 mg**
NDC: Valstar
IOM: 100-02, 15, 50

☙ **J9360** Injection, vinblastine sulfate, **1 mg**
Other: Alkaban-AQ, Velban, Velsar
IOM: 100-02, 15, 50

☙ **J9370** Vincristine sulfate, **1 mg**
NDC: Vincasar PFS
Other: Oncovin
IOM: 100-02, 15, 50

☙ **J9390** Injection, vinorelbine tartrate, **10 mg**
NDC: Navelbine
IOM: 100-02, 15, 50

✳ **J9395** Injection, fulvestrant, **25 mg**
NDC: Faslodex

☙ **J9600** Injection, porfimer sodium, **75 mg**
NDC: Photofrin
IOM: 100-02, 15, 50

☙ **J9999** Not otherwise classified, antineoplastic drugs
Bill on paper, bill one unit, and identify drug and total dosage in "Remarks" field. Include invoice of cost or NDC number in "Remarks" field.
Other: Allopurinol Sodium, Ifosfamide/Mesna
IOM: 100-02, 15, 50; 100-03, 2, 110.2

▶ New   → Revised   ✔ Reinstated   deleted Deleted
☙ Special coverage instructions   ◆ Not covered or valid by Medicare   ✳ Carrier discretion

TEMPORARY CODES ASSIGNED TO DME REGIONAL CARRIERS (K0000-K9999)

Wheelchairs and Accessories

NOTE: This section contains national codes assigned by CMS on a temporary basis and for the exclusive use of the durable medical equipment regional carriers (DMERC).

* **K0001**   Standard wheelchair

  Bill DME/MAC

  Capped rental

* **K0002**   Standard hemi (low seat) wheelchair

  Bill DME/MAC

  Capped rental

* **K0003**   Lightweight wheelchair

  Bill DME/MAC

  Capped rental

* **K0004**   High strength, lightweight wheelchair

  Bill DME/MAC

  Capped rental

* **K0005**   Ultralightweight wheelchair

  Bill DME/MAC

  Capped rental. Inexpensive and routinely purchased DME

* **K0006**   Heavy duty wheelchair

  Bill DME/MAC

  Capped rental

* **K0007**   Extra heavy duty wheelchair

  Bill DME/MAC

  Capped rental

* **K0009**   Other manual wheelchair/base

  Not Otherwise Classified.

* **K0010**   Standard - weight frame motorized/ power wheelchair

  Capped rental. Codes K0010-K0014 are not for manual wheelchairs with add-on power packs. Use the appropriate code for the manual wheelchair base provided (K0001-K0009) and code K0460

* **K0011**   Standard - weight frame motorized/ power wheelchair with programmable control parameters for speed adjustment, tremor dampening, acceleration control and braking

  Capped rental. A patient who requires a power wheelchair usually is totally nonambulatory and has severe weakness of the upper extremities due to a neurologic or muscular disease/ condition

* **K0012**   Lightweight portable motorized/power wheelchair

  Capped rental

* **K0014**   Other motorized/power wheelchair base

  Capped rental

* **K0015**   Detachable, non-adjustable height armrest, each

  Inexpensive and routinely purchased DME

* **K0017**   Detachable, adjustable height armrest, base, each

  Inexpensive and routinely purchased DME

* **K0018**   Detachable, adjustable height armrest, upper portion, each

  Inexpensive and routinely purchased DME

* **K0019**   Arm pad, each

  Inexpensive and routinely purchased DME

* **K0020**   Fixed, adjustable height armrest, pair

  Inexpensive and routinely purchased DME

* **K0037**   High mount flip-up footrest, each

  Inexpensive and routinely purchased DME

* **K0038**   Leg strap, each

  Inexpensive and routinely purchased DME

* **K0039**   Leg strap, H style, each

  Inexpensive and routinely purchased DME

* **K0040**   Adjustable angle footplate, each

  Inexpensive and routinely purchased DME

* **K0041**   Large size footplate, each

  Inexpensive and routinely purchased DME

▶ New   → Revised   ✔ Reinstated   ~~deleted~~ Deleted

☺ Special coverage instructions   ◆ Not covered or valid by Medicare   * Carrier discretion

* **K0042** Standard size footplate, each

Inexpensive and routinely purchased DME

* **K0043** Footrest, lower extension tube, each

Inexpensive and routinely purchased DME

* **K0044** Footrest, upper hanger bracket, each

Inexpensive and routinely purchased DME

* **K0045** Footrest, complete assembly

Inexpensive and routinely purchased DME

* **K0046** Elevating legrest, lower extension tube, each

Inexpensive and routinely purchased DME

* **K0047** Elevating legrest, upper hanger bracket, each

Inexpensive and routinely purchased DME

* **K0050** Ratchet assembly

Inexpensive and routinely purchased DME

* **K0051** Cam release assembly, footrest or legrests, each

Inexpensive and routinely purchased DME

* **K0052** Swing-away, detachable footrests, each

Inexpensive and routinely purchased DME

* **K0053** Elevating footrests, articulating (telescoping), each

Inexpensive and routinely purchased DME

* **K0056** Seat height less than 17″ or equal to or greater than 21″ for a high strength, lightweight, or ultralightweight wheelchair

Inexpensive and routinely purchased DME

* **K0065** Spoke protectors, each

Inexpensive and routinely purchased DME

* **K0069** Rear wheel assembly, complete, with solid tire, spokes or molded, each

Inexpensive and routinely purchased DME

* **K0070** Rear wheel assembly, complete, with pneumatic tire, spokes or molded, each

Inexpensive and routinely purchased DME

* **K0071** Front caster assembly, complete, with pneumatic tire, each

Caster assembly includes a caster fork (E2396), wheel rim, and tire. Inexpensive and routinely purchased DME

* **K0072** Front caster assembly, complete, with semi-pneumatic tire, each

Inexpensive and routinely purchased DME

* **K0073** Caster pin lock, each

Inexpensive and routinely purchased DME

* **K0077** Front caster assembly, complete, with solid tire, each

* **K0098** Drive belt for power wheelchair

Inexpensive and routinely purchased DME

* **K0105** IV hanger, each

Inexpensive and routinely purchased DME

* **K0108** Wheelchair component or accessory, not otherwise specified

☺ **K0195** Elevating leg rests, pair (for use with capped rental wheelchair base)

Bill DME/MAC

Medically necessary replacement items are covered if rollabout chair or transport chair covered

IOM: 100-03, 4, 280.1

☺ **K0455** Infusion pump used for uninterrupted parenteral administration of medication (e.g., epoprostenol or treprostinol)

Bill DME/MAC

An EIP may also be referred to as an external insulin pump, ambulatory pump, or mini-infuser. CMN/DIF required. Frequent and substantial service DME

IOM: 100-03, 1, 50.3

☺ **K0462** Temporary replacement for patient owned equipment being repaired, any type

Bill DME/MAC

Only report for maintenance and service for an item for which initial claim was paid. The term power mobility device (PMD) includes power operated vehicles (POVs) and power wheelchairs (PWCs). Not Otherwise Classified.

IOM: 100-04, 20, 40.1

▶ New   → Revised   ✔ Reinstated   ~~deleted~~ Deleted

☺ Special coverage instructions   ◆ Not covered or valid by Medicare   * Carrier discretion

⊚ **K0552**   Supplies for external drug infusion pump, syringe type cartridge, sterile, each

Bill DME/MAC

Supplies.

IOM: 100-03, 1, 50.3

✳ **K0601**   Replacement battery for external infusion pump owned by patient, silver oxide, 1.5 volt, each

Bill DME/MAC

Inexpensive and routinely purchased DME

✳ **K0602**   Replacement battery for external infusion pump owned by patient, silver oxide, 3 volt, each

Bill DME/MAC

Inexpensive and routinely purchased DME

✳ **K0603**   Replacement battery for external infusion pump owned by patient, alkaline, 1.5 volt, each

Bill DME/MAC

Inexpensive and routinely purchased DME

✳ **K0604**   Replacement battery for external infusion pump owned by patient, lithium, 3.6 volt, each

Bill DME/MAC

Inexpensive and routinely purchased DME

✳ **K0605**   Replacement battery for external infusion pump owned by patient, lithium, 4.5 volt, each

Bill DME/MAC

Inexpensive and routinely purchased DME

✳ **K0606**   Automatic external defibrillator, with integrated electrocardiogram analysis, garment type

Bill DME/MAC

Capped rental

✳ **K0607**   Replacement battery for automated external defibrillator, garment type only, each

Bill DME/MAC

Inexpensive and routinely purchased DME

✳ **K0608**   Replacement garment for use with automated external defibrillator, each

Bill DME/MAC

Inexpensive and routinely purchased DME

✳ **K0609**   Replacement electrodes for use with automated external defibrillator, garment type only, each

Bill DME/MAC

Supplies.

→ ✳ **K0669**   Wheelchair accessory, wheelchair seat or back cushion, does not meet specific code criteria or no written coding verification from DME PDAC

Bill DME/MAC

Inexpensive and routinely purchased DME

✳ **K0672**   Addition to lower extremity orthosis, removable soft interface, all components, replacement only, each

Bill DME/MAC

Prosthetics/Orthotics

→ ✳ **K0730**   Controlled dose inhalation drug delivery system

Bill DME/MAC

Inexpensive and routinely purchased DME

✳ **K0733**   Power wheelchair accessory, 12 to 24 amp hour sealed lead acid battery, each (e.g., gel cell, absorbed glassmat)

Bill DME/MAC

Inexpensive and routinely purchased DME

✳ **K0738**   Portable gaseous oxygen system, rental; home compressor used to fill portable oxygen cylinders; includes portable containers, regulator, flowmeter, humidifier, cannula or mask, and tubing

Bill DME/MAC

Oxygen and oxygen equipment

✳ **K0739**   Repair or nonroutine service for durable medical equipment other than oxygen equipment requiring the skill of a technician, labor component, per 15 minutes

Local carrier if used with implanted DME. If other, bill DME/MAC.

◆ **K0740**   Repair or nonroutine service for oxygen equipment requiring the skill of a technician, labor component, per 15 minutes

Bill DME/MAC

▶ New   → Revised   ✔ Reinstated   ~~deleted~~ Deleted

⊚ Special coverage instructions   ◆ Not covered or valid by Medicare   ✳ Carrier discretion

▶ ✪ **K0741** Portable gaseous oxygen system, rental, includes portable container, regulator, flowmeter, humidifier, cannula or mask, and tubing, for cluster headaches

▶ ✪ **K0742** Portable oxygen contents, gaseous, 1 month's supply = 1 unit, for cluster headaches, for initial months supply or to replace used contents

▶ ✳ **K0743** Suction pump, home model, portable, for use on wounds

Bill DME/MAC

▶ ✳ **K0744** Absorptive wound dressing for use with suction pump, home model, portable, pad size 16 square inches or less

Bill DME/MAC

▶ ✳ **K0745** Absorptive wound dressing for use with suction pump, home model, portable, pad size more than 16 square inches but less than or equal to 48 square inches

Bill DME/MAC

▶ ✳ **K0746** Absorptive wound dressing for use with suction pump, home model, portable, pad size greater than 48 square inches

Bill DME/MAC

✳ **K0800** Power operated vehicle, group 1 standard, patient weight capacity up to and including 300 pounds

Bill DME/MAC

Power mobility device (PMD) includes power operated vehicles (POVs) and power wheelchairs (PWCs). Inexpensive and routinely purchased DME

✳ **K0801** Power operated vehicle, group 1 heavy duty, patient weight capacity 301 to 450 pounds

Bill DME/MAC

Inexpensive and routinely purchased DME

✳ **K0802** Power operated vehicle, group 1 very heavy duty, patient weight capacity 451 to 600 pounds

Bill DME/MAC

Inexpensive and routinely purchased DME

✳ **K0806** Power operated vehicle, group 2 standard, patient weight capacity up to and including 300 pounds

Bill DME/MAC

Inexpensive and routinely purchased DME

✳ **K0807** Power operated vehicle, group 2 heavy duty, patient weight capacity 301 to 450 pounds

Bill DME/MAC

Inexpensive and routinely purchased DME

✳ **K0808** Power operated vehicle, group 2 very heavy duty, patient weight capacity 451 to 600 pounds

Bill DME/MAC

Inexpensive and routinely purchased DME

✳ **K0812** Power operated vehicle, not otherwise classified

Bill DME/MAC

Not Otherwise Classified.

✳ **K0813** Power wheelchair, group 1 standard, portable, sling/solid seat and back, patient weight capacity up to and including 300 pounds

Bill DME/MAC

Capped rental

✳ **K0814** Power wheelchair, group 1 standard, portable, captains chair, patient weight capacity up to and including 300 pounds

Bill DME/MAC

Capped rental

✳ **K0815** Power wheelchair, group 1 standard, sling/solid seat and back, patient weight capacity up to and including 300 pounds

Bill DME/MAC

Capped rental

✳ **K0816** Power wheelchair, group 1 standard, captains chair, patient weight capacity up to and including 300 pounds

Bill DME/MAC

Capped rental

✳ **K0820** Power wheelchair, group 2 standard, portable, sling/solid seat/back, patient weight capacity up to and including 300 pounds

Bill DME/MAC

Capped rental

✳ **K0821** Power wheelchair, group 2 standard, portable, captains chair, patient weight capacity up to and including 300 pounds

Bill DME/MAC

Capped rental

▶ New   → Revised   ✔ Reinstated   ~~deleted~~ Deleted

✪ Special coverage instructions   ◆ Not covered or valid by Medicare   ✳ Carrier discretion

✳ **K0822**   Power wheelchair, group 2 standard, sling/solid seat/back, patient weight capacity up to and including 300 pounds

Bill DME/MAC

Capped rental

✳ **K0823**   Power wheelchair, group 2 standard, captains chair, patient weight capacity up to and including 300 pounds

Bill DME/MAC

Capped rental

✳ **K0824**   Power wheelchair, group 2 heavy duty, sling/solid seat/back, patient weight capacity 301 to 450 pounds

Bill DME/MAC

Capped rental

✳ **K0825**   Power wheelchair, group 2 heavy duty, captains chair, patient weight capacity 301 to 450 pounds

Bill DME/MAC

Capped rental

✳ **K0826**   Power wheelchair, group 2 very heavy duty, sling/solid seat/back, patient weight capacity 451 to 600 pounds

Bill DME/MAC

Capped rental

✳ **K0827**   Power wheelchair, group 2 very heavy duty, captains chair, patient weight capacity 451 to 600 pounds

Bill DME/MAC

Capped rental

✳ **K0828**   Power wheelchair, group 2 extra heavy duty, sling/solid seat/back, patient weight capacity 601 pounds or more

Bill DME/MAC

Capped rental

✳ **K0829**   Power wheelchair, group 2 extra heavy duty, captains chair, patient weight 601 pounds or more

Bill DME/MAC

Capped rental

✳ **K0830**   Power wheelchair, group 2 standard, seat elevator, sling/solid seat/back, patient weight capacity up to and including 300 pounds

Bill DME/MAC

Capped rental

✳ **K0831**   Power wheelchair, group 2 standard, seat elevator, captains chair, patient weight capacity up to and including 300 pounds

Bill DME/MAC

✳ **K0835**   Power wheelchair, group 2 standard, single power option, sling/solid seat/back, patient weight capacity up to and including 300 pounds

Bill DME/MAC

Capped rental

✳ **K0836**   Power wheelchair, group 2 standard, single power option, captains chair, patient weight capacity up to and including 300 pounds

Bill DME/MAC

Capped rental

✳ **K0837**   Power wheelchair, group 2 heavy duty, single power option, sling/solid seat/back, patient weight capacity 301 to 450 pounds

Bill DME/MAC

Capped rental

✳ **K0838**   Power wheelchair, group 2 heavy duty, single power option, captains chair, patient weight capacity 301 to 450 pounds

Bill DME/MAC

Capped rental

✳ **K0839**   Power wheelchair, group 2 very heavy duty, single power option sling/solid seat/back, patient weight capacity 451 to 600 pounds

Bill DME/MAC

Capped rental

✳ **K0840**   Power wheelchair, group 2 extra heavy duty, single power option, sling/solid seat/back, patient weight capacity 601 pounds or more

Bill DME/MAC

Capped rental

✳ **K0841**   Power wheelchair, group 2 standard, multiple power option, sling/solid seat/back, patient weight capacity up to and including 300 pounds

Bill DME/MAC

Capped rental

✳ **K0842**   Power wheelchair, group 2 standard, multiple power option, captains chair, patient weight capacity up to and including 300 pounds

Bill DME/MAC

Capped rental

▶ New   → Revised   ✔ Reinstated   ~~deleted~~ Deleted

☼ Special coverage instructions   ◆ Not covered or valid by Medicare   ✳ Carrier discretion

220

* **K0843** Power wheelchair, group 2 heavy duty, multiple power option, sling/solid seat/back, patient weight capacity 301 to 450 pounds

Bill DME/MAC

Capped rental

* **K0848** Power wheelchair, group 3 standard, sling/solid seat/back, patient weight capacity up to and including 300 pounds

Bill DME/MAC

Capped rental

* **K0849** Power wheelchair, group 3 standard, captains chair, patient weight capacity up to and including 300 pounds

Bill DME/MAC

Capped rental

* **K0850** Power wheelchair, group 3 heavy duty, sling/solid seat/back, patient weight capacity 301 to 450 pounds

Bill DME/MAC

Capped rental

* **K0851** Power wheelchair, group 3 heavy duty, captains chair, patient weight capacity 301 to 450 pounds

Bill DME/MAC

Capped rental

* **K0852** Power wheelchair, group 3 very heavy duty, sling/solid seat/back, patient weight capacity 451 to 600 pounds

Bill DME/MAC

Capped rental

* **K0853** Power wheelchair, group 3 very heavy duty, captains chair, patient weight capacity 451 to 600 pounds

Bill DME/MAC

Capped rental

* **K0854** Power wheelchair, group 3 extra heavy duty, sling/solid seat/back, patient weight capacity 601 pounds or more

Bill DME/MAC

Capped rental

* **K0855** Power wheelchair, group 3 extra heavy duty, captains chair, patient weight capacity 601 pounds or more

Bill DME/MAC

Capped rental

* **K0856** Power wheelchair, group 3 standard, single power option, sling/solid seat/back, patient weight capacity up to and including 300 pounds

Bill DME/MAC

Capped rental

* **K0857** Power wheelchair, group 3 standard, single power option, captains chair, patient weight capacity up to and including 300 pounds

Bill DME/MAC

Capped rental

* **K0858** Power wheelchair, group 3 heavy duty, single power option, sling/solid seat/back, patient weight 301 to 450 pounds

Bill DME/MAC

Capped rental

* **K0859** Power wheelchair, group 3 heavy duty, single power option, captains chair, patient weight capacity 301 to 450 pounds

Bill DME/MAC

Capped rental

* **K0860** Power wheelchair, group 3 very heavy duty, single power option, sling/solid seat/back, patient weight capacity 451 to 600 pounds

Bill DME/MAC

Capped rental

* **K0861** Power wheelchair, group 3 standard, multiple power option, sling/solid seat/back, patient weight capacity up to and including 300 pounds

Bill DME/MAC

Capped rental

* **K0862** Power wheelchair, group 3 heavy duty, multiple power option, sling/solid seat/back, patient weight capacity 301 to 450 pounds

Bill DME/MAC

Capped rental

* **K0863** Power wheelchair, group 3 very heavy duty, multiple power option, sling/solid seat/back, patient weight capacity 451 to 600 pounds

Bill DME/MAC

Capped rental

* **K0864** Power wheelchair, group 3 extra heavy duty, multiple power option, sling/solid seat/back, patient weight capacity 601 pounds or more

Bill DME/MAC

Capped rental

▶ New   → Revised   ✔ Reinstated   deleted Deleted

☺ Special coverage instructions   ◆ Not covered or valid by Medicare   * Carrier discretion

* **K0868**   Power wheelchair, group 4 standard, sling/solid seat/back, patient weight capacity up to and including 300 pounds

Bill DME/MAC

Capped rental

* **K0869**   Power wheelchair, group 4 standard, captains chair, patient weight capacity up to and including 300 pounds

Bill DME/MAC

Capped rental

* **K0870**   Power wheelchair, group 4 heavy duty, sling/solid seat/back, patient weight capacity 301 to 450 pounds

Bill DME/MAC

Capped rental

* **K0871**   Power wheelchair, group 4 very heavy duty, sling/solid seat/back, patient weight capacity 451 to 600 pounds

Bill DME/MAC

Capped rental

* **K0877**   Power wheelchair, group 4 standard, single power option, sling/solid seat/back, patient weight capacity up to and including 300 pounds

Bill DME/MAC

Capped rental

* **K0878**   Power wheelchair, group 4 standard, single power option, captains chair, patient weight capacity up to and including 300 pounds

Bill DME/MAC

Capped rental

* **K0879**   Power wheelchair, group 4 heavy duty, single power option, sling/solid seat/back, patient weight capacity 301 to 450 pounds

Bill DME/MAC

Capped rental

* **K0880**   Power wheelchair, group 4 very heavy duty, single power option, sling/solid seat/back, patient weight 451 to 600 pounds

Bill DME/MAC

Capped rental

* **K0884**   Power wheelchair, group 4 standard, multiple power option, sling/solid seat/back, patient weight capacity up to and including 300 pounds

Bill DME/MAC

Capped rental

* **K0885**   Power wheelchair, group 4 standard, multiple power option, captains chair, patient weight capacity up to and including 300 pounds

Bill DME/MAC

Capped rental

* **K0886**   Power wheelchair, group 4 heavy duty, multiple power option, sling/solid seat/back, patient weight capacity 301 to 450 pounds

Bill DME/MAC

Capped rental

* **K0890**   Power wheelchair, group 5 pediatric, single power option, sling/solid seat/back, patient weight capacity up to and including 125 pounds

Bill DME/MAC

Capped rental

* **K0891**   Power wheelchair, group 5 pediatric, multiple power option, sling/solid seat/back, patient weight capacity up to and including 125 pounds

Bill DME/MAC

Capped rental

* **K0898**   Power wheelchair, not otherwise classified

Bill DME/MAC

→ * **K0899**   Power mobility device, not coded by DME PDAC or does not meet criteria

Bill DME/MAC

▶ New   → Revised   ✔ Reinstated   ~~deleted~~ Deleted

⊙ Special coverage instructions   ◆ Not covered or valid by Medicare   * Carrier discretion

ORTHOTICS (L0100-L4999)

DMEPOS fee schedule:
www.cms.gov/DMEPOSFeeSched/LSDMEPOSFEE/
list.asp#TopOfPage

Orthotic Devices: Spinal

Cervical

L0112-L0220:   Bill DME/MAC

* **L0112** Cranial cervical orthosis, congenital torticollis type, with or without soft interface material, adjustable range of motion joint, custom fabricated

* **L0113** Cranial cervical orthosis, torticollis type, with or without joint, with or without soft interface material, prefabricated, includes fitting and adjustment

* **L0120** Cervical, flexible, non-adjustable (foam collar)

Cervical orthoses, including soft and rigid devices may be used as nonoperative management for cervical trauma

* **L0130** Cervical, flexible, thermoplastic collar, molded to patient

* **L0140** Cervical, semi-rigid, adjustable (plastic collar)

* **L0150** Cervical, semi-rigid, adjustable molded chin cup (plastic collar with mandibular/occipital piece)

* **L0160** Cervical, semi-rigid, wire frame occipital/mandibular support

* **L0170** Cervical, collar, molded to patient model

* **L0172** Cervical, collar, semi-rigid thermoplastic foam, two piece

* **L0174** Cervical, collar, semi-rigid, thermoplastic foam, two piece with thoracic extension

Multiple Post Collar

* **L0180** Cervical, multiple post collar, occipital/mandibular supports, adjustable

* **L0190** Cervical, multiple post collar, occipital/mandibular supports, adjustable cervical bars (SOMI, Guilford, Taylor types)

* **L0200** Cervical, multiple post collar, occipital/mandibular supports, adjustable cervical bars, and thoracic extension

Thoracic

* **L0220** Thoracic, rib belt, custom fabricated

Thoracic-Lumbar-Sacral

Anterior-Posterior-Lateral Rotary-Control

L0430-L0492:   Bill DME/MAC

* **L0430** Spinal orthosis, anterior-posterior-lateral control, with interface material, custom fitted (Dewall posture protector only)

* **L0450** TLSO, flexible, provides trunk support, upper thoracic region, produces intracavitary pressure to reduce load on the intervertebral disks with rigid stays or panel(s), includes shoulder straps and closures, prefabricated, includes fitting and adjustment

Used to immobilize specified area of spine, and is generally worn under clothing

* **L0452** TLSO, flexible, provides trunk support, upper thoracic region, produces intracavitary pressure to reduce load on the intervertebral disks with rigid stays or panel(s), includes shoulder straps and closures, custom fabricated

* **L0454** TLSO flexible, provides trunk support, extends from sacrococcygeal junction to above T-9 vertebra, restricts gross trunk motion in the sagittal plane, produces intracavitary pressure to reduce load on the intervertebral disks with rigid stays or panel(s), includes shoulder straps and closures, prefabricated, includes fitting and adjustment

Used to immobilize specified areas of spine; and is generally designed to be worn under clothing; not specifically designed for patients in wheelchairs

* **L0456** TLSO, flexible, provides trunk support, thoracic region, rigid posterior panel and soft anterior apron, extends from the sacrococcygeal junction and terminates just inferior to the scapular spine, restricts gross trunk motion in the sagittal plane, produces intracavitary pressure to reduce load on the intervertebral disks, includes straps and closures, prefabricated, includes fitting and adjustment

▶ New   → Revised   ✔ Reinstated   ~~deleted~~ Deleted   ☺ Special coverage instructions   ◆ Not covered or valid by Medicare   * Carrier discretion

ORTHOTICS L0112 – L0456

223

* **L0458** TLSO, triplanar control, modular segmented spinal system, two rigid plastic shells, posterior extends from the sacrococcygeal junction and terminates just inferior to the scapular spine, anterior extends from the symphysis pubis to the xiphoid, soft liner, restricts gross trunk motion in the sagittal, coronal, and transverse planes, lateral strength is provided by overlapping plastic and stabilizing closures, includes straps and closures, prefabricated, includes fitting and adjustment

To meet Medicare's definition of body jacket, orthosis has to have rigid plastic shell that circles trunk with overlapping edges and stabilizing closures, and entire circumference of shell must be made of same rigid material

* **L0460** TLSO, triplanar control, modular segmented spinal system, two rigid plastic shells, posterior extends from the sacrococcygeal junction and terminates just inferior to the scapular spine, anterior extends from the symphysis pubis to the sternal notch, soft liner, restricts gross trunk motion in the sagittal, coronal, and transverse planes, lateral strength is provided by overlapping plastic and stabilizing closures, includes straps and closures, prefabricated, includes fitting and adjustment

* **L0462** TLSO, triplanar control, modular segmented spinal system, three rigid plastic shells, posterior extends from the sacrococcygeal junction and terminates just inferior to the scapular spine, anterior extends from the symphysis pubis to the sternal notch, soft liner, restricts gross trunk motion in the sagittal, coronal, and transverse planes, lateral strength is provided by overlapping plastic and stabilizing closures, includes straps and closures, prefabricated, includes fitting and adjustment

* **L0464** TLSO, triplanar control, modular segmented spinal system, four rigid plastic shells, posterior extends from sacrococcygeal junction and terminates just inferior to scapular spine, anterior extends from symphysis pubis to the sternal notch, soft liner, restricts gross trunk motion in sagittal, coronal, and transverse planes, lateral strength is provided by overlapping plastic and stabilizing closures, includes straps and closures, prefabricated, includes fitting and adjustment

* **L0466** TLSO, sagittal control, rigid posterior frame and flexible soft anterior apron with straps, closures and padding, restricts gross trunk motion in sagittal plane, produces intracavitary pressure to reduce load on intervertebral disks, includes fitting and shaping the frame, prefabricated, includes fitting and adjustment

* **L0468** TLSO, sagittal-coronal control, rigid posterior frame and flexible soft anterior apron with straps, closures and padding, extends from sacrococcygeal junction over scapulae, lateral strength provided by pelvic, thoracic, and lateral frame pieces, restricts gross trunk motion in sagittal, and coronal planes, produces intracavitary pressure to reduce load on intervertebral disks, includes fitting and shaping the frame, prefabricated, includes fitting and adjustment

* **L0470** TLSO, triplanar control, rigid posterior frame and flexible soft anterior apron with straps, closures and padding, extends from sacrococcygeal junction to scapula, lateral strength provided by pelvic, thoracic, and lateral frame pieces, rotational strength provided by subclavicular extensions, restricts gross trunk motion in sagittal, coronal, and transverse planes, provides intracavitary pressure to reduce load on the intervertebral disks, includes fitting and shaping the frame, prefabricated, includes fitting and adjustment

* **L0472** TLSO, triplanar control, hyperextension, rigid anterior and lateral frame extends from symphysis pubis to sternal notch with two anterior components (one pubic and one sternal), posterior and lateral pads with straps and closures, limits spinal flexion, restricts gross trunk motion in sagittal, coronal, and transverse planes, includes fitting and shaping the frame, prefabricated, includes fitting and adjustment

* **L0480** TLSO, triplanar control, one piece rigid plastic shell without interface liner, with multiple straps and closures, posterior extends from sacrococcygeal junction and terminates just inferior to scapular spine, anterior extends from symphysis pubis to sternal notch, anterior or posterior opening, restricts gross trunk motion in sagittal, coronal, and transverse planes, includes a carved plaster or CAD-CAM model, custom fabricated

▶ New   → Revised   ✔ Reinstated   deleted Deleted

☺ Special coverage instructions   ◆ Not covered or valid by Medicare   * Carrier discretion

* **L0482** TLSO, triplanar control, one piece rigid plastic shell with interface liner, multiple straps and closures, posterior extends from sacrococcygeal junction and terminates just inferior to scapular spine, anterior extends from symphysis pubis to sternal notch, anterior or posterior opening, restricts gross trunk motion in sagittal, coronal, and transverse planes, includes a carved plaster or CAD-CAM model, custom fabricated

* **L0484** TLSO, triplanar control, two piece rigid plastic shell without interface liner, with multiple straps and closures, posterior extends from sacrococcygeal junction and terminates just inferior to scapular spine, anterior extends from symphysis pubis to sternal notch, lateral strength is enhanced by overlapping plastic, restricts gross trunk motion in the sagittal, coronal, and transverse planes, includes a carved plaster or CAD-CAM model, custom fabricated

* **L0486** TLSO, triplanar control, two piece rigid plastic shell with interface liner, multiple straps and closures, posterior extends from sacrococcygeal junction and terminates just inferior to scapular spine, anterior extends from symphysis pubis to sternal notch, lateral strength is enhanced by overlapping plastic, restricts gross trunk motion in the sagittal, coronal, and transverse planes, includes a carved plaster or CAD-CAM model, custom fabricated

* **L0488** TLSO, triplanar control, one piece rigid plastic shell with interface liner, multiple straps and closures, posterior extends from sacrococcygeal junction and terminates just inferior to scapular spine, anterior extends from symphysis pubis to sternal notch, anterior or posterior opening, restricts gross trunk motion in sagittal, coronal, and transverse planes, prefabricated, includes fitting and adjustment

* **L0490** TLSO, sagittal-coronal control, one piece rigid plastic shell, with overlapping reinforced anterior, with multiple straps and closures, posterior extends from sacrococcygeal junction and terminates at or before the T-9 vertebra, anterior extends from symphysis pubis to xiphoid, anterior opening, restricts gross trunk motion in sagittal and coronal planes, prefabricated, includes fitting and adjustment

* **L0491** TLSO, sagittal-coronal control, modular segmented spinal system, two rigid plastic shells, posterior extends from the sacrococcygeal junction and terminates just inferior to the scapular spine, anterior extends from the symphysis pubis to the xiphoid, soft liner, restricts gross trunk motion in the sagittal and coronal planes, lateral strength is provided by overlapping plastic and stabilizing closures, includes straps and closures, prefabricated, includes fitting and adjustment

* **L0492** TLSO, sagittal-coronal control, modular segmented spinal system, three rigid plastic shells, posterior extends from the sacrococcygeal junction and terminates just inferior to the scapular spine, anterior extends from the symphysis pubis to the xiphoid, soft liner, restricts gross trunk motion in the sagittal and coronal planes, lateral strength is provided by overlapping plastic and stabilizing closures, includes straps and closures, prefabricated, includes fitting and adjustment

Sacroilliac, Lumbar, Sacral Orthosis

L0621-L0640:   Bill DME/MAC

* **L0621** Sacroiliac orthosis, flexible, provides pelvic-sacral support, reduces motion about the sacroiliac joint, includes straps, closures, may include pendulous abdomen design, prefabricated, includes fitting and adjustment

* **L0622** Sacroiliac orthosis, flexible, provides pelvic-sacral support, reduces motion about the sacroiliac joint, includes straps, closures, may include pendulous abdomen design, custom fabricated

Type of custom-fabricated device for which impression of specific body part is made (e.g., by means of plaster cast, or CAD-CAM [computer-aided design] technology); impression then used to make specific patient model

✳ **L0623** Sacroiliac orthosis, provides pelvic-sacral support, with rigid or semi-rigid panels over the sacrum and abdomen, reduces motion about the sacroiliac joint, includes straps, closures, may include pendulous abdomen design, prefabricated, includes fitting and adjustment

✳ **L0624** Sacroiliac orthosis, provides pelvic-sacral support, with rigid or semi-rigid panels placed over the sacrum and abdomen, reduces motion about the sacroiliac joint, includes straps, closures, may include pendulous abdomen design, custom fabricated

Custom fitted

✳ **L0625** Lumbar orthosis, flexible, provides lumbar support, posterior extends from L-1 to below L-5 vertebra, produces intracavitary pressure to reduce load on the intervertebral discs, includes straps, closures, may include pendulous abdomen design, shoulder straps, stays, prefabricated, includes fitting and adjustment

✳ **L0626** Lumbar orthosis, sagittal control, with rigid posterior panel(s), posterior extends from L-1 to below L-5 vertebra, produces intracavitary pressure to reduce load on the intervertebral discs, includes straps, closures, may include padding, stays, shoulder straps, pendulous abdomen design, prefabricated, includes fitting and adjustment

✳ **L0627** Lumbar orthosis, sagittal control, with rigid anterior and posterior panels, posterior extends from L-1 to below L-5 vertebra, produces intracavitary pressure to reduce load on the intervertebral discs, includes straps, closures, may include padding, shoulder straps, pendulous abdomen design, prefabricated, includes fitting and adjustment

✳ **L0628** Lumbar-sacral orthosis, flexible, provides lumbo-sacral support, posterior extends from sacrococcygeal junction to T-9 vertebra, produces intracavitary pressure to reduce load on the intervertebral discs, includes straps, closures, may include stays, shoulder straps, pendulous abdomen design, prefabricated, includes fitting and adjustment

✳ **L0629** Lumbar-sacral orthosis, flexible, provides lumbo-sacral support, posterior extends from sacrococcygeal junction to T-9 vertebra, produces intracavitary pressure to reduce load on the intervertebral discs, includes straps, closures, may include stays, shoulder straps, pendulous abdomen design, custom fabricated

Custom fitted

✳ **L0630** Lumbar-sacral orthosis, sagittal control, with rigid posterior panel(s), posterior extends from sacrococcygeal junction to T-9 vertebra, produces intracavitary pressure to reduce load on the intervertebral discs, includes straps, closures, may include padding, stays, shoulder straps, pendulous abdomen design, prefabricated, includes fitting and adjustment

✳ **L0631** Lumbar-sacral orthosis, sagittal control, with rigid anterior and posterior panels, posterior extends from sacrococcygeal junction to T-9 vertebra, produces intracavitary pressure to reduce load on the intervertebral discs, includes straps, closures, may include padding, shoulder straps, pendulous abdomen design, prefabricated, includes fitting and adjustment

✳ **L0632** Lumbar-sacral orthosis, sagittal control, with rigid anterior and posterior panels, posterior extends from sacrococcygeal junction to T-9 vertebra, produces intracavitary pressure to reduce load on the intervertebral discs, includes straps, closures, may include padding, shoulder straps, pendulous abdomen design, custom fabricated

Custom fitted

✳ **L0633** Lumbar-sacral orthosis, sagittal-coronal control, with rigid posterior frame/panel(s), posterior extends from sacrococcygeal junction to T-9 vertebra, lateral strength provided by rigid lateral frame/panels, produces intracavitary pressure to reduce load on intervertebral discs, includes straps, closures, may include padding, stays, shoulder straps, pendulous abdomen design, prefabricated, includes fitting and adjustment

---

▶ New   → Revised   ✔ Reinstated   ~~deleted~~ Deleted

☺ Special coverage instructions   ◆ Not covered or valid by Medicare   ✳ Carrier discretion

* **L0634** Lumbar-sacral orthosis, sagittal-coronal control, with rigid posterior frame/panel(s), posterior extends from sacrococcygeal junction to T-9 vertebra, lateral strength provided by rigid lateral frame/panel(s), produces intracavitary pressure to reduce load on intervertebral discs, includes straps, closures, may include padding, stays, shoulder straps, pendulous abdomen design, custom fabricated

Custom fitted

* **L0635** Lumbar-sacral orthosis, sagittal-coronal control, lumbar flexion, rigid posterior frame/panel(s), lateral articulating design to flex the lumbar spine, posterior extends from sacrococcygeal junction to T-9 vertebra, lateral strength provided by rigid lateral frame/panel(s), produces intracavitary pressure to reduce load on intervertebral discs, includes straps, closures, may include padding, anterior panel, pendulous abdomen design, prefabricated, includes fitting and adjustment

* **L0636** Lumbar sacral orthosis, sagittal-coronal control, lumbar flexion, rigid posterior frame/panels, lateral articulating design to flex the lumbar spine, posterior extends from sacrococcygeal junction to T-9 vertebra, lateral strength provided by rigid lateral frame/panels, produces intracavitary pressure to reduce load on intervertebral discs, includes straps, closures, may include padding, anterior panel, pendulous abdomen design, custom fabricated

Custom fitted

* **L0637** Lumbar-sacral orthosis, sagittal-coronal control, with rigid anterior and posterior frame/panels, posterior extends from sacrococcygeal junction to T-9 vertebra, lateral strength provided by rigid lateral frame/panels, produces intracavitary pressure to reduce load on intervertebral discs, includes straps, closures, may include padding, shoulder straps, pendulous abdomen design, prefabricated, includes fitting and adjustment

* **L0638** Lumbar-sacral orthosis, sagittal-coronal control, with rigid anterior and posterior frame/panels, posterior extends from sacrococcygeal junction to T-9 vertebra, lateral strength provided by rigid lateral frame/panels, produces intracavitary pressure to reduce load on intervertebral discs, includes straps, closures, may include padding, shoulder straps, pendulous abdomen design, custom fabricated

* **L0639** Lumbar-sacral orthosis, sagittal-coronal control, rigid shell(s)/panel(s), posterior extends from sacrococcygeal junction to T-9 vertebra, anterior extends from symphysis pubis to xyphoid, produces intracavitary pressure to reduce load on the intervertebral discs, overall strength is provided by overlapping rigid material and stabilizing closures, includes straps, closures may include soft interface, pendulous abdomen design, prefabricated, includes fitting and adjustment

Characterized by rigid plastic shell that encircles trunk with overlapping edges and stabilizing closures and provides high degree of immobility

* **L0640** Lumbar-sacral orthosis, sagittal-coronal control, rigid shell(s)/panel(s), posterior extends from sacrococcygeal junction to T-9 vertebra, anterior extends from symphysis pubis to xyphoid, produces intracavitary pressure to reduce load on the intervertebral discs, overall strength is provided by overlapping rigid material and stabilizing closures, includes straps, closures, may include soft interface, pendulous abdomen design, custom fabricated

Custom fitted

Cervical-Thoracic-Lumbar-Sacral

Anterior-Posterior-Lateral Control

L0700-L0710: Bill DME/MAC

* **L0700** Cervical-thoracic-lumbar-sacral-orthoses (CTLSO), anterior-posterior-lateral control, molded to patient model, (Minerva type)

* **L0710** CTLSO, anterior-posterior-lateral-control, molded to patient model, with interface material, (Minerva type)

▶ New   → Revised   ✔ Reinstated   deleted Deleted
☺ Special coverage instructions   ◆ Not covered or valid by Medicare   ✻ Carrier discretion

HALO Procedure

L0810-L0861: Bill DME/MAC

* ✱ **L0810** HALO procedure, cervical halo incorporated into jacket vest
* ✱ **L0820** HALO procedure, cervical halo incorporated into plaster body jacket
* ✱ **L0830** HALO procedure, cervical halo incorporated into Milwaukee type orthosis
* ✱ **L0859** Addition to HALO procedure, magnetic resonance image compatible systems, rings and pins, any material
* ✱ **L0861** Addition to HALO procedure, replacement liner/interface material

Additions to Spinal Orthoses

L0970-L0999: Bill DME/MAC

TLSO: Thoracic-lumbar-sacral orthoses
Spinal orthoses may be prefabricated, prefitted, or custom fabricated. Conservative treatment for back pain may include the use of spinal orthoses.

* ✱ **L0970** TLSO, corset front
* ✱ **L0972** LSO, corset front
* ✱ **L0974** TLSO, full corset
* ✱ **L0976** LSO, full corset
* ✱ **L0978** Axillary crutch extension
* ✱ **L0980** Peroneal straps, pair
* ✱ **L0982** Stocking supporter grips, set of four (4)

    Convenience item
* ✱ **L0984** Protective body sock, each

    Garment made of cloth or similar material that is worn under spinal orthosis and is not primarily medical in nature

    Convenience item
* ✱ **L0999** Addition to spinal orthosis, not otherwise specified

Orthotic Devices: Scoliosis Procedures (L1000-L1520)

NOTE: Orthotic care of scoliosis differs from other orthotic care in that the treatment is more dynamic in nature and uses ongoing continual modification of the orthosis to the patient's changing condition. This coding structure uses the proper names, or eponyms, of the procedures because they have historic and universal acceptance in the profession. It should be recognized that variations to the basic procedures described by the founders/developers are accepted in various medical and orthotic practices throughout the country. All procedures include a model of patient when indicated.

Scoliosis: Cervical-Thoracic-Lumbar-Sacral (CTLSO) (Milwaukee)

L1000-L1520: Bill DME/MAC

* ✱ **L1000** Cervical-thoracic-lumbar-sacral orthosis (CTLSO) (Milwaukee), inclusive of furnishing initial orthosis, including model
* ✱ **L1001** Cervical thoracic lumbar sacral orthosis, immobilizer, infant size, prefabricated, includes fitting and adjustment
* ✱ **L1005** Tension based scoliosis orthosis and accessory pads, includes fitting and adjustment
* ✱ **L1010** Addition to cervical-thoracic-lumbar-sacral orthosis (CTLSO) or scoliosis orthosis, axilla sling

Correction Pads

* ✱ **L1020** Addition to CTLSO or scoliosis orthosis, kyphosis pad
* ✱ **L1025** Addition to CTLSO or scoliosis orthosis, kyphosis pad, floating
* ✱ **L1030** Addition to CTLSO or scoliosis orthosis, lumbar bolster pad
* ✱ **L1040** Addition to CTLSO or scoliosis orthosis, lumbar or lumbar rib pad
* ✱ **L1050** Addition to CTLSO or scoliosis orthosis, sternal pad
* ✱ **L1060** Addition to CTLSO or scoliosis orthosis, thoracic pad
* ✱ **L1070** Addition to CTLSO or scoliosis orthosis, trapezius sling

---

▶ New   → Revised   ✔ Reinstated   ~~deleted~~ Deleted
☺ Special coverage instructions   ◆ Not covered or valid by Medicare   ✱ Carrier discretion

* **L1080** Addition to CTLSO or scoliosis orthosis, outrigger

* **L1085** Addition to CTLSO or scoliosis orthosis, outrigger, bilateral with vertical extensions

* **L1090** Addition to CTLSO or scoliosis orthosis, lumbar sling

* **L1100** Addition to CTLSO or scoliosis orthosis, ring flange, plastic or leather

* **L1110** Addition to CTLSO or scoliosis orthosis, ring flange, plastic or leather, molded to patient model

* **L1120** Addition to CTLSO, scoliosis orthosis, cover for upright, each

Scoliosis: Thoracic-Lumbar-Sacral (Low Profile)

* **L1200** Thoracic-lumbar-sacral-orthosis (TLSO), inclusive of furnishing initial orthosis only

* **L1210** Addition to TLSO, (low profile), lateral thoracic extension

* **L1220** Addition to TLSO, (low profile), anterior thoracic extension

* **L1230** Addition to TLSO, (low profile), Milwaukee type superstructure

* **L1240** Addition to TLSO, (low profile), lumbar derotation pad

* **L1250** Addition to TLSO, (low profile), anterior ASIS pad

* **L1260** Addition to TLSO, (low profile), anterior thoracic derotation pad

* **L1270** Addition to TLSO, (low profile), abdominal pad

* **L1280** Addition to TLSO, (low profile), rib gusset (elastic), each

* **L1290** Addition to TLSO, (low profile), lateral trochanteric pad

Other Scoliosis Procedures

* **L1300** Other scoliosis procedure, body jacket molded to patient model

* **L1310** Other scoliosis procedure, postoperative body jacket

* **L1499** Spinal orthosis, not otherwise specified

L1500 Thoracic-hip-knee-ankle orthosis (THKAO), mobility frame (Newington, Parapodium types) ✖

L1510 THKAO, standing frame, with or without tray and accessories ✖

L1520 THKAO, swivel walker ✖

Orthotic Devices: Lower Limb

NOTE: the procedures in L1600-L2999 are considered as *base* or *basic procedures* and may be modified by listing procedure from the Additions Sections and adding them to the base procedure.

Hip: Flexible

L1600-L2999: Bill DME/MAC

* **L1600** Hip orthosis (HO), abduction control of hip joints, flexible, Frejka type with cover, prefabricated, includes fitting and adjustment

* **L1610** Hip orthosis, abduction control of hip joints, flexible, (Frejka cover only) prefabricated, includes fitting and adjustment

* **L1620** Hip orthosis, abduction control of hip joints, flexible, (Pavlik harness), prefabricated, includes fitting and adjustment

* **L1630** Hip orthosis, abduction control of hip joints, semi-flexible (Von Rosen type), custom-fabricated

* **L1640** Hip orthosis, abduction control of hip joints, static, pelvic band or spreader bar, thigh cuffs, custom-fabricated

* **L1650** Hip orthosis, abduction control of hip joints, static, adjustable, (Ilfled type), prefabricated, includes fitting and adjustment

* **L1652** Hip orthosis, bilateral thigh cuffs with adjustable abductor spreader bar, adult size, prefabricated, includes fitting and adjustment, any type

* **L1660** Hip orthosis, abduction control of hip joints, static, plastic, prefabricated, includes fitting and adjustment

* **L1680** Hip orthosis, abduction control of hip joints, dynamic, pelvic control, adjustable hip motion control, thigh cuffs (Rancho hip action type), custom fabrication

* **L1685** Hip orthosis, abduction control of hip joint, postoperative hip abduction type, custom fabricated

▶ New → Revised ✔ Reinstated deleted Deleted
⊙ Special coverage instructions ◆ Not covered or valid by Medicare * Carrier discretion

* **L1686** Hip orthosis, abduction control of hip joint, postoperative hip abduction type, prefabricated, includes fitting and adjustment
* **L1690** Combination, bilateral, lumbo-sacral, hip, femur orthosis providing adduction and internal rotation control, prefabricated, includes fitting and adjustment

Legg Perthes

* **L1700** Legg-Perthes orthosis, (Toronto type), custom-fabricated
* **L1710** Legg-Perthes orthosis, (Newington type), custom-fabricated
* **L1720** Legg-Perthes orthosis, trilateral, (Tachdjian type), custom-fabricated
* **L1730** Legg-Perthes orthosis, (Scottish Rite type), custom-fabricated
* **L1755** Legg-Perthes orthosis, (Patten bottom type), custom-fabricated

Knee (KO)

* **L1810** Knee orthosis, elastic with joints, prefabricated, includes fitting and adjustment
* **L1820** Knee orthosis, elastic with condylar pads and joints, with or without patellar control, prefabricated, includes fitting and adjustment
* **L1830** Knee orthosis, immobilizer, canvas longitudinal, prefabricated, includes fitting and adjustment
* **L1831** Knee orthosis, locking knee joint(s), positional orthosis, prefabricated, includes fitting and adjustment
* **L1832** Knee orthrosis, adjustable knee joints (unicentric or polycentric), positional orthosis, rigid support, prefabricated, includes fitting and adjustment
* **L1834** Knee orthosis, without knee joint, rigid, custom-fabricated
* **L1836** Knee orthosis, rigid, without joint(s), includes soft interface material, prefabricated, includes fitting and adjustment
* **L1840** Knee orthosis, derotation, medial-lateral, anterior cruciate ligament, custom fabricated

* **L1843** Knee orthosis, single upright, thigh and calf, with adjustable flexion and extension joint (unicentric or polycentric), medial-lateral and rotation control, with or without varus/valgus adjustment; prefabricated, includes fitting and adjustment
* **L1844** Knee orthosis, single upright, thigh and calf, with adjustable flexion and extension joint (unicentric or polycentric), medial-lateral and rotation control, with or without varus/valgus adjustment, custom fabricated
* **L1845** Knee orthrosis, double upright, thigh and calf, with adjustable flexion and extension joint (unicentric or polycentric), medial-lateral and rotation control, with or without varus/valgus adjustment, prefabricated, includes fitting and adjustment
* **L1846** Knee orthrosis, double upright, thigh and calf, with adjustable flexion and extension joint (unicentric or polycentric), medial-lateral and rotation control, with or without varus/valgus adjustment, custom fabricated
* **L1847** Knee orthosis, double upright with adjustable joint, with inflatable air support chambers, prefabricated, includes fitting and adjustment
* **L1850** Knee orthosis, Swedish type, prefabricated, includes fitting and adjustment
* **L1860** Knee orthosis, modification of supracondylar prosthetic socket, custom fabricated (SK)

Ankle-Foot (AFO)

* **L1900** Ankle foot orthosis (AFO), spring wire, dorsiflexion assist calf band, custom-fabricated
* **L1902** Ankle foot orthosis, ankle gauntlet, prefabricated, includes fitting and adjustment
* **L1904** Ankle foot orthosis, molded ankle gauntlet, custom-fabricated
* **L1906** Ankle-foot orthosis, multiligamentus ankle support, prefabricated, includes fitting and adjustment
* **L1907** AFO, supramalleolar with straps, with or without interface/pads, custom fabricated

▶ New	→ Revised	✔ Reinstated	deleted Deleted
⊘ Special coverage instructions	◆ Not covered or valid by Medicare	* Carrier discretion	

* **L1910** Ankle foot orthosis, posterior, single bar, clasp attachment to shoe counter, prefabricated, includes fitting and adjustment

* **L1920** Ankle foot orthosis, single upright with static or adjustable stop (Phelps or Perlstein type), custom-fabricated

* **L1930** Ankle-foot orthosis, plastic or other material, prefabricated, includes fitting and adjustment

* **L1932** AFO, rigid anterior tibial section, total carbon fiber or equal material, prefabricated, includes fitting and adjustment

* **L1940** Ankle foot orthosis, plastic or other material, custom-fabricated

* **L1945** Ankle foot orthosis, plastic, rigid anterior tibial section (floor reaction), custom-fabricated

* **L1950** Ankle foot orthosis, spiral, (Institute of Rehabilitation Medicine type), plastic, custom-fabricated

* **L1951** Ankle foot orthosis, spiral, (Institute of Rehabilitative Medicine type), plastic or other material, prefabricated, includes fitting and adjustment

* **L1960** Ankle foot orthosis, posterior solid ankle, plastic, custom-fabricated

* **L1970** Ankle foot orthosis, plastic, with ankle joint, custom-fabricated

* **L1971** Ankle foot orthosis, plastic or other material with ankle joint, prefabricated, includes fitting and adjustment

* **L1980** Ankle foot orthosis, single upright free plantar dorsiflexion, solid stirrup, calf band/cuff (single bar 'BK' orthosis), custom-fabricated

* **L1990** Ankle foot orthosis, double upright free plantar dorsiflexion, solid stirrup, calf band/cuff (double bar 'BK' orthosis), custom-fabricated

Hip-Knee-Ankle-Foot (or Any Combination)

NOTE: L2000, L2020, and L2036 are base procedures to be used with any knee joint. L2010 and L2030 are to be used only with no knee joint.

* **L2000** Knee ankle foot orthosis, single upright, free knee, free ankle, solid stirrup, thigh and calf bands/cuffs (single bar 'AK' orthosis), custom-fabricated

→ * **L2005** Knee ankle foot orthosis, any material, single or double upright, stance control, automatic lock and swing phase release, any type activation; includes ankle joint, any type, custom fabricated

* **L2010** Knee ankle foot orthosis, single upright, free ankle, solid stirrup, thigh and calf bands/cuffs (single bar 'AK' orthosis), without knee joint, custom-fabricated

* **L2020** Knee ankle foot orthosis, double upright, free knee, free ankle, solid stirrup, thigh and calf bands/cuffs (double bar 'AK' orthosis), custom-fabricated

* **L2030** Knee ankle foot orthosis, double upright, free ankle, solid stirrup, thigh and calf bands/cuffs (double bar 'AK' orthosis), without knee joint, custom fabricated

* **L2034** Knee ankle foot orthosis, full plastic, single upright, with or without free motion knee, medial lateral rotation control, with or without free motion ankle, custom fabricated

* **L2035** Knee ankle foot orthosis, full plastic, static (pediatric size), without free motion ankle, prefabricated, includes fitting and adjustment

* **L2036** Knee ankle foot orthosis, full plastic, double upright, with or without free motion knee, with or without free motion ankle, custom fabricated

* **L2037** Knee ankle foot orthosis, full plastic, single upright, with or without free motion knee, with or without free motion ankle, custom fabricated

* **L2038** Knee ankle foot orthosis, full plastic, with or without free motion knee, multi-axis ankle, custom fabricated

Torsion Control

* **L2040** Hip knee ankle foot orthosis, torsion control, bilateral rotation straps, pelvic band/belt, custom fabricated

* **L2050** Hip knee ankle foot orthosis, torsion control, bilateral torsion cables, hip joint, pelvic band/belt, custom-fabricated

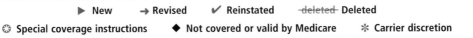

▶ New   → Revised   ✔ Reinstated   ̶d̶e̶l̶e̶t̶e̶d̶ Deleted
☺ Special coverage instructions   ◆ Not covered or valid by Medicare   ✳ Carrier discretion

* **L2060**   Hip knee ankle foot orthosis, torsion control, bilateral torsion cables, ball bearing hip joint, pelvic band/belt, custom-fabricated

* **L2070**   Hip knee ankle foot orthosis, torsion control, unilateral rotation straps, pelvic band/belt, custom-fabricated

* **L2080**   Hip knee ankle foot orthosis, torsion control, unilateral torsion cable, hip joint, pelvic band/belt, custom-fabricated

* **L2090**   Hip knee ankle foot orthosis, torsion control, unilateral torsion cable, ball bearing hip joint, pelvic band/belt, custom-fabricated

Fracture Orthoses

* **L2106**   Ankle foot orthosis, fracture orthosis, tibial fracture cast orthosis, thermoplastic type casting material, custom-fabricated

* **L2108**   Ankle foot orthosis, fracture orthosis, tibial fracture cast orthosis, custom-fabricated

* **L2112**   Ankle foot orthosis, fracture orthosis, tibial fracture orthosis, soft, prefabricated, includes fitting and adjustment

* **L2114**   Ankle foot orthosis, fracture orthosis, tibial fracture orthosis, semi-rigid, prefabricated, includes fitting and adjustment

* **L2116**   Ankle foot orthosis, fracture orthosis, tibial fracture orthosis, rigid, prefabricated, includes fitting and adjustment

* **L2126**   Knee ankle foot orthosis, fracture orthosis, femoral fracture cast orthosis, thermoplastic type casting material, custom-fabricated

* **L2128**   Knee ankle foot orthosis, fracture orthosis, femoral fracture cast orthosis, custom-fabricated

* **L2132**   KAFO, femoral fracture cast orthosis, soft, prefabricated, includes fitting and adjustment

* **L2134**   KAFO, femoral fracture cast orthosis, semi-rigid, prefabricated, includes fitting and adjustment

* **L2136**   KAFO, fracture orthosis, femoral fracture cast orthosis, rigid, prefabricated, includes fitting and adjustment

Additions to Fracture Orthosis

* **L2180**   Addition to lower extremity fracture orthosis, plastic shoe insert with ankle joints

* **L2182**   Addition to lower extremity fracture orthosis, drop lock knee joint

* **L2184**   Addition to lower extremity fracture orthosis, limited motion knee joint

* **L2186**   Addition to lower extremity fracture orthosis, adjustable motion knee joint, Lerman type

* **L2188**   Addition to lower extremity fracture orthosis, quadrilateral brim

* **L2190**   Addition to lower extremity fracture orthosis, waist belt

* **L2192**   Addition to lower extremity fracture orthosis, hip joint, pelvic band, thigh flange, and pelvic belt

Additions to Lower Extremity Orthosis
Shoe-Ankle-Shin-Knee

* **L2200**   Addition to lower extremity, limited ankle motion, each joint

* **L2210**   Addition to lower extremity, dorsiflexion assist (plantar flexion resist), each joint

* **L2220**   Addition to lower extremity, dorsiflexion and plantar flexion assist/resist, each joint

* **L2230**   Addition to lower extremity, split flat caliper stirrups and plate attachment

* **L2232**   Addition to lower extremity orthosis, rocker bottom for total contact ankle foot orthosis, for custom fabricated orthosis only

* **L2240**   Addition to lower extremity, round caliper and plate attachment

* **L2250**   Addition to lower extremity, foot plate, molded to patient model, stirrup attachment

* **L2260**   Addition to lower extremity, reinforced solid stirrup (Scott-Craig type)

* **L2265**   Addition to lower extremity, long tongue stirrup

---

▶ New   → Revised   ✔ Reinstated   ~~deleted~~ Deleted

☉ Special coverage instructions   ◆ Not covered or valid by Medicare   * Carrier discretion

* **L2270**   Addition to lower extremity, varus/valgus correction ('T') strap, padded/lined or malleolus pad

* **L2275**   Addition to lower extremity, varus/valgus correction, plastic modification, padded/lined

* **L2280**   Addition to lower extremity, molded inner boot

* **L2300**   Addition to lower extremity, abduction bar (bilateral hip involvement), jointed, adjustable

* **L2310**   Addition to lower extremity, abduction bar-straight

* **L2320**   Addition to lower extremity, non-molded lacer, for custom fabricated orthosis only

* **L2330**   Addition to lower extremity, lacer molded to patient model, for custom fabricated orthosis only

      Used whether closure is lacer or Velcro

* **L2335**   Addition to lower extremity, anterior swing band

* **L2340**   Addition to lower extremity, pre-tibial shell, molded to patient model

* **L2350**   Addition to lower extremity, prosthetic type, (BK) socket, molded to patient model, (used for 'PTB' and 'AFO' orthoses)

* **L2360**   Addition to lower extremity, extended steel shank

* **L2370**   Addition to lower extremity, Patten bottom

* **L2375**   Addition to lower extremity, torsion control, ankle joint and half solid stirrup

* **L2380**   Addition to lower extremity, torsion control, straight knee joint, each joint

* **L2385**   Addition to lower extremity, straight knee joint, heavy duty, each joint

* **L2387**   Addition to lower extremity, polycentric knee joint, for custom fabricated knee ankle foot orthosis, each joint

* **L2390**   Addition to lower extremity, offset knee joint, each joint

* **L2395**   Addition to lower extremity, offset knee joint, heavy duty, each joint

* **L2397**   Addition to lower extremity orthosis, suspension sleeve

Additions to Straight Knee or Offset Knee Joints

* **L2405**   Addition to knee joint, drop lock, each

* **L2415**   Addition to knee lock with integrated release mechanism (bail, cable, or equal), any material, each joint

* **L2425**   Addition to knee joint, disc or dial lock for adjustable knee flexion, each joint

* **L2430**   Addition to knee joint, ratchet lock for active and progressive knee extension, each joint

* **L2492**   Addition to knee joint, lift loop for drop lock ring

Additions to Thigh/Weight Bearing

Gluteal/Ischial Weight Bearing

* **L2500**   Addition to lower extremity, thigh/weight bearing, gluteal/ischial weight bearing, ring

* **L2510**   Addition to lower extremity, thigh/weight bearing, quadri-lateral brim, molded to patient model

* **L2520**   Addition to lower extremity, thigh/weight bearing, quadri-lateral brim, custom fitted

* **L2525**   Addition to lower extremity, thigh/weight bearing, ischial containment/narrow M-L brim molded to patient model

* **L2526**   Addition to lower extremity, thigh/weight bearing, ischial containment/narrow M-L brim, custom fitted

* **L2530**   Addition to lower extremity, thigh-weight bearing, lacer, non-molded

* **L2540**   Addition to lower extremity, thigh/weight bearing, lacer, molded to patient model

* **L2550**   Addition to lower extremity, thigh/weight bearing, high roll cuff

Additions to Pelvic and Thoracic Control

* **L2570**   Addition to lower extremity, pelvic control, hip joint, Clevis type two position joint, each

* **L2580**   Addition to lower extremity, pelvic control, pelvic sling

* **L2600**   Addition to lower extremity, pelvic control, hip joint, Clevis type, or thrust bearing, free, each

---

▶ New   → Revised   ✔ Reinstated   ~~deleted~~ Deleted

✪ Special coverage instructions   ◆ Not covered or valid by Medicare   * Carrier discretion

* **L2610**   Addition to lower extremity, pelvic control, hip joint, Clevis or thrust bearing, lock, each

* **L2620**   Addition to lower extremity, pelvic control, hip joint, heavy duty, each

* **L2622**   Addition to lower extremity, pelvic control, hip joint, adjustable flexion, each

* **L2624**   Addition to lower extremity, pelvic control, hip joint, adjustable flexion, extension, abduction control, each

* **L2627**   Addition to lower extremity, pelvic control, plastic, molded to patient model, reciprocating hip joint and cables

* **L2628**   Addition to lower extremity, pelvic control, metal frame, reciprocating hip joint and cables

* **L2630**   Addition to lower extremity, pelvic control, band and belt, unilateral

* **L2640**   Addition to lower extremity, pelvic control, band and belt, bilateral

* **L2650**   Addition to lower extremity, pelvic and thoracic control, gluteal pad, each

* **L2660**   Addition to lower extremity, thoracic control, thoracic band

* **L2670**   Addition to lower extremity, thoracic control, paraspinal uprights

* **L2680**   Addition to lower extremity, thoracic control, lateral support uprights

General Additions

* **L2750**   Addition to lower extremity orthosis, plating chrome or nickel, per bar

* **L2755**   Addition to lower extremity orthosis, high strength, lightweight material, all hybrid lamination/prepreg composite, per segment, for custom fabricated orthosis only

* **L2760**   Addition to lower extremity orthosis, extension, per extension, per bar (for lineal adjustment for growth)

* **L2768**   Orthotic side bar disconnect device, per bar

* **L2780**   Addition to lower extremity orthosis, non-corrosive finish, per bar

* **L2785**   Addition to lower extremity orthosis, drop lock retainer, each

* **L2795**   Addition to lower extremity orthosis, knee control, full kneecap

* **L2800**   Addition to lower extremity orthosis, knee control, knee cap, medial or lateral pull, for use with custom fabricated orthosis only

* **L2810**   Addition to lower extremity orthosis, knee control, condylar pad

* **L2820**   Addition to lower extremity orthosis, soft interface for molded plastic, below knee section

Only report if soft interface provided, either leather or other material

* **L2830**   Addition to lower extremity orthosis, soft interface for molded plastic, above knee section

* **L2840**   Addition to lower extremity orthosis, tibial length sock, fracture or equal, each

* **L2850**   Addition to lower extremity orthosis, femoral length sock, fracture or equal, each

◆ **L2861**   Addition to lower extremity joint, knee or ankle, concentric adjustable torsion style mechanism for custom fabricated orthotics only, each

* **L2999**   Lower extremity orthoses, not otherwise specified

Foot (Orthopedic Shoes)

Insert, Removable, Molded to Patient Model

L3000-L3649:   Bill DME/MAC

⊛ **L3000**   Foot, insert, removable, molded to patient model, 'UCB' type, Berkeley shell, each

If both feet casted and supplied with an orthosis, bill L3000-LT and L3000-RT

IOM: 100-02, 15, 290

⊛ **L3001**   Foot, insert, removable, molded to patient model, Spenco, each

IOM: 100-02, 15, 290

⊛ **L3002**   Foot, insert, removable, molded to patient model, Plastazote or equal, each

IOM: 100-02, 15, 290

⊛ **L3003**   Foot, insert, removable, molded to patient model, silicone gel, each

IOM: 100-02, 15, 290

⊛ **L3010**   Foot, insert, removable, molded to patient model, longitudinal arch support, each

IOM: 100-02, 15, 290

⊛ **L3020**   Foot, insert, removable, molded to patient model, longitudinal/metatarsal support, each

IOM: 100-02, 15, 290

▶ New   → Revised   ✔ Reinstated   ~~deleted~~ Deleted

⊛ Special coverage instructions   ◆ Not covered or valid by Medicare   * Carrier discretion

⊗ **L3030** Foot, insert, removable, formed to patient foot, each

IOM: 100-02, 15, 290

✳ **L3031** Foot, insert/plate, removable, addition to lower extremity orthosis, high strength, lightweight material, all hybrid lamination/prepreg composite, each

Arch Support, Removable, Premolded

⊗ **L3040** Foot, arch support, removable, premolded, longitudinal, each

IOM: 100-02, 15, 290

⊗ **L3050** Foot, arch support, removable, premolded, metatarsal, each

IOM: 100-02, 15, 290

⊗ **L3060** Foot, arch support, removable, premolded, longitudinal/metatarsal, each

IOM: 100-02, 15, 290

Arch Support, Non-removable, Attached to Shoe

⊗ **L3070** Foot, arch support, non-removable attached to shoe, longitudinal, each

IOM: 100-02, 15, 290

⊗ **L3080** Foot, arch support, non-removable attached to shoe, metatarsal, each

IOM: 100-02, 15, 290

⊗ **L3090** Foot, arch support, non-removable attached to shoe, longitudinal/metatarsal, each

IOM: 100-02, 15, 290

⊗ **L3100** Hallus-valgus night dynamic splint

IOM: 100-02, 15, 290

Abduction and Rotation Bars

⊗ **L3140** Foot, abduction rotation bar, including shoes

IOM: 100-02, 15, 290

⊗ **L3150** Foot, abduction rotation bar, without shoes

IOM: 100-02, 15, 290

✳ **L3160** Foot, adjustable shoe-styled positioning device

⊗ **L3170** Foot, plastic, silicone or equal, heel stabilizer, each

IOM: 100-02, 15, 290

Orthopedic Footwear

⊗ **L3201** Orthopedic shoe, oxford with supinator or pronator, infant

IOM: 100-02, 15, 290

⊗ **L3202** Orthopedic shoe, oxford with supinator or pronator, child

IOM: 100-02, 15, 290

⊗ **L3203** Orthopedic shoe, oxford with supinator or pronator, junior

IOM: 100-02, 15, 290

⊗ **L3204** Orthopedic shoe, hightop with supinator or pronator, infant

IOM: 100-02, 15, 290

⊗ **L3206** Orthopedic shoe, hightop with supinator or pronator, child

IOM: 100-02, 15, 290

⊗ **L3207** Orthopedic shoe, hightop with supinator or pronator, junior

IOM: 100-02, 15, 290

⊗ **L3208** Surgical boot, infant, each

IOM: 100-02, 15, 100

⊗ **L3209** Surgical boot, each, child

IOM: 100-02, 15, 100

⊗ **L3211** Surgical boot, each, junior

IOM: 100-02, 15, 100

⊗ **L3212** Benesch boot, pair, infant

IOM: 100-02, 15, 100

⊗ **L3213** Benesch boot, pair, child

IOM: 100-02, 15, 100

⊗ **L3214** Benesch boot, pair, junior

IOM: 100-02, 15, 100

◆ **L3215** Orthopedic footwear, ladies shoe, oxford, each

Medicare Statute 1862a8

◆ **L3216** Orthopedic footwear, ladies shoe, depth inlay, each

Medicare Statute 1862a8

◆ **L3217** Orthopedic footwear, ladies shoe, hightop, depth inlay, each

Medicare Statute 1862a8

◆ **L3219** Orthopedic footwear, mens shoe, oxford, each

Medicare Statute 1862a8

◆ **L3221** Orthopedic footwear, mens shoe, depth inlay, each

Medicare Statute 1862a8

▶ New   → Revised   ✔ Reinstated   ~~deleted~~ Deleted

⊗ Special coverage instructions   ◆ Not covered or valid by Medicare   ✳ Carrier discretion

◆ **L3222** Orthopedic footwear, mens shoe, hightop, depth inlay, each

Medicare Statute 1862a8

✪ **L3224** Orthopedic footwear, ladies shoe, oxford, used as an integral part of a brace (orthosis)

IOM: 100-02, 15, 290

✪ **L3225** Orthopedic footwear, mens shoe, oxford, used as an integral part of a brace (orthosis)

IOM: 100-02, 15, 290

✪ **L3230** Orthopedic footwear, custom shoe, depth inlay, each

IOM: 100-02, 15, 290

✪ **L3250** Orthopedic footwear, custom molded shoe, removable inner mold, prosthetic shoe, each

IOM: 100-02, 15, 290

✪ **L3251** Foot, shoe molded to patient model, silicone shoe, each

IOM: 100-02, 15, 290

✪ **L3252** Foot, shoe molded to patient model, Plastazote (or similar), custom fabricated, each

IOM: 100-02, 15, 290

✪ **L3253** Foot, molded shoe Plastazote (or similar), custom fitted, each

IOM: 100-02, 15, 290

✪ **L3254** Non-standard size or width

IOM: 100-02, 15, 290

✪ **L3255** Non-standard size or length

IOM: 100-02, 15, 290

✪ **L3257** Orthopedic footwear, additional charge for split size

IOM: 100-02, 15, 290

✪ **L3260** Surgical boot/shoe, each

IOM: 100-02, 15, 100

✳ **L3265** Plastazote sandal, each

Shoe Modifications

Lifts

✪ **L3300** Lift, elevation, heel, tapered to metatarsals, per inch

IOM: 100-02, 15, 290

✪ **L3310** Lift, elevation, heel and sole, Neoprene, per inch

IOM: 100-02, 15, 290

✪ **L3320** Lift, elevation, heel and sole, cork, per inch

IOM: 100-02, 15, 290

✪ **L3330** Lift, elevation, metal extension (skate)

IOM: 100-02, 15, 290

✪ **L3332** Lift, elevation, inside shoe, tapered, up to one-half inch

IOM: 100-02, 15, 290

✪ **L3334** Lift, elevation, heel, per inch

IOM: 100-02, 15, 290

Wedges

✪ **L3340** Heel wedge, SACH

IOM: 100-02, 15, 290

✪ **L3350** Heel wedge

IOM: 100-02, 15, 290

✪ **L3360** Sole wedge, outside sole

IOM: 100-02, 15, 290

✪ **L3370** Sole wedge, between sole

IOM: 100-02, 15, 290

✪ **L3380** Clubfoot wedge

IOM: 100-02, 15, 290

✪ **L3390** Outflare wedge

IOM: 100-02, 15, 290

✪ **L3400** Metatarsal bar wedge, rocker

IOM: 100-02, 15, 290

✪ **L3410** Metatarsal bar wedge, between sole

IOM: 100-02, 15, 290

✪ **L3420** Full sole and heel wedge, between sole

IOM: 100-02, 15, 290

Heels

✪ **L3430** Heel, counter, plastic reinforced

IOM: 100-02, 15, 290

✪ **L3440** Heel, counter, leather reinforced

IOM: 100-02, 15, 290

✪ **L3450** Heel, SACH cushion type

IOM: 100-02, 15, 290

✪ **L3455** Heel, new leather, standard

IOM: 100-02, 15, 290

✪ **L3460** Heel, new rubber, standard

IOM: 100-02, 15, 290

✪ **L3465** Heel, Thomas with wedge

IOM: 100-02, 15, 290

▶ New → Revised ✔ Reinstated deleted Deleted ✪ Special coverage instructions ◆ Not covered or valid by Medicare ✳ Carrier discretion

L3470   Heel, Thomas extended to ball
IOM: 100-02, 15, 290

L3480   Heel, pad and depression for spur
IOM: 100-02, 15, 290

L3485   Heel, pad, removable for spur
IOM: 100-02, 15, 290

Additions to Orthopedic Shoes

L3500   Orthopedic shoe addition, insole, leather
IOM: 100-02, 15, 290

L3510   Orthopedic shoe addition, insole, rubber
IOM: 100-02, 15, 290

L3520   Orthopedic shoe addition, insole, felt covered with leather
IOM: 100-02, 15, 290

L3530   Orthopedic shoe addition, sole, half
IOM: 100-02, 15, 290

L3540   Orthopedic shoe addition, sole, full
IOM: 100-02, 15, 290

L3550   Orthopedic shoe addition, toe tap standard
IOM: 100-02, 15, 290

L3560   Orthopedic shoe addition, toe tap, horseshoe
IOM: 100-02, 15, 290

L3570   Orthopedic shoe addition, special extension to instep (leather with eyelets)
IOM: 100-02, 15, 290

L3580   Orthopedic shoe addition, convert instep to Velcro closure
IOM: 100-02, 15, 290

L3590   Orthopedic shoe addition, convert firm shoe counter to soft counter
IOM: 100-02, 15, 290

L3595   Orthopedic shoe addition, March bar
IOM: 100-02, 15, 290

Transfer or Replacement

L3600   Transfer of an orthosis from one shoe to another, caliper plate, existing
IOM: 100-02, 15, 290

L3610   Transfer of an orthosis from one shoe to another, caliper plate, new
IOM: 100-02, 15, 290

L3620   Transfer of an orthosis from one shoe to another, solid stirrup, existing
IOM: 100-02, 15, 290

L3630   Transfer of an orthosis from one shoe to another, solid stirrup, new
IOM: 100-02, 15, 290

L3640   Transfer of an orthosis from one shoe to another, Dennis Browne splint (Riveton), both shoes
IOM: 100-02, 15, 290

L3649   Orthopedic shoe, modification, addition or transfer, not otherwise specified
IOM: 100-02, 15, 290

Orthotic Devices: Upper Limb

NOTE: The procedures in this section are considered as *base* or *basic procedures* and may be modified by listing procedures from the Additions section and adding them to the base procedure.

Shoulder

L3650-L3956:   Bill DME/MAC

* L3650   Shoulder orthosis, (SO), figure of eight design abduction restrainer, prefabricated, includes fitting and adjustment

* L3660   Shoulder orthosis, figure of eight design abduction restrainer, canvas and webbing, prefabricated, includes fitting and adjustment

* L3670   Shoulder orthosis, acromio/clavicular (canvas and webbing type), prefabricated includes fitting and adjustment

→ * L3671   Shoulder orthosis, shoulder joint design, without joints, may include soft interface, straps, custom fabricated, includes fitting and adjustment

▶ * L3674   Shoulder orthosis, abduction positioning (airplane design), thoracic component and support bar, with or without nontorsion joint/turnbuckle, may include soft interface, straps, custom fabricated, includes fitting and adjustment

* **L3675** Shoulder orthosis, vest type abduction restrainer, canvas webbing type or equal, prefabricated, includes fitting and adjustment

→ ☺ **L3677** Shoulder orthosis, shoulder joint design, without joints, may include soft interface, straps, pre-fabricated, includes fitting and adjustment

Elbow

* **L3702** Elbow orthosis, without joints, may include soft interface, straps, custom fabricated, includes fitting and adjustment

* **L3710** Elbow orthosis, elastic with metal joints, prefabricated, includes fitting and adjustment

* **L3720** Elbow orthosis, double upright with forearm/arm cuffs, free motion, custom-fabricated

* **L3730** Elbow orthosis, double upright with forearm/arm cuffs, extension/flexion assist, custom-fabricated

* **L3740** Elbow orthosis, double upright with forearm/arm cuffs, adjustable position lock with active control, custom-fabricated

* **L3760** Elbow orthosis, with adjustable position locking joint(s), prefabricated, includes fitting and adjustments, any type

* **L3762** Elbow orthosis, rigid, without joints, includes soft interface material, prefabricated, includes fitting and adjustment

* **L3763** Elbow wrist hand orthosis, rigid, without joints, may include soft interface, straps, custom fabricated, includes fitting and adjustment

* **L3764** Elbow wrist hand orthosis, includes one or more nontorsion joints, elastic bands, turnbuckles, may include soft interface, straps, custom fabricated, includes fitting and adjustment

* **L3765** Elbow wrist hand finger orthosis, rigid, without joints, may include soft interface, straps, custom fabricated, includes fitting and adjustment

* **L3766** Elbow wrist hand finger orthosis, includes one or more nontorsion joints, elastic bands, turnbuckles, may include soft interface, straps, custom fabricated, includes fitting and adjustment

Wrist-Hand-Finger Orthosis (WHFO)

* **L3806** Wrist hand finger orthosis, includes one or more nontorsion joint(s), turnbuckles, elastic bands/springs, may include soft interface material, straps, custom fabricated, includes fitting and adjustment

* **L3807** Wrist hand finger orthosis, without joint(s), prefabricated, includes fitting and adjustments, any type

* **L3808** Wrist hand finger orthosis, rigid without joints, may include soft interface material; straps, custom fabricated, includes fitting and adjustment

Additions and Extensions

◆ **L3891** Addition to upper extremity joint, wrist or elbow, concentric adjustable torsion style mechanism for custom fabricated orthotics only, each

* **L3900** Wrist hand finger orthosis, dynamic flexor hinge, reciprocal wrist extension/flexion, finger flexion/extension, wrist or finger driven, custom-fabricated

* **L3901** Wrist hand finger orthosis, dynamic flexor hinge, reciprocal wrist extension/flexion, finger flexion/extension, cable driven, custom-fabricated

External Power

* **L3904** Wrist hand finger orthosis, external powered, electric, custom-fabricated

* **L3905** Wrist hand orthosis, includes one or more nontorsion joints, elastic bands, turnbuckles, may include soft interface, straps, custom fabricated, includes fitting and adjustment

Other Wrist-Hand-Finger Orthoses: Custom Fitted

* **L3906** Wrist hand orthosis, without joints, may include soft interface, straps, custom fabricated, includes fitting and adjustment

* **L3908** Wrist hand orthosis, wrist extension control cock-up, non molded, prefabricated, includes fitting and adjustment

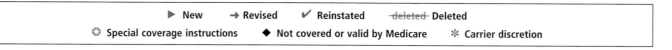

▶ New   → Revised   ✔ Reinstated   deleted Deleted

☺ Special coverage instructions   ◆ Not covered or valid by Medicare   * Carrier discretion

＊ **L3912** Hand finger orthosis, flexion glove with elastic finger control, prefabricated, includes fitting and adjustment

＊ **L3913** Hand finger orthosis, without joints, may include soft interface, straps, custom fabricated, includes fitting and adjustment

＊ **L3915** Wrist hand orthosis, includes one or more nontorsion joint(s), elastic bands, turnbuckles, may include soft interface, straps, prefabricated, includes fitting and adjustment

＊ **L3917** Hand orthosis, metacarpal fracture orthosis, prefabricated, includes fitting and adjustment

＊ **L3919** Hand orthosis, without joints, may include soft interface, straps, custom fabricated, includes fitting and adjustment

＊ **L3921** Hand finger orthosis, includes one or more nontorsion joints, elastic bands, turnbuckles, may include soft interface, straps, custom fabricated, includes fitting and adjustment

＊ **L3923** Hand finger orthosis, without joints, may include soft interface, straps, prefabricated, includes fitting and adjustments

＊ **L3925** Finger orthosis, proximal interphalangeal (PIP)/distal interphalangeal (DIP), non torsion joint/spring, extension/flexion, may include soft interface material, prefabricated, includes fitting and adjustment

＊ **L3927** Finger orthosis, proximal interphalangeal (PIP)/distal interphalangeal (DIP), without joint/spring, extension/flexion (e.g. static or ring type), may include soft interface material, prefabricated, includes fitting and adjustment

＊ **L3929** Hand finger orthosis, includes one or more nontorsion joint(s), turnbuckles, elastic bands/springs, may include soft interface material, straps, prefabricated, includes fitting and adjustment

＊ **L3931** Wrist hand finger orthosis, includes one or more nontorsion joint(s), turnbuckles, elastic bands/springs, may include soft interface material, straps, prefabricated, includes fitting and adjustment

＊ **L3933** Finger orthosis, without joints, may include soft interface, custom fabricated, includes fitting and adjustment

＊ **L3935** Finger orthosis, nontorsion joint, may include soft interface, custom fabricated, includes fitting and adjustment

＊ **L3956** Addition of joint to upper extremity orthosis, any material, per joint

Shoulder-Elbow-Wrist-Hand Orthosis (SEWHO)

Abduction Positioning: Custom Fitted

L3960-L4631: Bill DME/MAC

＊ **L3960** Shoulder elbow wrist hand orthosis, abduction positioning, airplane design, prefabricated, includes fitting and adjustment

＊ **L3961** Shoulder elbow wrist hand orthosis, shoulder cap design, without joints, may include soft interface, straps, custom fabricated, includes fitting and adjustment

＊ **L3962** Shoulder elbow wrist hand orthosis, abduction positioning, Erbs palsy design, prefabricated, includes fitting and adjustment

~~L3964~~ ~~Shoulder elbow orthosis, mobile arm support attached to wheelchair, balanced, adjustable, prefabricated, includes fitting and adjustment~~ ✖

~~L3965~~ ~~Shoulder elbow orthosis, mobile arm support attached to wheelchair, balanced, adjustable Rancho type, prefabricated, includes fitting and adjustment~~ ✖

~~L3966~~ ~~Shoulder elbow orthosis, mobile arm support attached to wheelchair, balanced, reclining, prefabricated, includes fitting and adjustment~~ ✖

＊ **L3967** Shoulder elbow wrist hand orthosis, abduction positioning (airplane design), thoracic component and support bar, without joints, may include soft interface, straps, custom fabricated, includes fitting and adjustment

~~L3968~~ ~~Shoulder elbow orthosis, mobile arm support attached to wheelchair, balanced, friction arm support (friction dampening to proximal and distal joints), prefabricated, includes fitting and adjustment~~ ✖

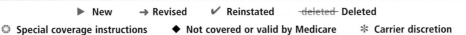

▶ New   → Revised   ✔ Reinstated   ~~deleted~~ Deleted
☉ Special coverage instructions   ◆ Not covered or valid by Medicare   ＊ Carrier discretion

L3969 Shoulder elbow orthosis, mobile arm ✖
support, monosuspension arm and
hand support, overhead elbow forearm
hand sling support, yoke type
suspension support, prefabricated,
includes fitting and adjustment

Additions to Mobile Arm Supports and SEWHO

L3970 SEO, addition to mobile arm support, ✖
elevating proximal arm

✳ **L3971** Shoulder elbow wrist hand orthosis,
shoulder cap design, includes one or
more nontorsion joints, elastic bands,
turnbuckles, may include soft interface,
straps, custom fabricated, includes
fitting and adjustment

L3972 SEO, addition to mobile arm support, ✖
offset or lateral rocker arm with elastic
balance control

✳ **L3973** Shoulder elbow wrist hand orthosis,
abduction positioning (airplane design),
thoracic component and support bar,
includes one or more nontorsion joints,
elastic bands, turnbuckles, may include
soft interface, straps, custom
fabricated, includes fitting and
adjustment

L3974 SEO, addition to mobile arm support, ✖
supinator

✳ **L3975** Shoulder elbow wrist hand finger
orthosis, shoulder cap design, without
joints, may include soft interface,
straps, custom fabricated, includes
fitting and adjustment

✳ **L3976** Shoulder elbow wrist hand finger
orthosis, abduction positioning
(airplane design), thoracic component
and support bar, without joints, may
include soft interface, straps, custom
fabricated, includes fitting and
adjustment

✳ **L3977** Shoulder elbow wrist hand finger
orthosis, shoulder cap design, includes
one or more nontorsion joints, elastic
bands, turnbuckles, may include
soft interface, straps, custom
fabricated, includes fitting and
adjustment

✳ **L3978** Shoulder elbow wrist hand finger
orthosis, abduction positioning
(airplane design), thoracic component
and support bar, includes one or more
nontorsion joints, elastic bands,
turnbuckles, may include soft interface,
straps, custom fabricated, includes
fitting and adjustment

Fracture Orthoses

✳ **L3980** Upper extremity fracture orthosis,
humeral, prefabricated, includes fitting
and adjustment

✳ **L3982** Upper extremity fracture orthosis,
radius/ulnar, prefabricated, includes
fitting and adjustment

✳ **L3984** Upper extremity fracture orthosis,
wrist, prefabricated, includes fitting
and adjustment

✳ **L3995** Addition to upper extremity orthosis,
sock, fracture or equal, each

✳ **L3999** Upper limb orthosis, not otherwise
specified

Specific Repair

✳ **L4000** Replace girdle for spinal orthosis
(CTLSO or SO)

✳ **L4002** Replacement strap, any orthosis,
includes all components, any length,
any type

✳ **L4010** Replace trilateral socket brim

✳ **L4020** Replace quadrilateral socket brim,
molded to patient model

✳ **L4030** Replace quadrilateral socket brim,
custom fitted

✳ **L4040** Replace molded thigh lacer, for custom
fabricated orthosis only

✳ **L4045** Replace non-molded thigh lacer, for
custom fabricated orthosis only

✳ **L4050** Replace molded calf lacer, for custom
fabricated orthosis only

✳ **L4055** Replace non-molded calf lacer, for
custom fabricated orthosis only

✳ **L4060** Replace high roll cuff

✳ **L4070** Replace proximal and distal upright
for KAFO

✳ **L4080** Replace metal bands KAFO, proximal
thigh

✳ **L4090** Replace metal bands KAFO-AFO, calf
or distal thigh

✳ **L4100** Replace leather cuff KAFO, proximal
thigh

✳ **L4110** Replace leather cuff KAFO-AFO,
calf or distal thigh

✳ **L4130** Replace pretibial shell

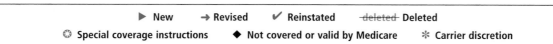

▶ New   → Revised   ✔ Reinstated   deleted Deleted

☉ Special coverage instructions   ◆ Not covered or valid by Medicare   ✳ Carrier discretion

Repairs

⊘ **L4205** Repair of orthotic device, labor component, per 15 minutes
IOM: 100-02, 15, 110.2

⊘ **L4210** Repair of orthotic device, repair or replace minor parts
IOM: 100-02, 15, 110.2; 100-02, 15, 120

Ancillary Orthotic Services

✳ **L4350** Ankle control orthosis, stirrup style, rigid, includes any type interface (e.g., pneumatic, gel), prefabricated, includes fitting and adjustment

✳ **L4360** Walking boot, pneumatic, and/or vacuum, with or without joints, with or without interface material, prefabricated, includes fitting and adjustment

Noncovered when walking boots used primarily to relieve pressure, especially on sole of foot, or are used for patients with foot ulcers

✳ **L4370** Pneumatic full leg splint, prefabricated, includes fitting and adjustment

~~L4380 Pneumatic knee splint, prefabricated, includes fitting and adjustment~~ ✖

✳ **L4386** Walking boot, non-pneumatic, with or without joints, with or without interface material, prefabricated, includes fitting and adjustment

✳ **L4392** Replacement, soft interface material, static AFO

✳ **L4394** Replace soft interface material, foot drop splint

✳ **L4396** Static or dynamic ankle foot orthosis, including soft interface material, adjustable for fit, for positioning, may be used for minimal ambulation, prefabricated, includes fitting and adjustment

✳ **L4398** Foot drop splint, recumbent positioning device, prefabricated, includes fitting and adjustment

▶ ✳ **L4631** Ankle foot orthosis, walking boot type, varus/valgus correction, rocker bottom, anterior tibial shell, soft interface, custom arch support, plastic or other material, includes straps and closures, custom fabricated

PROSTHETICS (L5000-L9999)

Lower Limb (L5000-L5999)

NOTE: The procedures in this section are considered as *base* or *basic procedures* and may be modified by listing items/procedures or special materials from the Additions section and adding them to the base procedure.

Partial Foot

L5000-L5999:   Bill DME/MAC

⊘ **L5000** Partial foot, shoe insert with longitudinal arch, toe filler
IOM: 100-02, 15, 290

⊘ **L5010** Partial foot, molded socket, ankle height, with toe filler
IOM: 100-02, 15, 290

⊘ **L5020** Partial foot, molded socket, tibial tubercle height, with toe filler
IOM: 100-02, 15, 290

Ankle

✳ **L5050** Ankle, Symes, molded socket, SACH foot

✳ **L5060** Ankle, Symes, metal frame, molded leather socket, articulated ankle/foot

Below Knee

✳ **L5100** Below knee, molded socket, shin, SACH foot

✳ **L5105** Below knee, plastic socket, joints and thigh lacer, SACH foot

Knee Disarticulation

✳ **L5150** Knee disarticulation (or through knee), molded socket, external knee joints, shin, SACH foot

✳ **L5160** Knee disarticulation (or through knee), molded socket, bent knee configuration, external knee joints, shin, SACH foot

Above Knee

✳ **L5200** Above knee, molded socket, single axis constant friction knee, shin, SACH foot

✳ **L5210** Above knee, short prosthesis, no knee joint ('stubbies'), with foot blocks, no ankle joints, each

---

▶ New   → Revised   ✔ Reinstated   ~~deleted~~ Deleted

⊘ Special coverage instructions   ◆ Not covered or valid by Medicare   ✳ Carrier discretion

* **L5220** Above knee, short prosthesis, no knee joint ('stubbies'), with articulated ankle/foot, dynamically aligned, each

* **L5230** Above knee, for proximal femoral focal deficiency, constant friction knee, shin, SACH foot

Hip Disarticulation

* **L5250** Hip disarticulation, Canadian type; molded socket, hip joint, single axis constant friction knee, shin, SACH foot

* **L5270** Hip disarticulation, tilt table type; molded socket, locking hip joint, single axis constant friction knee, shin, SACH foot

Hemipelvectomy

* **L5280** Hemipelvectomy, Canadian type; molded socket, hip joint, single axis constant friction knee, shin, SACH foot

Endoskeleton: Below Knee

* **L5301** Below knee, molded socket, shin, SACH foot, endoskeletal system

~~L5311~~ ~~Knee disarticulation (or through knee), molded socket, external knee joints, shin, SACH foot, endoskeletal system~~ ✖

▶ * **L5312** Knee disarticulation (or through knee), molded socket, single axis knee, pylon, sach foot, endoskeletal system

Endoskeletal: Above Knee

* **L5321** Above knee, molded socket, open end, SACH foot, endoskeletal system, single axis knee

Endoskeletal: Hip Disarticulation

* **L5331** Hip disarticulation, Canadian type, molded socket, endoskeletal system, hip joint, single axis knee, SACH foot

Endoskeletal: Hemipelvectomy

* **L5341** Hemipelvectomy, Canadian type, molded socket, endoskeletal system, hip joint, single axis knee, SACH foot

Immediate Postsurgical or Early Fitting Procedures

* **L5400** Immediate post surgical or early fitting, application of initial rigid dressing, including fitting, alignment, suspension, and one cast change, below knee

* **L5410** Immediate post surgical or early fitting, application of initial rigid dressing, including fitting, alignment and suspension, below knee, each additional cast change and realignment

* **L5420** Immediate post surgical or early fitting, application of initial rigid dressing, including fitting, alignment and suspension and one cast change 'AK' or knee disarticulation

* **L5430** Immediate postsurgical or early fitting, application of initial rigid dressing, including fitting, alignment, and suspension, 'AK' or knee disarticulation, each additional cast change and realignment

* **L5450** Immediate post surgical or early fitting, application of non-weight bearing rigid dressing, below knee

* **L5460** Immediate post surgical or early fitting, application of non-weight bearing rigid dressing, above knee

Initial Prosthesis

* **L5500** Initial, below knee 'PTB' type socket, non-alignable system, pylon, no cover, SACH foot, plaster socket, direct formed

* **L5505** Initial, above knee–knee disarticulation, ischial level socket, non-alignable system, pylon, no cover, SACH foot, plaster socket, direct formed

Preparatory Prosthesis

* **L5510** Preparatory, below knee 'PTB' type socket, non-alignable system, pylon, no cover, SACH foot, plaster socket, molded to model

* **L5520** Preparatory, below knee 'PTB' type socket, non-alignable system, pylon, no cover, SACH foot, thermoplastic or equal, direct formed

* **L5530** Preparatory, below knee 'PTB' type socket, non-alignable system, pylon, no cover, SACH foot, thermoplastic or equal, molded to model

* **L5535** Preparatory, below knee 'PTB' type socket, non-alignable system, no cover, SACH foot, prefabricated, adjustable open end socket

---

▶ New   → Revised   ✔ Reinstated   ~~deleted~~ Deleted
⊘ Special coverage instructions   ◆ Not covered or valid by Medicare   * Carrier discretion

* **L5540** Preparatory, below knee 'PTB' type socket, non-alignable system, pylon, no cover, SACH foot, laminated socket, molded to model

* **L5560** Preparatory, above knee - knee disarticulation, ischial level socket, non-alignable system, pylon, no cover, SACH foot, plaster socket, molded to model

* **L5570** Preparatory, above knee - knee disarticulation, ischial level socket, non-alignable system, pylon, no cover, SACH foot, thermoplastic or equal, direct formed

* **L5580** Preparatory, above knee - knee disarticulation, ischial level socket, non-alignable system, pylon, no cover, SACH foot, thermoplastic or equal, molded to model

* **L5585** Preparatory, above knee - knee disarticulation, ischial level socket, non-alignable system, pylon, no cover, SACH foot, prefabricated adjustable open end socket

* **L5590** Preparatory, above knee - knee disarticulation, ischial level socket, non-alignable system, pylon, no cover, SACH foot, laminated socket, molded to model

* **L5595** Preparatory, hip disarticulation-hemipelvectomy, pylon, no cover, SACH foot, thermoplastic or equal, molded to patient model

* **L5600** Preparatory, hip disarticulation-hemipelvectomy, pylon, no cover, SACH foot, laminated socket, molded to patient model

Additions to Lower Extremity

* **L5610** Addition to lower extremity, endoskeletal system, above knee, hydracadence system

* **L5611** Addition to lower extremity, endoskeletal system, above knee-knee disarticulation, 4 bar linkage, with friction swing phase control

* **L5613** Addition to lower extremity, endoskeletal system, above knee-knee disarticulation, 4 bar linkage, with hydraulic swing phase control

* **L5614** Addition to lower extremity, exoskeletal system, above knee-knee disarticulation, 4 bar linkage, with pneumatic swing phase control

* **L5616** Addition to lower extremity, endoskeletal system, above knee, universal multiplex system, friction swing phase control

* **L5617** Addition to lower extremity, quick change self-aligning unit, above knee or below knee, each

Additions to Test Sockets

* **L5618** Addition to lower extremity, test socket, Symes

* **L5620** Addition to lower extremity, test socket, below knee

* **L5622** Addition to lower extremity, test socket, knee disarticulation

* **L5624** Addition to lower extremity, test socket, above knee

* **L5626** Addition to lower extremity, test socket, hip disarticulation

* **L5628** Addition to lower extremity, test socket, hemipelvectomy

* **L5629** Addition to lower extremity, below knee, acrylic socket

Additions to Socket Variations

* **L5630** Addition to lower extremity, Symes type, expandable wall socket

* **L5631** Addition to lower extremity, above knee or knee disarticulation, acrylic socket

* **L5632** Addition to lower extremity, Symes type, 'PTB' brim design socket

* **L5634** Addition to lower extremity, Symes type, posterior opening (Canadian) socket

* **L5636** Addition to lower extremity, Symes type, medial opening socket

* **L5637** Addition to lower extremity, below knee, total contact

* **L5638** Addition to lower extremity, below knee, leather socket

* **L5639** Addition to lower extremity, below knee, wood socket

* **L5640** Addition to lower extremity, knee disarticulation, leather socket

* **L5642** Addition to lower extremity, above knee, leather socket

* **L5643** Addition to lower extremity, hip disarticulation, flexible inner socket, external frame

* **L5644** Addition to lower extremity, above knee, wood socket

---

▶ New → Revised ✔ Reinstated ~~deleted~~ Deleted

☉ Special coverage instructions ◆ Not covered or valid by Medicare ✳ Carrier discretion

* **L5645** Addition to lower extremity, below knee, flexible inner socket, external frame

* **L5646** Addition to lower extremity, below knee, air, fluid, gel or equal, cushion socket

* **L5647** Addition to lower extremity, below knee, suction socket

* **L5648** Addition to lower extremity, above knee, air, fluid, gel or equal, cushion socket

* **L5649** Addition to lower extremity, ischial containment/narrow M-L socket

* **L5650** Additions to lower extremity, total contact, above knee or knee disarticulation socket

* **L5651** Addition to lower extremity, above knee, flexible inner socket, external frame

* **L5652** Addition to lower extremity, suction suspension, above knee or knee disarticulation socket

* **L5653** Addition to lower extremity, knee disarticulation, expandable wall socket

Additions to Socket Insert and Suspension

* **L5654** Addition to lower extremity, socket insert, Symes, (Kemblo, Pelite, Aliplast, Plastazote or equal)

* **L5655** Addition to lower extremity, socket insert, below knee (Kemblo, Pelite, Aliplast, Plastazote or equal)

* **L5656** Addition to lower extremity, socket insert, knee disarticulation (Kemblo, Pelite, Aliplast, Plastazote or equal)

* **L5658** Addition to lower extremity, socket insert, above knee (Kemblo, Pelite, Aliplast, Plastazote or equal)

* **L5661** Addition to lower extremity, socket insert, multi-durometer Symes

* **L5665** Addition to lower extremity, socket insert, multi-durometer, below knee

* **L5666** Addition to lower extremity, below knee, cuff suspension

* **L5668** Addition to lower extremity, below knee, molded distal cushion

* **L5670** Addition to lower extremity, below knee, molded supracondylar suspension ('PTS' or similar)

* **L5671** Addition to lower extremity, below knee/above knee suspension locking mechanism (shuttle, lanyard or equal), excludes socket insert

* **L5672** Addition to lower extremity, below knee, removable medial brim suspension

* **L5673** Addition to lower extremity, below knee/above knee, custom fabricated from existing mold or prefabricated, socket insert, silicone gel, elastomeric or equal, for use with locking mechanism

* **L5676** Additions to lower extremity, below knee, knee joints, single axis, pair

* **L5677** Additions to lower extremity, below knee, knee joints, polycentric, pair

* **L5678** Additions to lower extremity, below knee, joint covers, pair

* **L5679** Addition to lower extremity, below knee/above knee, custom fabricated from existing mold or prefabricated, socket insert, silicone gel, elastomeric or equal, not for use with locking mechanism

* **L5680** Addition to lower extremity, below knee, thigh lacer, nonmolded

* **L5681** Addition to lower extremity, below knee/above knee, custom fabricated socket insert for congenital or atypical traumatic amputee, silicone gel, elastomeric or equal, for use with or without locking mechanism, initial only (for other than initial, use code L5673 or L5679)

* **L5682** Addition to lower extremity, below knee, thigh lacer, gluteal/ischial, molded

* **L5683** Addition to lower extremity, below knee/above knee, custom fabricated socket insert for other than congenital or atypical traumatic amputee, silicone gel, elastomeric, or equal, for use with or without locking mechanism, initial only (for other than initial, use code L5673 or L5679)

* **L5684** Addition to lower extremity, below knee, fork strap

* **L5685** Addition to lower extremity prosthesis, below knee, suspension/sealing sleeve, with or without valve, any material, each

* **L5686** Addition to lower extremity, below knee, back check (extension control)

* **L5688** Addition to lower extremity, below knee, waist belt, webbing

* **L5690** Addition to lower extremity, below knee, waist belt, padded and lined

* **L5692** Addition to lower extremity, above knee, pelvic control belt, light

* **L5694** Addition to lower extremity, above knee, pelvic control belt, padded and lined

* **L5695** Addition to lower extremity, above knee, pelvic control, sleeve suspension, neoprene or equal, each

▶ New → Revised ✔ Reinstated deleted Deleted

⊘ Special coverage instructions ◆ Not covered or valid by Medicare * Carrier discretion

* **L5696** Addition to lower extremity, above knee or knee disarticulation, pelvic joint

* **L5697** Addition to lower extremity, above knee or knee disarticulation, pelvic band

* **L5698** Addition to lower extremity, above knee or knee disarticulation, Silesian bandage

* **L5699** All lower extremity prostheses, shoulder harness

Additions/Replacements to Feet-Ankle Units

* **L5700** Replacement, socket, below knee, molded to patient model

* **L5701** Replacement, socket, above knee/knee disarticulation, including attachment plate, molded to patient model

* **L5702** Replacement, socket, hip disarticulation, including hip joint, molded to patient model

* **L5703** Ankle, Symes, molded to patient model, socket without solid ankle cushion heel (SACH) foot, replacement only

* **L5704** Custom shaped protective cover, below knee

* **L5705** Custom shaped protective cover, above knee

* **L5706** Custom shaped protective cover, knee disarticulation

* **L5707** Custom shaped protective cover, hip disarticulation

Additions to Exoskeletal–Knee-Shin System

* **L5710** Addition, exoskeletal knee-shin system, single axis, manual lock

* **L5711** Additions exoskeletal knee-shin system, single axis, manual lock, ultra-light material

* **L5712** Addition, exoskeletal knee-shin system, single axis, friction swing and stance phase control (safety knee)

* **L5714** Addition, exoskeletal knee-shin system, single axis, variable friction swing phase control

* **L5716** Addition, exoskeletal knee-shin system, polycentric, mechanical stance phase lock

* **L5718** Addition, exoskeletal knee-shin system, polycentric, friction swing and stance phase control

* **L5722** Addition, exoskeletal knee-shin system, single axis, pneumatic swing, friction stance phase control

* **L5724** Addition, exoskeletal knee-shin system, single axis, fluid swing phase control

* **L5726** Addition, exoskeletal knee-shin system, single axis, external joints, fluid swing phase control

* **L5728** Addition, exoskeletal knee-shin system, single axis, fluid swing and stance phase control

* **L5780** Addition, exoskeletal knee-shin system, single axis, pneumatic/hydra pneumatic swing phase control

* **L5781** Addition to lower limb prosthesis, vacuum pump, residual limb volume management and moisture evacuation system

* **L5782** Addition to lower limb prosthesis, vacuum pump, residual limb volume management and moisture evacuation system, heavy duty

Component Modification

* **L5785** Addition, exoskeletal system, below knee, ultra-light material (titanium, carbon fiber, or equal)

* **L5790** Addition, exoskeletal system, above knee, ultra-light material (titanium, carbon fiber, or equal)

* **L5795** Addition, exoskeletal system, hip disarticulation, ultra-light material (titanium, carbon fiber, or equal)

Endoskeletal

* **L5810** Addition, endoskeletal knee-shin system, single axis, manual lock

* **L5811** Addition, endoskeletal knee-shin system, single axis, manual lock, ultralight material

* **L5812** Addition, endoskeletal knee-shin system, single axis, friction swing and stance phase control (safety knee)

* **L5814** Addition, endoskeletal knee-shin system, polycentric, hydraulic swing phase control, mechanical stance phase lock

* **L5816** Addition, endoskeletal knee-shin system, polycentric, mechanical stance phase lock

* **L5818** Addition, endoskeletal knee-shin system, polycentric, friction swing, and stance phase control

* **L5822** Addition, endoskeletal knee-shin system, single axis, pneumatic swing, friction stance phase control

* **L5824** Addition, endoskeletal knee-shin system, single axis, fluid swing phase control

* **L5826** Addition, endoskeletal knee-shin system, single axis, hydraulic swing phase control, with miniature high activity frame

---

▶ New   → Revised   ✔ Reinstated   deleted Deleted
☺ Special coverage instructions   ◆ Not covered or valid by Medicare   * Carrier discretion

✳ **L5828** Addition, endoskeletal knee-shin system, single axis, fluid swing and stance phase control

✳ **L5830** Addition, endoskeletal knee-shin system, single axis, pneumatic/swing phase control

✳ **L5840** Addition, endoskeletal knee/shin system, 4-bar linkage or multiaxial, pneumatic swing phase control

✳ **L5845** Addition, endoskeletal, knee-shin system, stance flexion feature, adjustable

✳ **L5848** Addition to endoskeletal, knee-shin system, fluid stance extension, dampening feature, with or without adjustability

✳ **L5850** Addition, endoskeletal system, above knee or hip disarticulation, knee extension assist

✳ **L5855** Addition, endoskeletal system, hip disarticulation, mechanical hip extension assist

✳ **L5856** Addition to lower extremity prosthesis, endoskeletal knee-shin system, microprocessor control feature, swing and stance phase; includes electronic sensor(s), any type

✳ **L5857** Addition to lower extremity prosthesis, endoskeletal knee-shin system, microprocessor control feature, swing phase only; includes electronic sensor(s), any type

✳ **L5858** Addition to lower extremity prosthesis, endoskeletal knee shin system, microprocessor control feature, stance phase only, includes electronic sensor(s), any type

✳ **L5910** Addition, endoskeletal system, below knee, alignable system

✳ **L5920** Addition, endoskeletal system, above knee or hip disarticulation, alignable system

✳ **L5925** Addition, endoskeletal system, above knee, knee disarticulation or hip disarticulation, manual lock

✳ **L5930** Addition, endoskeletal system, high activity knee control frame

✳ **L5940** Addition, endoskeletal system, below knee, ultra-light material (titanium, carbon fiber or equal)

✳ **L5950** Addition, endoskeletal system, above knee, ultra-light material (titanium, carbon fiber or equal)

✳ **L5960** Addition, endoskeletal system, hip disarticulation, ultra-light material (titanium, carbon fiber, or equal)

▶ ✳ **L5961** Addition, endoskeletal system, polycentric hip joint, pneumatic or hydraulic control, rotation control, with or without flexion, and/or extension control

✳ **L5962** Addition, endoskeletal system, below knee, flexible protective outer surface covering system

✳ **L5964** Addition, endoskeletal system, above knee, flexible protective outer surface covering system

✳ **L5966** Addition, endoskeletal system, hip disarticulation, flexible protective outer surface covering system

✳ **L5968** Addition to lower limb prosthesis, multiaxial ankle with swing phase active dorsiflexion feature

✳ **L5970** All lower extremity prostheses, foot, external keel, SACH foot

✳ **L5971** All lower extremity prosthesis, solid ankle cushion keel (SACH) foot, replacement only

✳ **L5972** All lower extremity prostheses, flexible heel foot (Safe, Sten, Bock Dynamic or equal)

✳ **L5973** Endoskeletal ankle foot system, microprocessor controlled feature, dorsiflexion and/or plantar flexion control, includes power source

✳ **L5974** All lower extremity prostheses, foot, single axis ankle/foot

✳ **L5975** All lower extremity prostheses, combination single axis ankle and flexible keel foot

✳ **L5976** All lower extremity prostheses, energy storing foot (Seattle Carbon Copy II or equal)

✳ **L5978** All lower extremity prostheses, foot, multiaxial ankle/foot

✳ **L5979** All lower extremity prostheses, multiaxial ankle, dynamic response foot, one piece system

✳ **L5980** All lower extremity prostheses, flex foot system

✳ **L5981** All lower extremity prostheses, flexwalk system or equal

✳ **L5982** All exoskeletal lower extremity prostheses, axial rotation unit

✳ **L5984** All endoskeletal lower extremity prostheses, axial rotation unit, with or without adjustability

✳ **L5985** All endoskeletal lower extremity prostheses, dynamic prosthetic pylon

✳ **L5986** All lower extremity prostheses, multiaxial rotation unit ('MCP' or equal)

▶ New   → Revised   ✔ Reinstated   ~~deleted~~ Deleted
⊙ Special coverage instructions   ◆ Not covered or valid by Medicare   ✳ Carrier discretion

* **L5987** All lower extremity prostheses, shank foot system with vertical loading pylon
* **L5988** Addition to lower limb prosthesis, vertical shock reducing pylon feature
* **L5990** Addition to lower extremity prosthesis, user adjustable heel height
* **L5999** Lower extremity prosthesis, not otherwise specified

Upper Limb

NOTE: The procedures in L6000-L6599 are considered as base or basic procedures and may be modified by listing procedures from the additions sections. The base procedures include only standard friction wrist and control cable system unless otherwise specified.

Partial Hand

L6000-L6698:   Bill DME/MAC

→ * **L6000** Partial hand, thumb remaining
→ * **L6010** Partial hand, little and/or ring finger remaining
→ * **L6020** Partial hand, no finger remaining
  * **L6025** Transcarpal/metacarpal or partial hand disarticulation prosthesis, external power, self-suspended, inner socket with removable forearm section, electrodes and cables, two batteries, charger, myoelectric control of terminal device

Wrist Disarticulation

* **L6050** Wrist disarticulation, molded socket, flexible elbow hinges, triceps pad
* **L6055** Wrist disarticulation, molded socket with expandable interface, flexible elbow hinges, triceps pad

Below Elbow

* **L6100** Below elbow, molded socket, flexible elbow hinge, triceps pad
* **L6110** Below elbow, molded socket, (Muenster or Northwestern suspension types)
* **L6120** Below elbow, molded double wall split socket, step-up hinges, half cuff
* **L6130** Below elbow, molded double wall split socket, stump activated locking hinge, half cuff

Elbow Disarticulation

* **L6200** Elbow disarticulation, molded socket, outside locking hinge, forearm

* **L6205** Elbow disarticulation, molded socket with expandable interface, outside locking hinges, forearm

Above Elbow

* **L6250** Above elbow, molded double wall socket, internal locking elbow, forearm

Shoulder Disarticulation

* **L6300** Shoulder disarticulation, molded socket, shoulder bulkhead, humeral section, internal locking elbow, forearm
* **L6310** Shoulder disarticulation, passive restoration (complete prosthesis)
* **L6320** Shoulder disarticulation, passive restoration (shoulder cap only)

Interscapular Thoracic

* **L6350** Interscapular thoracic, molded socket, shoulder bulkhead, humeral section, internal locking elbow, forearm
* **L6360** Interscapular thoracic, passive restoration (complete prosthesis)
* **L6370** Interscapular thoracic, passive restoration (shoulder cap only)

Immediate and Early Postsurgical Procedures

* **L6380** Immediate post surgical or early fitting, application of initial rigid dressing, including fitting alignment and suspension of components, and one cast change, wrist disarticulation or below elbow
* **L6382** Immediate post surgical or early fitting, application of initial rigid dressing including fitting alignment and suspension of components, and one cast change, elbow disarticulation or above elbow
* **L6384** Immediate post surgical or early fitting, application of initial rigid dressing including fitting alignment and suspension of components, and one cast change, shoulder disarticulation or interscapular thoracic
* **L6386** Immediate post surgical or early fitting, each additional cast change and realignment
* **L6388** Immediate post surgical or early fitting, application of rigid dressing only

---

▶ New   → Revised   ✔ Reinstated   ~~deleted~~ Deleted

☺ Special coverage instructions   ◆ Not covered or valid by Medicare   * Carrier discretion

Endoskeletal: Below Elbow

✳ **L6400** Below elbow, molded socket, endoskeletal system, including soft prosthetic tissue shaping

Endoskeletal: Elbow Disarticulation

✳ **L6450** Elbow disarticulation, molded socket, endoskeletal system, including soft prosthetic tissue shaping

Endoskeletal: Above Elbow

✳ **L6500** Above elbow, molded socket, endoskeletal system, including soft prosthetic tissue shaping

Endoskeletal: Shoulder Disarticulation

✳ **L6550** Shoulder disarticulation, molded socket, endoskeletal system, including soft prosthetic tissue shaping

Endoskeletal: Interscapular Thoracic

✳ **L6570** Interscapular thoracic, molded socket, endoskeletal system, including soft prosthetic tissue shaping

✳ **L6580** Preparatory, wrist disarticulation or below elbow, single wall plastic socket, friction wrist, flexible elbow hinges, figure of eight harness, humeral cuff, Bowden cable control, USMC or equal pylon, no cover, molded to patient model

✳ **L6582** Preparatory, wrist disarticulation or below elbow, single wall socket, friction wrist, flexible elbow hinges, figure of eight harness, humeral cuff, Bowden cable control, USMC or equal pylon, no cover, direct formed

✳ **L6584** Preparatory, elbow disarticulation or above elbow, single wall plastic socket, friction wrist, locking elbow, figure of eight harness, fair lead cable control, USMC or equal pylon, no cover, molded to patient model

✳ **L6586** Preparatory, elbow disarticulation or above elbow, single wall socket, friction wrist, locking elbow, figure of eight harness, fair lead cable control, USMC or equal pylon, no cover, direct formed

✳ **L6588** Preparatory, shoulder disarticulation or interscapular thoracic, single wall plastic socket, shoulder joint, locking elbow, friction wrist, chest strap, fair lead cable control, USMC or equal pylon, no cover, molded to patient model

✳ **L6590** Preparatory, shoulder disarticulation or interscapular thoracic, single wall socket, shoulder joint, locking elbow, friction wrist, chest strap, fair lead cable control, USMC or equal pylon, no cover, direct formed

Additions to Upper Limb

NOTE: The following procedures/modifications/components may be added to other base procedures. The items in this section should reflect the additional complexity of each modification procedure, in addition to base procedure, at the time of the original order.

✳ **L6600** Upper extremity additions, polycentric hinge, pair

✳ **L6605** Upper extremity additions, single pivot hinge, pair

✳ **L6610** Upper extremity additions, flexible metal hinge, pair

✳ **L6611** Addition to upper extremity prosthesis, external powered, additional switch, any type

✳ **L6615** Upper extremity addition, disconnect locking wrist unit

✳ **L6616** Upper extremity addition, additional disconnect insert for locking wrist unit, each

✳ **L6620** Upper extremity addition, flexion/extension wrist unit, with or without friction

✳ **L6621** Upper extremity prosthesis addition, flexion/extension wrist with or without friction, for use with external powered terminal device

✳ **L6623** Upper extremity addition, spring assisted rotational wrist unit with latch release

✳ **L6624** Upper extremity addition, flexion/extension and rotation wrist unit

✳ **L6625** Upper extremity addition, rotation wrist unit with cable lock

✳ **L6628** Upper extremity addition, quick disconnect hook adapter, Otto Bock or equal

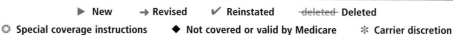

L6400 – L6628 PROSTHETICS

* **L6629** Upper extremity addition, quick disconnect lamination collar with coupling piece, Otto Bock or equal

* **L6630** Upper extremity addition, stainless steel, any wrist

* **L6632** Upper extremity addition, latex suspension sleeve, each

* **L6635** Upper extremity addition, lift assist for elbow

* **L6637** Upper extremity addition, nudge control elbow lock

* **L6638** Upper extremity addition to prosthesis, electric locking feature, only for use with manually powered elbow

* **L6640** Upper extremity additions, shoulder abduction joint, pair

* **L6641** Upper extremity addition, excursion amplifier, pulley type

* **L6642** Upper extremity addition, excursion amplifier, lever type

* **L6645** Upper extremity addition, shoulder flexion-abduction joint, each

* **L6646** Upper extremity addition, shoulder joint, multipositional locking, flexion, adjustable abduction friction control, for use with body powered or external powered system

* **L6647** Upper extremity addition, shoulder lock mechanism, body powered actuator

* **L6648** Upper extremity addition, shoulder lock mechanism, external powered actuator

* **L6650** Upper extremity addition, shoulder universal joint, each

* **L6655** Upper extremity addition, standard control cable, extra

* **L6660** Upper extremity addition, heavy duty control cable

* **L6665** Upper extremity addition, Teflon, or equal, cable lining

* **L6670** Upper extremity addition, hook to hand, cable adapter

* **L6672** Upper extremity addition, harness, chest or shoulder, saddle type

* **L6675** Upper extremity addition, harness, (e.g. figure of eight type), single cable design

* **L6676** Upper extremity addition, harness, (e.g. figure of eight type), dual cable design

* **L6677** Upper extremity addition, harness, triple control, simultaneous operation of terminal device and elbow

* **L6680** Upper extremity addition, test socket, wrist disarticulation or below elbow

* **L6682** Upper extremity addition, test socket, elbow disarticulation or above elbow

* **L6684** Upper extremity addition, test socket, shoulder disarticulation or interscapular thoracic

* **L6686** Upper extremity addition, suction socket

* **L6687** Upper extremity addition, frame type socket, below elbow or wrist disarticulation

* **L6688** Upper extremity addition, frame type socket, above elbow or elbow disarticulation

* **L6689** Upper extremity addition, frame type socket, shoulder disarticulation

* **L6690** Upper extremity addition, frame type socket, interscapular-thoracic

* **L6691** Upper extremity addition, removable insert, each

* **L6692** Upper extremity addition, silicone gel insert or equal, each

* **L6693** Upper extremity addition, locking elbow, forearm counterbalance

* **L6694** Addition to upper extremity prosthesis, below elbow/above elbow, custom fabricated from existing mold or prefabricated, socket insert, silicone gel, elastomeric or equal, for use with locking mechanism

* **L6695** Addition to upper extremity prosthesis, below elbow/above elbow, custom fabricated from existing mold or prefabricated, socket insert, silicone gel, elastomeric or equal, not for use with locking mechanism

* **L6696** Addition to upper extremity prosthesis, below elbow/above elbow, custom fabricated socket insert for congenital or atypical traumatic amputee, silicone gel, elastomeric or equal, for use with or without locking mechanism, initial only (for other than initial, use code L6694 or L6695)

* **L6697** Addition to upper extremity prosthesis, below elbow/above elbow, custom fabricated socket insert for other than congenital or atypical traumatic amputee, silicone gel, elastomeric or equal, for use with or without locking mechanism, initial only (for other than initial, use code L6694 or L6695)

* **L6698** Addition to upper extremity prosthesis, below elbow/above elbow, lock mechanism, excludes socket insert

---

▶ New   → Revised   ✔ Reinstated   ~~deleted~~ Deleted

○ **Special coverage instructions**   ◆ **Not covered or valid by Medicare**   ✳ **Carrier discretion**

Terminal Devices

Hooks

L6703-L6915:   Bill DME/MAC

  * **L6703**   Terminal device, passive hand/mitt, any material, any size

  * **L6704**   Terminal device, sport/recreational/work attachment, any material, any size

  * **L6706**   Terminal device, hook, mechanical, voluntary opening, any material, any size, lined or unlined

  * **L6707**   Terminal device, hook, mechanical, voluntary closing, any material, any size, lined or unlined

  * **L6708**   Terminal device, hand, mechanical, voluntary opening, any material, any size

  * **L6709**   Terminal device, hand, mechanical, voluntary closing, any material, any size

  * **L6711**   Terminal device, hook, mechanical, voluntary opening, any material, any size, lined or unlined, pediatric

  * **L6712**   Terminal device, hook, mechanical, voluntary closing, any material, any size, lined or unlined, pediatric

  * **L6713**   Terminal device, hand, mechanical, voluntary opening, any material, any size, pediatric

  * **L6714**   Terminal device, hand, mechanical, voluntary closing, any material, any size, pediatric

▶ * **L6715**   Terminal device, multiple articulating digit, includes motor(s), initial issue or replacement

  * **L6721**   Terminal device, hook or hand, heavy duty, mechanical, voluntary opening, any material, any size, lined or unlined

  * **L6722**   Terminal device, hook or hand, heavy duty, mechanical, voluntary closing, any material, any size, lined or unlined

  ☉ **L6805**   Addition to terminal device, modifier wrist unit

        IOM: 100-02, 15, 120; 100-04, 3, 10.4

  ☉ **L6810**   Addition to terminal device, precision pinch device

        IOM: 100-02, 15, 120; 100-04, 3, 10.4

Hands

▶ * **L6880**   Electric hand, switch or myoelectric controlled, independently articulating digits, any grasp pattern or combination of grasp patterns, includes motor(s)

  * **L6881**   Automatic grasp feature, addition to upper limb electric prosthetic terminal device

  ☉ **L6882**   Microprocessor control feature, addition to upper limb prosthetic terminal device

        IOM: 100-02, 15, 120; 100-04, 3, 10.4

Replacement Sockets

  * **L6883**   Replacement socket, below elbow/wrist disarticulation, molded to patient model, for use with or without external power

  * **L6884**   Replacement socket, above elbow/elbow disarticulation, molded to patient model, for use with or without external power

  * **L6885**   Replacement socket, shoulder disarticulation/interscapular thoracic, molded to patient model, for use with or without external power

Gloves for Above Hands

  * **L6890**   Addition to upper extremity prosthesis, glove for terminal device, any material, prefabricated, includes fitting and adjustment

  * **L6895**   Addition to upper extremity prosthesis, glove for terminal device, any material, custom fabricated

Hand Restoration

  * **L6900**   Hand restoration (casts, shading and measurements included), partial hand, with glove, thumb or one finger remaining

  * **L6905**   Hand restoration (casts, shading and measurements included), partial hand, with glove, multiple fingers remaining

  * **L6910**   Hand restoration (casts, shading and measurements included), partial hand, with glove, no fingers remaining

  * **L6915**   Hand restoration (shading, and measurements included), replacement glove for above

---

▶ New   → Revised   ✔ Reinstated   ~~deleted~~ Deleted

☉ Special coverage instructions   ◆ Not covered or valid by Medicare   * Carrier discretion

External Power

Base Devices

* **L6920** Wrist disarticulation, external power, self-suspended inner socket, removable forearm shell, Otto Bock or equal switch, cables, two batteries and one charger, switch control of terminal device

Bill DME/MAC

* **L6925** Wrist disarticulation, external power, self-suspended inner socket, removable forearm shell, Otto Bock or equal electrodes, cables, two batteries and one charger, myoelectronic control of terminal device

Bill DME/MAC

* **L6930** Below elbow, external power, self-suspended inner socket, removable forearm shell, Otto Bock or equal switch, cables, two batteries and one charger, switch control of terminal device

Bill DME/MAC

* **L6935** Below elbow, external power, self-suspended inner socket, removable forearm shell, Otto Bock or equal electrodes, cables, two batteries and one charger, myoelectronic control of terminal device

Bill DME/MAC

* **L6940** Elbow disarticulation, external power, molded inner socket, removable humeral shell, outside locking hinges, forearm, Otto Bock or equal switch, cables, two batteries and one charger, switch control of terminal device

Bill DME/MAC

* **L6945** Elbow disarticulation, external power, molded inner socket, removable humeral shell, outside locking hinges, forearm, Otto Bock or equal electrodes, cables, two batteries and one charger, myoelectronic control of terminal device

Bill DME/MAC

* **L6950** Above elbow, external power, molded inner socket, removable humeral shell, internal locking elbow, forearm, Otto Bock or equal switch, cables, two batteries and one charger, switch control of terminal device

Bill DME/MAC

* **L6955** Above elbow, external power, molded inner socket, removable humeral shell, internal locking elbow, forearm, Otto Bock or equal electrodes, cables, two batteries and one charger, myoelectronic control of terminal device

Bill DME/MAC

* **L6960** Shoulder disarticulation, external power, molded inner socket, removable shoulder shell, shoulder bulkhead, humeral section, mechanical elbow, forearm, Otto Bock or equal switch, cables, two batteries and one charger, switch control of terminal device

Bill DME/MAC

* **L6965** Shoulder disarticulation, external power, molded inner socket, removable shoulder shell, shoulder bulkhead, humeral section, mechanical elbow, forearm, Otto Bock or equal electrodes, cables, two batteries and one charger, myoelectronic control of terminal device

Bill DME/MAC

* **L6970** Interscapular-thoracic, external power, molded inner socket, removable shoulder shell, shoulder bulkhead, humeral section, mechanical elbow, forearm, Otto Bock or equal switch, cables, two batteries and one charger, switch control of terminal device

Bill DME/MAC

* **L6975** Interscapular-thoracic, external power, molded inner socket, removable shoulder shell, shoulder bulkhead, humeral section, mechanical elbow, forearm, Otto Bock or equal electrodes, cables, two batteries and one charger, myoelectronic control of terminal device

Bill DME/MAC

Terminal Devices

* **L7007** Electric hand, switch or myoelectric controlled, adult

Bill DME/MAC

* **L7008** Electric hand, switch or myoelectric controlled, pediatric

Bill DME/MAC

* **L7009** Electric hook, switch or myoelectric controlled, adult

Bill DME/MAC

* **L7040** Prehensile actuator, switch controlled

Bill DME/MAC

▶ New   → Revised   ✔ Reinstated   ~~deleted~~ Deleted

⊙ Special coverage instructions   ◆ Not covered or valid by Medicare   * Carrier discretion

* **L7045** Electric hook, switch or myoelectric controlled, pediatric

    Bill DME/MAC

Elbow

* **L7170** Electronic elbow, Hosmer or equal, switch controlled

    Bill DME/MAC

* **L7180** Electronic elbow, microprocessor sequential control of elbow and terminal device

    Bill DME/MAC

* **L7181** Electronic elbow, microprocessor simultaneous control of elbow and terminal device

    Bill DME/MAC

* **L7185** Electronic elbow, adolescent, Variety Village or equal, switch controlled

    Bill DME/MAC

* **L7186** Electronic elbow, child, Variety Village or equal, switch controlled

    Bill DME/MAC

* **L7190** Electronic elbow, adolescent, Variety Village or equal, myoelectronically controlled

    Bill DME/MAC

* **L7191** Electronic elbow, child, Variety Village or equal, myoelectronically controlled

    Bill DME/MAC

* **L7260** Electronic wrist rotator, Otto Bock or equal

    Bill DME/MAC

* **L7261** Electronic wrist rotator, for Utah arm

    Bill DME/MAC

~~L7266~~ ~~Servo control, Steeper or equal~~ ✖

~~L7272~~ ~~Analogue control, UNB or equal~~ ✖

~~L7274~~ ~~Proportional control, 6-12 volt, Liberty, Utah or equal~~ ✖

Battery Components

* **L7360** Six volt battery, each

    Bill DME/MAC

* **L7362** Battery charger, six volt, each

    Bill DME/MAC

* **L7364** Twelve volt battery, each

    Bill DME/MAC

* **L7366** Battery charger, twelve volt, each

    Bill DME/MAC

* **L7367** Lithium ion battery, replacement

    Bill DME/MAC

→ * **L7368** Lithium ion battery charger, replacement only

    Bill DME/MAC

Other/Repair

* **L7400** Addition to upper extremity prosthesis, below elbow/wrist disarticulation, ultralight material (titanium, carbon fiber or equal)

    Bill DME/MAC

* **L7401** Addition to upper extremity prosthesis, above elbow disarticulation, ultralight material (titanium, carbon fiber or equal)

    Bill DME/MAC

* **L7402** Addition to upper extremity prosthesis, shoulder disarticulation/interscapular thoracic, ultralight material (titanium, carbon fiber or equal)

    Bill DME/MAC

* **L7403** Addition to upper extremity prosthesis, below elbow/wrist disarticulation, acrylic material

    Bill DME/MAC

* **L7404** Addition to upper extremity prosthesis, above elbow disarticulation, acrylic material

    Bill DME/MAC

* **L7405** Addition to upper extremity prosthesis, shoulder disarticulation/interscapular thoracic, acrylic material

    Bill DME/MAC

* **L7499** Upper extremity prosthesis, not otherwise specified

    Bill DME/MAC

~~L7500~~ ~~Repair of prosthetic device, hourly rate (excludes V5335 repair of oral or laryngeal prosthesis or artificial larynx)~~ ✖

⊙ **L7510** Repair of prosthetic device, repair or replace minor parts

    Bill local carrier if repair of implanted prosthetic device. If other, bill DME/MAC

    IOM: 100-02, 15, 110.2; 100-02, 15, 120; 100-04, 32, 100

▶ New   → Revised   ✔ Reinstated   ~~deleted~~ Deleted   ⊙ Special coverage instructions   ◆ Not covered or valid by Medicare   * Carrier discretion

✳ **L7520** Repair prosthetic device, labor component, per 15 minutes

Bill local carrier if repair of implanted prosthetic device. If other, bill DME/MAC

◆ **L7600** Prosthetic donning sleeve, any material, each

Bill DME/MAC

Medicare Statute 1862(1)(a)

General

✳ **L7900** Male vacuum erection system

Bill DME/MAC

Breast Prostheses

☺ **L8000** Breast prosthesis, mastectomy bra

Bill DME/MAC

IOM: 100-02, 15, 120

☺ **L8001** Breast prosthesis, mastectomy bra, with integrated breast prosthesis form, unilateral

Bill DME/MAC

IOM: 100-02, 15, 120

☺ **L8002** Breast prosthesis, mastectomy bra, with integrated breast prosthesis form, bilateral

Bill DME/MAC

IOM: 100-02, 15, 120

☺ **L8010** Breast prosthesis, mastectomy sleeve

Bill DME/MAC

IOM: 100-02, 15, 120

☺ **L8015** External breast prosthesis garment, with mastectomy form, post mastectomy

Bill DME/MAC

IOM: 100-02, 15, 120

☺ **L8020** Breast prosthesis, mastectomy form

Bill DME/MAC

IOM: 100-02, 15, 120

✳ **L8030** Breast prosthesis, silicone or equal, without integral adhesive

Bill DME/MAC

IOM: 100-02, 15, 120

☺ **L8031** Breast prosthesis, silicone or equal, with integral adhesive

Bill DME/MAC

IOM: 100-02, 15, 120

✳ **L8032** Nipple prosthesis, reusable, any type, each

Bill DME/MAC

☺ **L8035** Custom breast prosthesis, post mastectomy, molded to patient model

Bill DME/MAC

IOM: 100-02, 15, 120

✳ **L8039** Breast prosthesis, not otherwise specified

Bill DME/MAC

Nasal, Orbital, Auricular Prosthesis

✳ **L8040** Nasal prosthesis, provided by a non-physician

Bill DME/MAC

✳ **L8041** Midfacial prosthesis, provided by a non-physician

Bill DME/MAC

✳ **L8042** Orbital prosthesis, provided by a non-physician

Bill DME/MAC

✳ **L8043** Upper facial prosthesis, provided by a non-physician

Bill DME/MAC

✳ **L8044** Hemi-facial prosthesis, provided by a non-physician

Bill DME/MAC

✳ **L8045** Auricular prosthesis, provided by a non-physician

Bill DME/MAC

✳ **L8046** Partial facial prosthesis, provided by a non-physician

Bill DME/MAC

✳ **L8047** Nasal septal prosthesis, provided by a non-physician

Bill DME/MAC

✳ **L8048** Unspecified maxillofacial prosthesis, by report, provided by a non-physician

Bill DME/MAC

✳ **L8049** Repair or modification of maxillofacial prosthesis, labor component, 15 minute increments, provided by a non-physician

Bill DME/MAC

▶ New   → Revised   ✔ Reinstated   ~~deleted~~ Deleted
☺ Special coverage instructions   ◆ Not covered or valid by Medicare   ✳ Carrier discretion

PROSTHETICS L7520 – L8049

253

Trusses

⚙ **L8300** Truss, single with standard pad

Bill DME/MAC

IOM: 100-02, 15, 120; 100-03, 4, 280.11; 100-03, 4, 280.12; 100-04, 4, 240

⚙ **L8310** Truss, double with standard pads

Bill DME/MAC

IOM: 100-02, 15, 120; 100-03, 4, 280.11; 100-03, 4, 280.12; 100-04, 4, 240

⚙ **L8320** Truss, addition to standard pad, water pad

Bill DME/MAC

IOM: 100-02, 15, 120; 100-03, 4, 280.11; 100-03, 4, 280.12; 100-04, 4, 240

⚙ **L8330** Truss, addition to standard pad, scrotal pad

Bill DME/MAC

IOM: 100-02, 15, 120; 100-03, 4, 280.11; 100-03, 4, 280.12; 100-04, 4, 240

Prosthetic Socks

⚙ **L8400** Prosthetic sheath, below knee, each

Bill DME/MAC

IOM: 100-02, 15, 200

⚙ **L8410** Prosthetic sheath, above knee, each

Bill DME/MAC

IOM: 100-02, 15, 200

⚙ **L8415** Prosthetic sheath, upper limb, each

Bill DME/MAC

IOM: 100-02, 15, 200

✳ **L8417** Prosthetic sheath/sock, including a gel cushion layer, below knee or above knee, each

Bill DME/MAC

⚙ **L8420** Prosthetic sock, multiple ply, below knee, each

Bill DME/MAC

IOM: 100-02, 15, 200

⚙ **L8430** Prosthetic sock, multiple ply, above knee, each

Bill DME/MAC

IOM: 100-02, 15, 200

⚙ **L8435** Prosthetic sock, multiple ply, upper limb, each

Bill DME/MAC

IOM: 100-02, 15, 200

⚙ **L8440** Prosthetic shrinker, below knee, each

Bill DME/MAC

IOM: 100-02, 15, 200

⚙ **L8460** Prosthetic shrinker, above knee, each

Bill DME/MAC

IOM: 100-02, 15, 200

⚙ **L8465** Prosthetic shrinker, upper limb, each

Bill DME/MAC

IOM: 100-02, 15, 200

⚙ **L8470** Prosthetic sock, single ply, fitting, below knee, each

Bill DME/MAC

IOM: 100-02, 15, 200

⚙ **L8480** Prosthetic sock, single ply, fitting, above knee, each

Bill DME/MAC

IOM: 100-02, 15, 200

⚙ **L8485** Prosthetic sock, single ply, fitting, upper limb, each

Bill DME/MAC

IOM: 100-02, 15, 200

✳ **L8499** Unlisted procedure for miscellaneous prosthetic services

Bill local carrier if repair of implanted prosthetic device. If other, bill DME/MAC

Prosthetic Implants

Larynx, Tracheoesophageal

⚙ **L8500** Artificial larynx, any type

Bill DME/MAC

IOM: 100-02, 15, 120; 100-03, 1, 50.2; 100-04, 4, 240

⚙ **L8501** Tracheostomy speaking valve

Bill DME/MAC

IOM: 100-03, 1, 50.4

✳ **L8505** Artificial larynx replacement battery/accessory, any type

Bill DME/MAC

✳ **L8507** Tracheo-esophageal voice prosthesis, patient inserted, any type, each

Bill DME/MAC

✳ **L8509** Tracheo-esophageal voice prosthesis, inserted by a licensed health care provider, any type

Bill DME/MAC

▶ New   → Revised   ✔ Reinstated   -deleted- Deleted
⚙ Special coverage instructions   ◆ Not covered or valid by Medicare   ✳ Carrier discretion

✪ **L8510**   Voice amplifier

Bill DME/MAC

IOM: 100-03, 1, 50.2

✳ **L8511**   Insert for indwelling tracheoesophageal prosthesis, with or without valve, replacement only, each

Bill DME/MAC

✳ **L8512**   Gelatin capsules or equivalent, for use with tracheoesophageal voice prosthesis, replacement only, per 10

Bill DME/MAC

✳ **L8513**   Cleaning device used with tracheoesophageal voice prosthesis, pipet, brush, or equal, replacement only, each

Bill DME/MAC

✳ **L8514**   Tracheoesophageal puncture dilator, replacement only, each

Bill DME/MAC

✳ **L8515**   Gelatin capsule, application device for use with tracheoesophageal voice prosthesis, each

Bill DME/MAC

Breast

✪ **L8600**   Implantable breast prosthesis, silicone or equal

Bill local carrier

IOM: 100-02, 15, 120; 100-3, 2, 140.2

Urinary System

✪ **L8603**   Injectable bulking agent, collagen implant, urinary tract, 2.5 ml syringe, includes shipping and necessary supplies

Bill local carrier

Bill on paper, acquisition cost invoice required

IOM: 100-03, 4, 280.1

✳ **L8604**   Injectable bulking agent, dextranomer/hyaluronic acid copolymer implant, urinary tract, 1 ml, includes shipping and necessary supplies1

Bill local carrier

✪ **L8606**   Injectable bulking agent, synthetic implant, urinary tract, 1 ml syringe, includes shipping and necessary supplies

Bill local carrier

Bill on paper, acquisition cost invoice required

IOM: 100-03, 4, 280.1

Head (Skull, Facial Bones, and Temporomandibular Joint)

✳ **L8609**   Artificial cornea

Bill local carrier

✪ **L8610**   Ocular implant

Bill local carrier

IOM: 100-02, 15, 120

✪ **L8612**   Aqueous shunt

Bill local carrier

IOM: 100-02, 15, 120

Cross Reference Q0074

✪ **L8613**   Ossicula implant

Bill local carrier

IOM: 100-02, 15, 120

✪ **L8614**   Cochlear device, includes all internal and external components

Bill local carrier

IOM: 100-02, 15, 120; 100-03, 1, 50.3

✪ **L8615**   Headset/headpiece for use with cochlear implant device, replacement

Bill local carrier

IOM: 100-03, 1, 50.3

✪ **L8616**   Microphone for use with cochlear implant device, replacement

Bill local carrier

IOM: 100-03, 1, 50.3

✪ **L8617**   Transmitting coil for use with cochlear implant device, replacement

Bill local carrier

IOM: 100-03, 1, 50.3

✪ **L8618**   Transmitter cable for use with cochlear implant device, replacement

Bill local carrier

IOM: 100-03, 1, 50.3

✳ **L8619**   Cochlear implant, external speech processor and controller, integrated system, replacement

Bill local carrier

IOM: 100-03, 1, 50.3

▶ New   → Revised   ✔ Reinstated   ~~deleted~~ Deleted

✪ Special coverage instructions   ◆ Not covered or valid by Medicare   ✳ Carrier discretion

✳ **L8621**   Zinc air battery for use with cochlear implant device, replacement, each

Bill local carrier

✳ **L8622**   Alkaline battery for use with cochlear implant device, any size, replacement, each

Bill local carrier

✳ **L8623**   Lithium ion battery for use with cochlear implant device speech processor, other than ear level, replacement, each

Bill local carrier

✳ **L8624**   Lithium ion battery for use with cochlear implant device speech processor, ear level, replacement, each

Bill local carrier

☺ **L8627**   Cochlear implant, external speech processor, component, replacement

Bill local carrier

IOM: 103-03, Part 1, 50.3

☺ **L8628**   Cochlear implant, external controller component, replacement

Bill local carrier

IOM: 103-03, Part 1, 50.3

☺ **L8629**   Transmitting coil and cable, integrated, for use with cochlear implant device, replacement

Bill local carrier

IOM: 103-03, Part 1, 50.3

Upper Extremity

☺ **L8630**   Metacarpophalangeal joint implant

Bill local carrier

IOM: 100-02, 15, 120

☺ **L8631**   Metacarpal phalangeal joint replacement, two or more pieces, metal (e.g., stainless steel or cobalt chrome), ceramic-like material (e.g., pyrocarbon), for surgical implantation (all sizes, includes entire system)

Bill local carrier

IOM: 100-02, 15, 120

Lower Extremity (Joint: Knee, Ankle, Toe)

☺ **L8641**   Metatarsal joint implant

Bill local carrier

IOM: 100-02, 15, 120

☺ **L8642**   Hallux implant

Bill local carrier

May be billed by ambulatory surgical center or surgeon

IOM: 100-02, 15, 120

Cross Reference CPT Q0073

Miscellaneous Muscular-Skeletal

☺ **L8658**   Interphalangeal joint spacer, silicone or equal, each

Bill local carrier

IOM: 100-02, 15, 120

☺ **L8659**   Interphalangeal finger joint replacement, 2 or more pieces, metal (e.g., stainless steel or cobalt chrome), ceramic-like material (e.g., pyrocarbon) for surgical implantation, any size

Bill local carrier

IOM: 100-02, 15, 120

Cardiovascular System

☺ **L8670**   Vascular graft material, synthetic, implant

Bill local carrier

IOM: 100-02, 15, 120

Neurostimulator

☺ **L8680**   Implantable neurostimulator electrode, each

Bill local carrier

Related CPT codes: 43647, 63650, 63655, 64553, 64555, 64560, 64561, 64565, 64573, 64575, 64577, 64580, 64581.

IOM: 100-03, 4, 280.4

☺ **L8681**   Patient programmer (external) for use with implantable programmable neurostimulator pulse generator, replacement only

Bill local carrier

IOM: 100-03, 4, 280.4

☺ **L8682**   Implantable neurostimulator radiofrequency receiver

Bill local carrier

IOM: 100-03, 4, 280.4

▶ New　　→ Revised　　✔ Reinstated　　deleted Deleted

☺ Special coverage instructions　　◆ Not covered or valid by Medicare　　✳ Carrier discretion

⊘ **L8683** Radiofrequency transmitter (external) for use with implantable neurostimulator radiofrequency receiver

Bill local carrier

IOM: 100-03, 4, 280.4

⊘ **L8684** Radiofrequency transmitter (external) for use with implantable sacral root neurostimulator receiver for bowel and bladder management, replacement

Bill local carrier

IOM: 100-03, 4, 280.4

⊘ **L8685** Implantable neurostimulator pulse generator, single array, rechargeable, includes extension

Bill local carrier

Related CPT codes: 61885, 64590, 63685.

IOM: 100-03, 4, 280.4

⊘ **L8686** Implantable neurostimulator pulse generator, single array, non-rechargeable, includes extension

Bill local carrier

Related CPT codes: 61885, 64590, 63685.

IOM: 100-03, 4, 280.4

⊘ **L8687** Implantable neurostimulator pulse generator, dual array, rechargeable, includes extension

Bill local carrier

Related CPT codes: 64590, 63685, 61886.

IOM: 100-03, 4, 280.4

⊘ **L8688** Implantable neurostimulator pulse generator, dual array, non-rechargeable, includes extension

Bill local carrier

Related CPT codes: 61885, 64590, 63685.

IOM: 100-03, 4, 280.4

⊘ **L8689** External recharging system for battery (internal) for use with implantable neurostimulator, replacement only

Bill local carrier

IOM: 100-03, 4, 280.4

✳ **L8690** Auditory osseointegrated device, includes all internal and external components

Bill local carrier

Related CPT codes: 69714, 69715, 69717, 69718.

✳ **L8691** Auditory osseointegrated device, external sound processor, replacement

Bill local carrier

◆ **L8692** Auditory osseointegrated device, external sound processor, used without osseointegration, body worn, includes headband or other means of external attachment

Bill local carrier

Medicare Statute 1862(a)(7)

▶ ✳ **L8693** Auditory osseointegrated device abutment, any length, replacement only

Bill local carrier

⊘ **L8695** External recharging system for battery (external) for use with implantable neurostimulator, replacement only

Bill local carrier

IOM: 100-03, 4, 280.4

Genital

✳ **L8699** Prosthetic implant, not otherwise specified

Bill local carrier

✳ **L9900** Orthotic and prosthetic supply, accessory, and/or service component of another HCPCS "L" code

Bill local carrier if repair of implanted prosthetic device. If other, bill DME/MAC

▶ New　　→ Revised　　✔ Reinstated　　deleted Deleted
⊘ Special coverage instructions　　◆ Not covered or valid by Medicare　　✳ Carrier discretion

OTHER MEDICAL SERVICES (M0000-M0301)

M0064-M0301: Bill local carrier

⊛ **M0064** Brief office visit for the sole purpose of monitoring or changing drug prescriptions used in the treatment of mental psychoneurotic and personality disorders

Not to be reported separately from CPT codes 90801-90857

◆ **M0075** Cellular therapy

◆ **M0076** Prolotherapy

Prolotherapy stimulates production of new ligament tissue. Not covered by Medicare

◆ **M0100** Intragastric hypothermia using gastric freezing

◆ **M0300** IV chelation therapy (chemical endarterectomy)

Non-covered by Medicare

◆ **M0301** Fabric wrapping of abdominal aneurysm

Treatment for abdominal aneurysms that involves wrapping aneurysms with cellophane or fascia lata. Fabric wrapping of abdominal aneurysms is not a covered Medicare procedure.

▶ New   → Revised   ✔ Reinstated   ̶d̶e̶l̶e̶t̶e̶d̶ Deleted
⊛ Special coverage instructions   ◆ Not covered or valid by Medicare   ✳ Carrier discretion

LABORATORY SERVICES (P0000-P9999)

Chemistry and Toxicology Tests

P2028-P2038:   Bill local carrier

⊛ **P2028**   Cephalin floculation, blood

IOM: 100-03, 4, 300.1

⊛ **P2029**   Congo red, blood

IOM: 100-03, 4, 300.1

◆ **P2031**   Hair analysis (excluding arsenic)

IOM: 100-03, 4, 300.1

⊛ **P2033**   Thymol turbidity, blood

IOM: 100-03, 4, 300.1

⊛ **P2038**   Mucoprotein, blood (seromucoid) (medical necessity procedure)

IOM: 100-03, 4, 300.1

Pathology Screening Tests

P3000-P7001:   Bill local carrier

⊛ **P3000**   Screening Papanicolaou smear, cervical or vaginal, up to three smears, by technician under physician supervision

Co-insurance and deductible waived

Assign for Pap smear ordered for screening purposes only, conventional method, performed by technician

IOM: 100-03, 3, 190.2,

Laboratory Certification: Cytology

⊛ **P3001**   Screening Papanicolaou smear, cervical or vaginal, up to three smears, requiring interpretation by physician

Co-insurance and deductible waived

Report professional component for Pap smears requiring physician interpretation. There are CPT codes assigned for diagnostic Paps, such as, 88141; HCPCS are for screening Paps

IOM: 100-03, 3, 190.2

Laboratory Certification: Cytology

Microbiology Tests

◆ **P7001**   Culture, bacterial, urine; quantitative, sensitivity study

Cross Reference CPT

Laboratory Certification: Bacteriology

Miscellaneous Pathology

P9010-P9615:   Bill local carrier

⊛ **P9010**   Blood (whole), for transfusion, per unit

Blood furnished on an outpatient basis, subject to Medicare Part B blood deductible; applicable to first 3 pints of whole blood or equivalent units of packed red cells in calendar year

IOM: 100-01, 3, 20.5; 100-02, 1, 10

OPPS recognized blood/blood products

⊛ **P9011**   Blood, split unit

Reports all splitting activities of any blood component

IOM: 100-01, 3, 20.5; 100-02, 1, 10

OPPS recognized blood/blood products

⊛ **P9012**   Cryoprecipitate, each unit

IOM: 100-01, 3, 20.5; 100-02, 1, 10

OPPS recognized blood/blood products

⊛ **P9016**   Red blood cells, leukocytes reduced, each unit

IOM: 100-01, 3, 20.5; 100-02, 1, 10

OPPS recognized blood/blood products

⊛ **P9017**   Fresh frozen plasma (single donor), frozen within 8 hours of collection, each unit

IOM: 100-01, 3, 20.5; 100-02, 1, 10

OPPS recognized blood/blood products

⊛ **P9019**   Platelets, each unit

IOM: 100-01, 3, 20.5; 100-02, 1, 10

OPPS recognized blood/blood products

⊛ **P9020**   Platelet rich plasma, each unit

IOM: 100-01, 3, 20.5; 100-02, 1, 10

OPPS recognized blood/blood products

⊛ **P9021**   Red blood cells, each unit

IOM: 100-01, 3, 20.5; 100-02, 1, 10

OPPS recognized blood/blood products

⊛ **P9022**   Red blood cells, washed, each unit

IOM: 100-01, 3, 20.5; 100-02, 1, 10

OPPS recognized blood/blood products

▶ New   → Revised   ✔ Reinstated   ~~deleted~~ Deleted

⊛ Special coverage instructions   ◆ Not covered or valid by Medicare   ✳ Carrier discretion

⚙ **P9023** Plasma, pooled multiple donor, solvent/detergent treated, frozen, each unit

IOM: 100-01, 3, 20.5; 100-02, 1, 10

OPPS recognized blood/blood products

⚙ **P9031** Platelets, leukocytes reduced, each unit

IOM: 100-01, 3, 20.5; 100-02, 1, 10

OPPS recognized blood/blood products

⚙ **P9032** Platelets, irradiated, each unit

IOM: 100-01, 3, 20.5; 100-02, 1, 10

OPPS recognized blood/blood products

⚙ **P9033** Platelets, leukocytes reduced, irradiated, each unit

IOM: 100-01, 3, 20.5; 100-02, 1, 10

OPPS recognized blood/blood products

⚙ **P9034** Platelets, pheresis, each unit

IOM: 100-01, 3, 20.5; 100-02, 1, 10

OPPS recognized blood/blood products

⚙ **P9035** Platelets, pheresis, leukocytes reduced, each unit

IOM: 100-01, 3, 20.5; 100-02, 1, 10

OPPS recognized blood/blood products

⚙ **P9036** Platelets, pheresis, irradiated, each unit

IOM: 100-01, 3, 20.5; 100-02, 1, 10

OPPS recognized blood/blood products

⚙ **P9037** Platelets, pheresis, leukocytes reduced, irradiated, each unit

IOM: 100-01, 3, 20.5; 100-02, 1, 10

OPPS recognized blood/blood products

⚙ **P9038** Red blood cells, irradiated, each unit

IOM: 100-01, 3, 20.5; 100-02, 1, 10

OPPS recognized blood/blood products

⚙ **P9039** Red blood cells, deglycerolized, each unit

IOM: 100-01, 3, 20.5; 100-02, 1, 10

OPPS recognized blood/blood products

⚙ **P9040** Red blood cells, leukocytes reduced, irradiated, each unit

IOM: 100-01, 3, 20.5; 100-02, 1, 10

OPPS recognized blood/blood products

✳ **P9041** Infusion, albumin (human), 5%, 50 ml

✳ **P9043** Infusion, plasma protein fraction (human), 5%, 50 ml

IOM: 100-01, 3, 20.5; 100-02, 1, 10

OPPS recognized blood/blood products

⚙ **P9044** Plasma, cryoprecipitate reduced, each unit

IOM: 100-01, 3, 20.5; 100-02, 1, 10

OPPS recognized blood/blood products

✳ **P9045** Infusion, albumin (human), 5%, 250 ml

✳ **P9046** Infusion, albumin (human), 25%, 20 ml

✳ **P9047** Infusion, albumin (human), 25%, 50 ml

✳ **P9048** Infusion, plasma protein fraction (human), 5%, 250 ml

OPPS recognized blood/blood products

✳ **P9050** Granulocytes, pheresis, each unit

OPPS recognized blood/blood products

⚙ **P9051** Whole blood or red blood cells, leukocytes reduced, CMV-negative, each unit

Medicare Statute 1833(t)

OPPS recognized blood/blood products

⚙ **P9052** Platelets, HLA-matched leukocytes reduced, apheresis/pheresis, each unit

Medicare Statute 1833(t)

OPPS recognized blood/blood products

⚙ **P9053** Platelets, pheresis, leukocytes reduced, CMV-negative, irradiated, each unit

Freezing and thawing are reported separately, see Transmittal 1487 (Hospital outpatient)

Medicare Statute 1833(t)

OPPS recognized blood/blood products

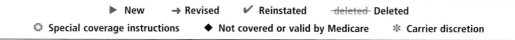

▶ New → Revised ✔ Reinstated ~~deleted~~ Deleted
⚙ Special coverage instructions ◆ Not covered or valid by Medicare ✳ Carrier discretion

⊛ **P9054** Whole blood or red blood cells, leukocytes reduced, frozen, deglycerol, washed, each unit

Medicare Statute 1833(t)

OPPS recognized blood/blood products

⊛ **P9055** Platelets, leukocytes reduced, CMV-negative, apheresis/pheresis, each unit

Medicare Statute 1833(t)

OPPS recognized blood/blood products

⊛ **P9056** Whole blood, leukocytes reduced, irradiated, each unit

Medicare Statute 1833(t)

OPPS recognized blood/blood products

⊛ **P9057** Red blood cells, frozen/deglycerolized/washed, leukocytes reduced, irradiated, each unit

Medicare Statute 1833(t)

OPPS recognized blood/blood products

⊛ **P9058** Red blood cells, leukocytes reduced, CMV-negative, irradiated, each unit

Medicare Statute 1833(t)

OPPS recognized blood/blood products

⊛ **P9059** Fresh frozen plasma between 8-24 hours of collection, each unit

Medicare Statute 1833(t)

OPPS recognized blood/blood products

⊛ **P9060** Fresh frozen plasma, donor retested, each unit

Medicare Statute 1833(t)

OPPS recognized blood/blood products

⊛ **P9603** Travel allowance one way in connection with medically necessary laboratory specimen collection drawn from home bound or nursing home bound patient; prorated miles actually traveled

Fee for clinical laboratory travel (P9603) is $0.96 per mile for CY2011

IOM: 100-04, 16, 60

⊛ **P9604** Travel allowance one way in connection with medically necessary laboratory specimen collection drawn from home bound or nursing home bound patient; prorated trip charge

Fee for clinical laboratory travel is $9.60 per flat rate trip for CY2011

IOM: 100-04, 16, 60

⊛ **P9612** Catheterization for collection of specimen, single patient, all places of service

NCCI edits indicate that when 51701 is comprehensive or is a Column 1 code, P9612 cannot be reported. When the catheter insertion is a component of another procedure, do not report straight catheterization separately.

IOM: 100-04, 16, 60

⊛ **P9615** Catheterization for collection of specimen(s) (multiple patients)

IOM: 100-04, 16, 60

▶ New   → Revised   ✔ Reinstated   deleted Deleted
⊛ Special coverage instructions   ◆ Not covered or valid by Medicare   ✳ Carrier discretion

LABORATORY SERVICES   P9054 – P9615

261

TEMPORARY CODES ASSIGNED BY CMS (Q0000-Q9999)

Cardiokymography

⊙ **Q0035**   Cardiokymography

Bill local carrier

Report modifier 26 if professional component only

IOM: 100-03, 1, 20.24

Chemotherapy

Q0081-Q0085:   Bill local carrier

⊙ **Q0081**   Infusion therapy, using other than chemotherapeutic drugs, per visit

IV piggyback only assigned one time per patient encounter per day. Report for hydration or the intravenous administration of antibiotics, anti-emetics, or analgesics. Bill on paper. Requires a report.

IOM: 100-03, 4, 280.14

✻ **Q0083**   Chemotherapy administration by other than infusion technique only (e.g., subcutaneous, intramuscular, push), per visit

⊙ **Q0084**   Chemotherapy administration by infusion technique only, per visit

IOM: 100-03, 4, 280.14

✻ **Q0085**   Chemotherapy administration by both infusion technique and other technique(s) (e.g., subcutaneous, intramuscular, push), per visit

Smear, Papanicolaou

⊙ **Q0091**   Screening Papanicolaou smear; obtaining, preparing and conveyance of cervical or vaginal smear to laboratory

Bill local carrier

Medicare does not cover comprehensive preventive medicine services; however, services described by G0101 and Q0091 (only for Medicare patients) are covered. Includes the services necessary to procure and transport the specimen to the laboratory.

IOM: 100-03, 3, 190.2

Equipment, X-Ray, Portable

⊙ **Q0092**   Set-up portable x-ray equipment

Bill local carrier

IOM: 100-04, 13, 90

Laboratory

Q0111-Q0115:   Bill local carrier

✻ **Q0111**   Wet mounts, including preparations of vaginal, cervical or skin specimens

Laboratory Certification: Bacteriology, Mycology, Parasitology

✻ **Q0112**   All potassium hydroxide (KOH) preparations

Laboratory Certification: Mycology

✻ **Q0113**   Pinworm examinations

Laboratory Certification: Parasitology

✻ **Q0114**   Fern test

Laboratory certification: Routine chemistry

✻ **Q0115**   Post-coital direct, qualitative examinations of vaginal or cervical mucous

Laboratory Certification: Hematology

Drugs

✻ **Q0138**   Injection, ferumoxytol, for treatment of iron deficiency anemia, 1 mg (non-ESRD use)

Feraheme is FDA approved for chronic kidney disease

NDC: Feraheme

✻ **Q0139**   Injection, ferumoxytol, for treatment of iron deficiency anemia, 1 mg (for ESRD on dialysis)

NDC: Feraheme

◆ **Q0144**   Azithromycin dihydrate, oral, capsules/powder, 1 gm

If "incident to" a physician's service, do not bill; otherwise, bill DME/MAC.

Other: Zithromax

▶ ⊙ **Q0162**   Ondansetron 1 mg, oral, FDA-approved prescription anti-emetic, for use as a complete therapeutic substitute for an IV anti-emetic at the time of chemotherapy treatment, not to exceed a 48 hour dosage regimen

Medicare Statute 4557

▶ New	→ Revised	✔ Reinstated	~~deleted~~ Deleted
⊙ Special coverage instructions	◆ Not covered or valid by Medicare		✻ Carrier discretion

⊛ **Q0163** Diphenhydramine hydrochloride, 50 mg, oral, FDA approved prescription anti-emetic, for use as a complete therapeutic substitute for an IV anti-emetic at time of chemotherapy treatment not to exceed a 48 hour dosage regimen

Bill DME/MAC

NDC: Compoz, Dytuss

Other: Alercap, Aler-Dryl, Allergy Children's, Allergy Relief Intense Strength, Allergy Relief Medicine, Allermax, Alertab, Anti-Hist, Antihistamine, Banophen, Complete Allergy Medication, Complete Allergy medicine, Diphedryl, Diphen, Diphenhist, Diphenyl, Dormin Sleep Aid, Geridryl, Good Sense Antihistamine Allergy Relief, Good Sense Nighttime Sleep Aid, Genahist, Hydramine, Medicine Shoppe Medi-Phedryl, Medicine Shoppe Nite Time Sleep, Mediphedryl, Night Time Sleep Aid, Nytol Quickcaps, Nytol Quickgels maximum strength, Q-Dryl, Quality Choice dye-free allergy medicine, Quality Choice Sleep Aid, Quality Choice Rest Simply, Quenalin, Rite Aid Allergy, Serabrina La France, Siladryl Allergy, Silphen, Simply Sleep, Sleep Formula, Sleep Tabs, Sleep-ettes D, Sleepinal, Sominex, Twilite, Valu-Dryl Allergy

Medicare Statute 4557

⊛ **Q0164** Prochlorperazine maleate, 5 mg, oral, FDA approved prescription anti-emetic, for use as a complete therapeutic substitute for an IV anti-emetic at the time of chemotherapy treatment, not to exceed a 48 hour dosage regimen

Bill DME/MAC

NDC: Compazine

Medicare Statute 4557

⊛ **Q0165** Prochlorperazine maleate, 10 mg, oral, FDA approved prescription anti-emetic, for use as a complete therapeutic substitute for an IV anti-emetic at the time of chemotherapy treatment, not to exceed a 48 hour dosage regimen

Bill DME/MAC

NDC: Compazine

Medicare Statute 4557

⊛ **Q0166** Granisetron hydrochloride, 1 mg, oral, FDA approved prescription anti-emetic, for use as a complete therapeutic substitute for an IV anti-emetic at the time of chemotherapy treatment, not to exceed a 24 hour dosage regimen

Bill DME/MAC

NDC: Kytril

Medicare Statute 4557

⊛ **Q0167** Dronabinol, 2.5 mg, oral, FDA approved prescription anti-emetic, for use as a complete therapeutic substitute for an IV anti-emetic at the time of chemotherapy treatment, not to exceed a 48 hour dosage regimen

Bill DME/MAC

NDC: Marinol

Medicare Statute 4557

⊛ **Q0168** Dronabinol, 5 mg, oral, FDA approved prescription anti-emetic, for use as a complete therapeutic substitute for an IV anti-emetic at the time of chemotherapy treatment, not to exceed a 48 hour dosage regimen

Bill DME/MAC

NDC: Marinol

Medicare Statute 4557

⊛ **Q0169** Promethazine hydrochloride, 12.5 mg, oral, FDA approved prescription anti-emetic, for use as a complete therapeutic substitute for an IV anti-emetic at the time of chemotherapy treatment, not to exceed a 48 hour dosage regimen

Bill DME/MAC

NDC: Phenergan

Medicare Statute 4557

⊛ **Q0170** Promethazine hydrochloride, 25 mg, oral, FDA approved prescription anti-emetic, for use as a complete therapeutic substitute for an IV anti-emetic at the time of chemotherapy treatment, not to exceed a 48 hour dosage regimen

Bill DME/MAC

Other: Phenergan, Promacot

Medicare Statute 4557

▶ New　→ Revised　✔ Reinstated　~~deleted~~ Deleted

⊛ Special coverage instructions　◆ Not covered or valid by Medicare　✳ Carrier discretion

⊗ **Q0171**   Chlorpromazine hydrochloride, 10 mg, oral, FDA approved prescription anti-emetic, for use as a complete therapeutic substitute for an IV anti-emetic at the time of chemotherapy treatment, not to exceed a 48 hour dosage regimen

Bill DME/MAC

Medicare Statute 4557

⊗ **Q0172**   Chlorpromazine hydrochloride, 25 mg, oral, FDA approved prescription anti-emetic, for use as a complete therapeutic substitute for an IV anti-emetic at the time of chemotherapy treatment, not to exceed a 48 hour dosage regimen

Bill DME/MAC

Medicare Statute 4557

⊗ **Q0173**   Trimethobenzamide hydrochloride, 250 mg, oral, FDA approved prescription anti-emetic, for use as a complete therapeutic substitute for an IV anti-emetic at the time of chemotherapy treatment, not to exceed a 48 hour dosage regimen

Bill DME/MAC

Other: Tigan

Medicare Statute 4557

⊗ **Q0174**   Thiethylperazine maleate, 10 mg, oral, FDA approved prescription anti-emetic, for use as a complete therapeutic substitute for an IV anti-emetic at the time of chemotherapy treatment, not to exceed a 48 hour dosage regimen

Bill DME/MAC

Other: Torecan

Medicare Statute 4557

⊗ **Q0175**   Perphenazine, 4 mg, oral, FDA approved prescription anti-emetic, for use as a complete therapeutic substitute for an IV anti-emetic at the time of chemotherapy treatment, not to exceed a 48 hour dosage regimen

Bill DME/MAC

Medicare Statute 4557

⊗ **Q0176**   Perphenazine, 8mg, oral, FDA approved prescription anti-emetic, for use as a complete therapeutic substitute for an IV anti-emetic at the time of chemotherapy treatment, not to exceed a 48 hour dosage regimen

Bill DME/MAC

Medicare Statute 4557

⊗ **Q0177**   Hydroxyzine pamoate, 25 mg, oral, FDA approved prescription anti-emetic, for use as a complete therapeutic substitute for an IV anti-emetic at the time of chemotherapy treatment, not to exceed a 48 hour dosage regimen

Bill DME/MAC

Other: Vistaril

Medicare Statute 4557

⊗ **Q0178**   Hydroxyzine pamoate, 50 mg, oral, FDA approved prescription anti-emetic, for use as a complete therapeutic substitute for an IV anti-emetic at the time of chemotherapy treatment, not to exceed a 48 hour dosage regimen

Bill DME/MAC

Other: Vistaril

Medicare Statute 4557

~~Q0179   Ondansetron hydrochloride, 8 mg, oral, FDA approved prescription anti-emetic, for use as a complete therapeutic substitute for an IV anti-emetic at the time of chemotherapy treatment, not to exceed a 48 hour dosage regimen~~   ✱

⊗ **Q0180**   Dolasetron mesylate, 100 mg, oral, FDA approved prescription anti-emetic, for use as a complete therapeutic substitute for an IV anti-emetic at the time of chemotherapy treatment, not to exceed a 24 hour dosage regimen

Bill DME/MAC

NDC: Anzemet

Medicare Statute 4557

⊗ **Q0181**   Unspecified oral dosage form, FDA approved prescription anti-emetic, for use as a complete therapeutic substitute for a IV anti-emetic at the time of chemotherapy treatment, not to exceed a 48 hour dosage regimen

Bill DME/MAC

Medicare Statute 4557

Miscellaneous Devices

▶ ⊗ **Q0478**   Power adapter for use with electric or electric/pneumatic ventricular assist device, vehicle type

CMS has determined the reasonable useful lifetime is one year. Add modifier -RA to claims to report when battery is replaced because it was lost, stolen, or irreparably damaged. (http://www.wpsmedicare.com/part_b/publications/communique/archived/_files/winter-2011-comm.pdf)

▶ New   → Revised   ✔ Reinstated   ~~deleted~~ Deleted

⊗ Special coverage instructions   ◆ Not covered or valid by Medicare   ✱ Carrier discretion

264

▶ ۞ **Q0479** Power module for use with electric or electric/pneumatic ventricular assist device, replacement only

CMS has determined the reasonable useful lifetime is one year. Add modifier -RA in cases where the battery is replaced because it was lost, stolen, or irreparably damaged. (http://www.wpsmedicare.com/part_b/publications/communique/archived/_files/winter-2011-comm.pdf)

۞ **Q0480** Driver for use with pneumatic ventricular assist device, replacement only

Bill local carrier

۞ **Q0481** Microprocessor control unit for use with electric ventricular assist device, replacement only

Bill local carrier

۞ **Q0482** Microprocessor control unit for use with electric/pneumatic combination ventricular assist device, replacement only

Bill local carrier

۞ **Q0483** Monitor/display module for use with electric ventricular assist device, replacement only

Bill local carrier

۞ **Q0484** Monitor/display module for use with electric or electric/pneumatic ventricular assist device, replacement only

Bill local carrier

۞ **Q0485** Monitor control cable for use with electric ventricular assist device, replacement only

Bill local carrier

۞ **Q0486** Monitor control cable for use with electric/pneumatic ventricular assist device, replacement only

Bill local carrier

۞ **Q0487** Leads (pneumatic/electrical) for use with any type electric/pneumatic ventricular assist device, replacement only

Bill local carrier

۞ **Q0488** Power pack base for use with electric ventricular assist device, replacement only

Bill local carrier

۞ **Q0489** Power pack base for use with electric/pneumatic ventricular assist device, replacement only

Bill local carrier

۞ **Q0490** Emergency power source for use with electric ventricular assist device, replacement only

Bill local carrier

۞ **Q0491** Emergency power source for use with electric/pneumatic ventricular assist device, replacement only

Bill local carrier

۞ **Q0492** Emergency power supply cable for use with electric ventricular assist device, replacement only

Bill local carrier

۞ **Q0493** Emergency power supply cable for use with electric/pneumatic ventricular assist device, replacement only

Bill local carrier

۞ **Q0494** Emergency hand pump for use with electric or electric/pneumatic ventricular assist device, replacement only

Bill local carrier

۞ **Q0495** Battery/power pack charger for use with electric or electric/pneumatic ventricular assist device, replacement only

Bill local carrier

✷ **Q0496** Battery, other than lithium-ion, for use with electric or electric/pneumatic ventricular assist device, replacement only

Bill local carrier

Reasonable useful lifetime is 6 months (CR3931).

۞ **Q0497** Battery clips for use with electric or electric/pneumatic ventricular assist device, replacement only

Bill local carrier

۞ **Q0498** Holster for use with electric or electric/pneumatic ventricular assist device, replacement only

Bill local carrier

→ ✷ **Q0499** Belt/vest/bag for use to carry external peripheral components of any type ventricular assist device, replacement only

Bill local carrier

۞ **Q0500** Filters for use with electric or electric/pneumatic ventricular assist device, replacement only

Bill local carrier

۞ **Q0501** Shower cover for use with electric or electric/pneumatic ventricular assist device, replacement only

Bill local carrier

▶ New → Revised ✔ Reinstated deleted Deleted

۞ Special coverage instructions ◆ Not covered or valid by Medicare ✷ Carrier discretion

☼ **Q0502**   Mobility cart for pneumatic ventricular assist device, replacement only

Bill local carrier

☼ **Q0503**   Battery for pneumatic ventricular assist device, replacement only, each

Bill local carrier

Reasonable useful lifetime is 6 months (CR3931).

☼ **Q0504**   Power adapter for pneumatic ventricular assist device, replacement only, vehicle type

Bill local carrier

☼ **Q0505**   Miscellaneous supply or accessory for use with ventricular assist device

Bill local carrier

☼ **Q0506**   Battery, lithium-ion, for use with electric or electric/pneumatic, ventricular assist device, replacement only

Bill local carrier

Reasonable useful lifetime is 12 months. Add -RA for replacement if lost, stolen, or irreparable damage.

Fee, Pharmacy

Q0510-Q0515:   Bill DME/MAC

☼ **Q0510**   Pharmacy supply fee for initial immunosuppressive drug(s), first month following transplant

☼ **Q0511**   Pharmacy supply fee for oral anti-cancer, oral anti-emetic or immunosuppressive drug(s); for the first prescription in a 30-day period

☼ **Q0512**   Pharmacy supply fee for oral anti-cancer, oral anti-emetic or immunosuppressive drug(s); for a subsequent prescription in a 30-day period

☼ **Q0513**   Pharmacy dispensing fee for inhalation drug(s); per 30 days

☼ **Q0514**   Pharmacy dispensing fee for inhalation drug(s); per 90 days

☼ **Q0515**   Injection, sermorelin acetate, 1 microgram

NDC: Geref Diagnostic

IOM: 100-02, 15, 50

Lens, Intraocular

Q1004-Q1005:   Bill local carrier

~~Q1003~~   ~~New technology intraocular lens category 3 (reduced spherical aberration)~~   ✖

☼ **Q1004**   New technology intraocular lens category 4 as defined in Federal Register notice

☼ **Q1005**   New technology intraocular lens category 5 as defined in Federal Register notice

Solutions and Drugs

☼ **Q2004**   Irrigation solution for treatment of bladder calculi, for example renacidin, per 500 ml

Bill local carrier

IOM: 100-02, 15, 50

Medicare Statute 1861S2B

✳ **Q2009**   Injection, fosphenytoin, 50 mg phenytoin equivalent

Bill local carrier

NDC: Cerebyx

IOM: 100-02, 15, 50

Medicare Statute 1861S2B

☼ **Q2017**   Injection, teniposide, 50 mg

Bill local carrier

NDC: Vumon

IOM: 100-02, 15, 50

Medicare Statute 1861S2B

▶ ☼ **Q2026**   Injection, radiesse, 0.1 ml

▶ ☼ **Q2027**   Injection, sculptra, 0.1 ml

▶ ☼ **Q2035**   Influenza virus vaccine, split virus, when administered to individuals 3 years of age and older, for intramuscular use (Afluria)

IOM: 100-02, 15, 50

▶ ☼ **Q2036**   Influenza virus vaccine, split virus, when administered to individuals 3 years of age and older, for intramuscular use (Flulaval)

IOM: 100-02, 15, 50

▶ ☼ **Q2037**   Influenza virus vaccine, split virus, when administered to individuals 3 years of age and older, for intramuscular use (Fluvirin)

IOM: 100-02, 15, 50

▶ ☼ **Q2038**   Influenza virus vaccine, split virus, when administered to individuals 3 years of age or older, for intramuscular use (Fluzone)

IOM: 100-02, 15, 50

▶ ☼ **Q2039**   Influenza virus vaccine, split virus, when administered to individuals 3 years of age and older, for intramuscular use (not otherwise specified)

IOM: 100-02, 15, 50

▶ New   → Revised   ✔ Reinstated   ~~deleted~~ Deleted

☼ Special coverage instructions   ◆ Not covered or valid by Medicare   ✳ Carrier discretion

~~Q2040   Injection, incobotulinumtoxin A, 1 unit~~ ✖

~~Q2041   Injection, von Willebrand factor complex (human), Wilate, 1 I.U.,VWF: RCO~~ ✖

~~Q2042   Injection, hydroxyprojesterone caproate, 1 mg~~ ✖

▶ ⊘ **Q2043**   Sipuleucel-T, minimum of 50 million autologous CD54+ cells activated with PAP-GM-CSF, includng leukapheresis and all other preparatory procedures, per infusion

~~Q2044   Injection, belimumab, 10 mg~~ ✖

Brachytherapy Radioelements

⊘ **Q3001**   Radioelements for brachytherapy, any type, each
Bill local carrier
IOM: 100-04, 12, 70; 100-04, 13, 20

Telehealth

✳ **Q3014**   Telehealth originating site facility fee
Bill local carrier
Effective January of each year, the fee for telehealth services is increased by the Medicare Economic Index (MEI). The telehealth originating facility site fee (HCPCS code Q3014) for 2011 was 80 percent of the lesser of the actual charge or $24.10.

Drugs

Q3025-Q3026:   Bill local carrier

⊘ **Q3025**   Injection, interferon beta-1a, 11 mcg for intramuscular use
NDC: Avonex
IOM: 100-02, 15, 50

◆ **Q3026**   Injection, interferon beta-1a, 11 mcg for subcutaneous use
Other: Rebif

Test, Skin

⊘ **Q3031**   Collagen skin test
Bill local carrier
IOM: 100-03, 4, 280.1

Supplies, Cast

Q4001-Q4051:   Bill local carrier
Payment on a reasonable charge basis is required for splints, casts by regulations contained in 42 CFR 405.501.

✳ **Q4001**   Casting supplies, body cast adult, with or without head, plaster

✳ **Q4002**   Cast supplies, body cast adult, with or without head, fiberglass

✳ **Q4003**   Cast supplies, shoulder cast, adult (11 years +), plaster

✳ **Q4004**   Cast supplies, shoulder cast, adult (11 years +), fiberglass

✳ **Q4005**   Cast supplies, long arm cast, adult (11 years +), plaster

✳ **Q4006**   Cast supplies, long arm cast, adult (11 years +), fiberglass

✳ **Q4007**   Cast supplies, long arm cast, pediatric (0-10 years), plaster

✳ **Q4008**   Cast supplies, long arm cast, pediatric (0-10 years), fiberglass

✳ **Q4009**   Cast supplies, short arm cast, adult (11 years +), plaster

✳ **Q4010**   Cast supplies, short arm cast, adult (11 years +), fiberglass

✳ **Q4011**   Cast supplies, short arm cast, pediatric (0-10 years), plaster

✳ **Q4012**   Cast supplies, short arm cast, pediatric (0-10 years), fiberglass

✳ **Q4013**   Cast supplies, gauntlet cast (includes lower forearm and hand), adult (11 years +), plaster

✳ **Q4014**   Cast supplies, gauntlet cast (includes lower forearm and hand), adult (11 years +), fiberglass

✳ **Q4015**   Cast supplies, gauntlet cast (includes lower forearm and hand), pediatric (0-10 years), plaster

✳ **Q4016**   Cast supplies, gauntlet cast (includes lower forearm and hand), pediatric (0-10 years), fiberglass

✳ **Q4017**   Cast supplies, long arm splint, adult (11 years +), plaster

✳ **Q4018**   Cast supplies, long arm splint, adult (11 years +), fiberglass

✳ **Q4019**   Cast supplies, long arm splint, pediatric (0-10 years), plaster

✳ **Q4020**   Cast supplies, long arm splint, pediatric (0-10 years), fiberglass

✳ **Q4021**   Cast supplies, short arm splint, adult (11 years +), plaster

▶ New   → Revised   ✔ Reinstated   ~~deleted~~ Deleted
⊘ Special coverage instructions   ◆ Not covered or valid by Medicare   ✳ Carrier discretion

✳ **Q4022**   Cast supplies, short arm splint, adult (11 years +), fiberglass

✳ **Q4023**   Cast supplies, short arm splint, pediatric (0-10 years), plaster

✳ **Q4024**   Cast supplies, short arm splint, pediatric (0-10 years), fiberglass

✳ **Q4025**   Cast supplies, hip spica (one or both legs), adult (11 years +), plaster

✳ **Q4026**   Cast supplies, hip spica (one or both legs), adult (11 years +), fiberglass

✳ **Q4027**   Cast supplies, hip spica (one or both legs), pediatric (0-10 years), plaster

✳ **Q4028**   Cast supplies, hip spica (one or both legs), pediatric (0-10 years), fiberglass

✳ **Q4029**   Cast supplies, long leg cast, adult (11 years +), plaster

✳ **Q4030**   Cast supplies, long leg cast, adult (11 years +), fiberglass

✳ **Q4031**   Cast supplies, long leg cast, pediatric (0-10 years), plaster

✳ **Q4032**   Cast supplies, long leg cast, pediatric (0-10 years), fiberglass

✳ **Q4033**   Cast supplies, long leg cylinder cast, adult (11 years +), plaster

✳ **Q4034**   Cast supplies, long leg cylinder cast, adult (11 years +), fiberglass

✳ **Q4035**   Cast supplies, long leg cylinder cast, pediatric (0-10 years), plaster

✳ **Q4036**   Cast supplies, long leg cylinder cast, pediatric (0-10 years), fiberglass

✳ **Q4037**   Cast supplies, short leg cast, adult (11 years +), plaster

✳ **Q4038**   Cast supplies, short leg cast, adult (11 years +), fiberglass

✳ **Q4039**   Cast supplies, short leg cast, pediatric (0-10 years), plaster

✳ **Q4040**   Cast supplies, short leg cast, pediatric (0-10 years), fiberglass

✳ **Q4041**   Cast supplies, long leg splint, adult (11 years +), plaster

✳ **Q4042**   Cast supplies, long leg splint, adult (11 years +), fiberglass

✳ **Q4043**   Cast supplies, long leg splint, pediatric (0-10 years), plaster

✳ **Q4044**   Cast supplies, long leg splint, pediatric (0-10 years), fiberglass

✳ **Q4045**   Cast supplies, short leg splint, adult (11 years +), plaster

✳ **Q4046**   Cast supplies, short leg splint, adult (11 years +), fiberglass

✳ **Q4047**   Cast supplies, short leg splint, pediatric (0-10 years), plaster

✳ **Q4048**   Cast supplies, short leg splint, pediatric (0-10 years), fiberglass

✳ **Q4049**   Finger splint, static

✳ **Q4050**   Cast supplies, for unlisted types and materials of casts

✳ **Q4051**   Splint supplies, miscellaneous (includes thermoplastics, strapping, fasteners, padding and other supplies)

Drugs

✳ **Q4074**   Iloprost, inhalation solution, FDA-approved final product, non-compounded, administered through DME, unit dose form, up to 20 micrograms

NDC: Ventavis

☺ **Q4081**   Injection, epoetin alfa, 100 units (for ESRD on dialysis)

Bill DME/MAC for method II home dialysis. If other, bill DME/MAC.

NDC: Epogen, Procrit

✳ **Q4082**   Drug or biological, not otherwise classified, Part B drug competitive acquisition program (CAP)

Bill local carrier

Skin Substitutes

✳ **Q4100**   Skin substitute, not otherwise specified

Bill local carrier

Other: Orcel, Surgimend collagen matrix

→ ✳ **Q4101**   Apligraf, per square centimeter

Bill local carrier

→ ✳ **Q4102**   Oasis Wound Matrix, per square centimeter

Bill local carrier

→ ✳ **Q4103**   Oasis Burn Matrix, per square centimeter

Bill local carrier

→ ✳ **Q4104**   Integra Bilayer Matrix Wound Dressing (BMWD), per square centimeter

Bill local carrier

→ ✳ **Q4105**   Integra Dermal Regeneration Template (DRT), per square centimeter

Bill local carrier

→ ✳ **Q4106**   Dermagraft, per square centimeter

Bill local carrier

→ ✳ **Q4107**   Graftjacket, per square centimeter

Bill local carrier

NDC: Graftjacket Maxstrip, Graftjacket Small Ligament Repair Matrix, Graftjacket STD, Handjacket Scaffold Thin, Maxforce Thick, Ulcerjacket Scaffold, Ultra Maxforce

Other: Graftjacket SLR

▶ New   → Revised   ✔ Reinstated   ~~deleted~~ Deleted

☺ Special coverage instructions   ◆ Not covered or valid by Medicare   ✳ Carrier discretion

→ ✳ **Q4108** Integra Matrix, per square centimeter
Bill local carrier
NDC: Integra Matrix Wound Dressing

→ ✳ **Q4110** Primatrix, per square centimeter
Bill local carrier
Other: Primatrix dermal repair scaffold

→ ✳ **Q4111** GammaGraft, per square centimeter
Bill local carrier

→ ✳ **Q4112** Cymetra, injectable, 1cc
Bill local carrier

→ ✳ **Q4113** GraftJacket Xpress, injectable, 1cc
Bill local carrier

✳ **Q4114** Integra Flowable Wound Matrix, injectable, 1cc
Bill local carrier

→ ✳ **Q4115** Alloskin, per square centimeter
Bill local carrier

→ ✳ **Q4116** Alloderm, per square centimeter
Bill local carrier

▶ ✳ **Q4117** Hyalomatrix, per square centimeter
IOM: 100-02, 15, 50

▶ ✳ **Q4118** Matristem micromatrix, 1 mg

▶ ✳ **Q4119** Matristem wound matrix, per square centimeter

▶ ✳ **Q4120** Matristem burn matrix, per square centimeter

▶ ✳ **Q4121** Theraskin, per square centimeter

▶ ✳ **Q4122** Dermacell, per square centimeter

▶ ✳ **Q4123** AlloSkin RT, per square centimeter

▶ ✳ **Q4124** Oasis Ultra Tri-layer Wound Matrix, per square centimeter

▶ ✳ **Q4125** Arthroflex, per square centimeter

▶ ✳ **Q4126** Memoderm, per square centimeter

▶ ✳ **Q4127** Talymed, per square centimeter

▶ ✳ **Q4128** FlexHD or Allopatch HD, per square centimeter

▶ ✳ **Q4129** Unite Biomatrix, per square centimeter

▶ ✳ **Q4130** Strattice TM, per square centimeter

Hospice Care

☺ **Q5001** Hospice care provided in patient's home/residence
Bill local carrier

☺ **Q5002** Hospice care provided in assisted living facility
Bill local carrier

☺ **Q5003** Hospice care provided in nursing long term care facility (LTC) or non-skilled nursing facility (NF)
Bill local carrier

☺ **Q5004** Hospice care provided in skilled nursing facility (SNF)
Bill local carrier

☺ **Q5005** Hospice care provided in inpatient hospital
Bill local carrier

☺ **Q5006** Hospice care provided in inpatient hospice facility
Bill local carrier

Hospice care provided in an inpatient hospice facility. These are residential facilities, which are places for patients to live while receiving routine home care or continuous home care. These hospice residential facilities are not certified by Medicare or Medicaid for provision of General Inpatient (GIP) or respite care, and regulations at 42 CFR 418.202(e) do not allow provision of GIP or respite care at hospice residential facilities. (http://www.palmettogba.com/Palmetto/Providers.Nsf/files/Hospice_Coalition_QAs_03-2011.pdf/$File/Hospice_Coalition_QAs_03-2011.pdf)

☺ **Q5007** Hospice care provided in long term care facility
Bill local carrier

☺ **Q5008** Hospice care provided in inpatient psychiatric facility
Bill local carrier

☺ **Q5009** Hospice care provided in place not otherwise specified (NOS)
Bill local carrier

▶ ☺ **Q5010** Hospice home care provided in a hospice facility

Contrast

☺ **Q9951** Low osmolar contrast material, 400 or greater mg/ml iodine concentration, per ml
Bill local carrier
IOM: 100-04, 12, 70; 100-04, 13, 20; 100-04, 13, 90

☺ **Q9953** Injection, iron-based magnetic resonance contrast agent, per ml
Bill local carrier
NDC: Feridex IV
IOM: 100-04, 12, 70; 100-04, 13, 20; 100-04, 13, 90

▶ New   → Revised   ✔ Reinstated   ~~deleted~~ Deleted

☺ Special coverage instructions   ◆ Not covered or valid by Medicare   ✳ Carrier discretion

⊙ **Q9954**   Oral magnetic resonance contrast agent, per 100 ml

Bill local carrier

NDC: Gastromark

IOM: 100-04, 12, 70; 100-04, 13, 20; 100-04, 13, 90

⁎ **Q9955**   Injection, perflexane lipid microspheres, per ml

Bill local carrier

⁎ **Q9956**   Injection, octafluoropropane microspheres, per ml

Bill local carrier

NDC: Optison

⁎ **Q9957**   Injection, perflutren lipid microspheres, per ml

Bill local carrier

NDC: Definity

⊙ **Q9958**   High osmolar contrast material, up to 149 mg/ml iodine concentration, per ml

Bill local carrier

NDC: Conray 30, Cysto-Conray II, Cystografin, Cystografin-Dilute, Hypaque Sodium Oral, Reno-30, Reno-Dip

IOM: 100-04, 12, 70; 100-04, 13, 20; 100-04, 13, 90

⊙ **Q9959**   High osmolar contrast material, 150-199 mg/ml iodine concentration, per ml

Bill local carrier

IOM: 100-04, 12, 70; 100-04, 13, 20; 100-04, 13, 90

⊙ **Q9960**   High osmolar contrast material, 200-249 mg/ml iodine concentration, per ml

Bill local carrier

NDC: Conray 43

IOM: 100-04, 12, 70; 100-04, 13, 20; 100-04, 13, 90

⊙ **Q9961**   High osmolar contrast material, 250-299 mg/ml iodine concentration, per ml

Bill local carrier

NDC: Conray, Cholografin Meglumine, Renografin-60, Reno-M60

IOM: 100-04, 12, 70; 100-04, 13, 20; 100-04, 13, 90

⊙ **Q9962**   High osmolar contrast material, 300-349 mg/ml iodine concentration, per ml

Bill local carrier

IOM: 100-04, 12, 70; 100-04, 13, 20; 100-04, 13, 90

⊙ **Q9963**   High osmolar contrast material, 350-399 mg/ml iodine concentration, per ml

Bill local carrier

NDC: Gastrografin, Hypaque, Md-76R, Md Gastroview, Renocal-76, Sinografin

IOM: 100-04, 12, 70; 100-04, 13, 20; 100-04, 13, 90

⊙ **Q9964**   High osmolar contrast material, 400 or greater mg/ml iodine concentration, per ml

Bill local carrier

IOM: 100-04, 12, 70; 100-04, 13, 20; 100-04, 13, 90

⊙ **Q9965**   Low osmolar contrast material, 100-199 mg/ml iodine concentration, per ml

Bill local carrier

NDC: Omnipaque, Ultravist 150

IOM: 100-04, 12, 70; 100-04, 13, 20; 100-04, 13, 90

⊙ **Q9966**   Low osmolar contrast material, 200-299 mg/ml iodine concentration, per ml

Bill local carrier

NDC: Isovue-200, Isovue-250, Omnipaque, Optiray, Ultravist, Visipaque

IOM: 100-04, 12, 70; 100-04, 13, 20; 100-04, 13, 90

⊙ **Q9967**   Low osmolar contrast material, 300-399 mg/ml iodine concentration, per ml

Bill local carrier

NDC: Hexabrix 320, Isovue-300, Isovue-370, Omnipaque 300, Omnipaque 350, Optiray, Oxilan, Ultravist, Vispaque

IOM: 100-04, 12, 70; 100-04, 13, 20; 100-04, 13, 90

⁎ **Q9968**   Injection, non-radioactive, non-contrast, visualization adjunct (e.g., Methylene Blue, Isosulfan Blue), 1 mg

---

▶ New   → Revised   ✔ Reinstated   ~~deleted~~ Deleted

⊙ Special coverage instructions   ◆ Not covered or valid by Medicare   ⁎ Carrier discretion

DIAGNOSTIC RADIOLOGY SERVICES (R0000-R9999)

Transportation/Setup of Portable Equipment

R0070-R0076: Bill local carrier

⊛ **R0070** Transportation of portable x-ray equipment and personnel to home or nursing home, per trip to facility or location, one patient seen

CMS Transmittal B03-049; specific instructions to contractors on pricing

IOM: 100-04, 13, 90; 100-04, 13, 90.3

⊛ **R0075** Transportation of portable x-ray equipment and personnel to home or nursing home, per trip to facility or location, more than one patient seen

IOM: 100-04, 13, 90; 100-04, 13, 90.3

This code would not apply to the x-ray equipment if stored at the location where the x-ray was performed (e.g., a nursing home).

⊛ **R0076** Transportation of portable ECG to facility or location, per patient

EKG procedure code 93000 or 93005 must be submitted on same claim as transportation code. Bundled status on physician fee schedule

IOM: 100-01, 5, 90.2; 100-02, 15, 80; 100-03, 1, 20.15; 100-04, 13, 90; 100-04, 16, 10; 100-04, 16, 110.4

▶ New　→ Revised　✔ Reinstated　deleted Deleted
⊛ Special coverage instructions　◆ Not covered or valid by Medicare　✳ Carrier discretion

TEMPORARY NATIONAL CODES ESTABLISHED BY PRIVATE PAYERS (S0000-S9999)

Medicare and other federal payers do not recognize "S" codes; however, S codes may be useful for claims to some private insurers.

◆ **S0012** Butorphanol tartrate, nasal spray, **25 mg**

◆ **S0014** Tacrine hydrochloride, **10 mg**

◆ **S0017** Injection, aminocaproic acid, **5 grams**

◆ **S0020** Injection, bupivacaine hydrochloride, **30 ml**

◆ **S0021** Injection, cefoperazone sodium, **1 gram**

◆ **S0023** Injection, cimetidine hydrochloride, **300 mg**

◆ **S0028** Injection, famotidine, **20 mg**

◆ **S0030** Injection, metronidazole, **500 mg**

◆ **S0032** Injection, nafcillin sodium, **2 grams**

◆ **S0034** Injection, ofloxacin, **400 mg**

◆ **S0039** Injection, sulfamethoxazole and trimethoprim, **10 ml**

◆ **S0040** Injection, ticarcillin disodium and clavulanate potassium, **3.1 grams**

◆ **S0073** Injection, aztreonam, **500 mg**

◆ **S0074** Injection, cefotetan disodium, **500 mg**

◆ **S0077** Injection, clindamycin phosphate, **300 mg**

◆ **S0078** Injection, fosphenytoin sodium, **750 mg**

◆ **S0080** Injection, pentamidine isethionate, **300 mg**

◆ **S0081** Injection, piperacillin sodium, **500 mg**

◆ **S0088** Imatinib, **100 mg**

◆ **S0090** Sildenafil citrate, **25 mg**

◆ **S0091** Granisetron hydrochloride, **1 mg** (for circumstances falling under the Medicare Statute, use Q0166)

◆ **S0092** Injection, hydromorphone hydrochloride, **250 mg** (loading dose for infusion pump)

◆ **S0093** Injection, morphine sulfate, **500 mg** (loading dose for infusion pump)

◆ **S0104** Zidovudine, oral, **100 mg**

◆ **S0106** Bupropion HCl sustained release tablet, **150 mg,** per bottle of 60 tablets

◆ **S0108** Mercaptopurine, oral, **50 mg**

◆ **S0109** Methadone, oral, **5 mg**

◆ **S0117** Tretinoin, topical, **5 grams**

▶ ◆ **S0119** Ondansetron, oral, 4 mg (for circumstances falling under the medicare statute, use HCPCS Q code)

◆ **S0122** Injection, menotropins, **75 IU**

◆ **S0126** Injection, follitropin alfa, **75 IU**

◆ **S0128** Injection, follitropin beta, **75 IU**

◆ **S0132** Injection, ganirelix acetate, **250 mcg**

◆ **S0136** Clozapine, **25 mg**

◆ **S0137** Didanosine (DDI), **25 mg**

◆ **S0138** Finasteride, **5 mg**

◆ **S0139** Minoxidil, **10 mg**

◆ **S0140** Saquinavir, **200 mg**

◆ **S0142** Colistimethate sodium, inhalation solution administered through DME, concentrated form, **per mg**

◆ **S0145** Injection, pegylated interferon alfa-2a, **180 mcg per ml**

▶ ◆ **S0148** Injection, pegylated interferon ALFA-2b, **10 mcg**

◆ **S0155** Sterile dilutant for epoprostenol, **50 ml**

◆ **S0156** Exemestane, **25 mg**

◆ **S0157** Becaplermin gel 0.01%, **0.5 gm**

◆ **S0160** Dextroamphetamine sulfate, **5 mg**

◆ **S0164** Injection, pantoprazole sodium, **40 mg**

◆ **S0166** Injection, olanzapine, **2.5 mg**

▶ ◆ **S0169** Calcitrol, **0.25 microgram**

◆ **S0170** Anastrozole, oral, **1mg**

◆ **S0171** Injection, bumetanide, **0.5 mg**

◆ **S0172** Chlorambucil, oral, **2 mg**

◆ **S0174** Dolasetron mesylate, oral **50 mg** (for circumstances falling under the Medicare Statute, use Q0180)

◆ **S0175** Flutamide, oral, **125 mg**

◆ **S0176** Hydroxyurea, oral, **500 mg**

◆ **S0177** Levamisole hydrochloride, oral, **50 mg**

◆ **S0178** Lomustine, oral, **10 mg**

◆ **S0179** Megestrol acetate, oral, **20 mg**

~~S0181~~ ~~Ondansetron hydrochloride, oral, 4 mg (for circumstances falling under the Medicare Statute, use Q0179)~~ ✻

▶ New	→ Revised	✔ Reinstated	~~deleted~~ Deleted
✪ Special coverage instructions		◆ Not covered or valid by Medicare	✻ Carrier discretion

◆ **S0182** Procarbazine hydrochloride, oral, **50 mg**

◆ **S0183** Prochlorperazine maleate, oral, **5 mg** (for circumstances falling under the Medicare Statute, use Q0164-Q0165)

◆ **S0187** Tamoxifen citrate, oral, **10 mg**

◆ **S0189** Testosterone pellet, **75 mg**

◆ **S0190** Mifepristone, oral, **200 mg**

◆ **S0191** Misoprostol, oral **200 mcg**

◆ **S0194** Dialysis/stress vitamin supplement, oral, **100 capsules**

◆ **S0195** Pneumococcal conjugate vaccine, polyvalent, intramuscular, for children from five years to nine years of age who have not previously received the vaccine

◆ **S0197** Prenatal vitamins, 30-day supply

◆ **S0199** Medically induced abortion by oral ingestion of medication including all associated services and supplies (e.g., patient counseling, office visits, confirmation of pregnancy by HCG, ultrasound to confirm duration of pregnancy, ultrasound to confirm completion of abortion) except drugs

◆ **S0201** Partial hospitalization services, less than 24 hours, per diem

◆ **S0207** Paramedic intercept, non-hospital-based ALS service (non-voluntary), non-transport

◆ **S0208** Paramedic intercept, hospital-based ALS service (non-voluntary), non-transport

◆ **S0209** Wheelchair van, mileage, per mile

◆ **S0215** Non-emergency transportation; mileage per mile

◆ **S0220** Medical conference by a physician with interdisciplinary team of health professionals or representatives of community agencies to coordinate activities of patient care (patient is present); approximately 30 minutes

◆ **S0221** Medical conference by a physician with interdisciplinary team of health professionals or representatives of community agencies to coordinate activities of patient care (patient is present); approximately 60 minutes

◆ **S0250** Comprehensive geriatric assessment and treatment planning performed by assessment team

◆ **S0255** Hospice referral visit (advising patient and family of care options) performed by nurse, social worker, or other designated staff

◆ **S0257** Counseling and discussion regarding advance directives or end of life care planning and decisions, with patient and/or surrogate (list separately in addition to code for appropriate evaluation and management service)

◆ **S0260** History and physical (outpatient or office) related to surgical procedure (list separately in addition to code for appropriate evaluation and management service)

◆ **S0265** Genetic counseling, under physician supervision, each 15 minutes

◆ **S0270** Physician management of patient home care, standard monthly case rate (per 30 days)

◆ **S0271** Physician management of patient home care, hospice monthly case rate (per 30 days)

◆ **S0272** Physician management of patient home care, episodic care monthly case rate (per 30 days)

◆ **S0273** Physician visit at member's home, outside of a capitation arrangement

◆ **S0274** Nurse practitioner visit at member's home, outside of a capitation arrangement

◆ **S0280** Medical home program, comprehensive care coordination and planning, initial plan

◆ **S0281** Medical home program, comprehensive care coordination and planning, maintenance of plan

◆ **S0302** Completed Early Periodic Screening Diagnosis and Treatment (EPSDT) service (list in addition to code for appropriate evaluation and management service)

◆ **S0310** Hospitalist services (list separately in addition to code for appropriate evaluation and management service)

◆ **S0315** Disease management program; initial assessment and initiation of the program

◆ **S0316** Disease management program; follow-up/reassessment

◆ **S0317** Disease management program; per diem

▶ New → Revised ✔ Reinstated ~~deleted~~ Deleted
◎ Special coverage instructions ◆ Not covered or valid by Medicare ✱ Carrier discretion

◆ **S0320** Telephone calls by a registered nurse to a disease management program member for monitoring purposes; per month

◆ **S0340** Lifestyle modification program for management of coronary artery disease, including all supportive services; first quarter/stage

◆ **S0341** Lifestyle modification program for management of coronary artery disease, including all supportive services; second or third quarter/stage

◆ **S0342** Lifestyle modification program for management of coronary artery disease, including all supportive services; fourth quarter/stage

◆ **S0390** Routine foot care; removal and/or trimming of corns, calluses and/or nails and preventive maintenance in specific medical conditions (e.g. diabetes), per visit

◆ **S0395** Impression casting of a foot performed by a practitioner other than the manufacturer of the orthotic

◆ **S0400** Global fee for extracorporeal shock wave lithotripsy treatment of kidney stone(s)

◆ **S0500** Disposable contact lens, per lens

◆ **S0504** Single vision prescription lens (safety, athletic, or sunglass), per lens

◆ **S0506** Bifocal vision prescription lens (safety, athletic, or sunglass), per lens

◆ **S0508** Trifocal vision prescription lens (safety, athletic, or sunglass), per lens

◆ **S0510** Non-prescription lens (safety, athletic, or sunglass), per lens

◆ **S0512** Daily wear specialty contact lens, per lens

◆ **S0514** Color contact lens, per lens

◆ **S0515** Scleral lens, liquid bandage device, per lens

◆ **S0516** Safety eyeglass frames

◆ **S0518** Sunglasses frames

◆ **S0580** Polycarbonate lens (list this code in addition to the basic code for the lens)

◆ **S0581** Nonstandard lens (list this code in addition to the basic code for the lens)

◆ **S0590** Integral lens service, miscellaneous services reported separately

◆ **S0592** Comprehensive contact lens evaluation

◆ **S0595** Dispensing new spectacle lenses for patient supplied frame

◆ **S0601** Screening proctoscopy

◆ **S0610** Annual gynecological examination, new patient

◆ **S0612** Annual gynecological examination, established patient

◆ **S0613** Annual gynecological examination; clinical breast examination without pelvic evaluation

◆ **S0618** Audiometry for hearing aid evaluation to determine the level and degree of hearing loss

◆ **S0620** Routine ophthalmological examination including refraction; new patient

Many non-Medicare vision plans may require code for routine encounter, no complaints

◆ **S0621** Routine ophthalmological examination including refraction; established patient

Many non-Medicare vision plans may require code for routine encounter, no complaints

◆ **S0622** Physical exam for college, new or established patient (list separately) in addition to appropriate evaluation and management code

~~S0625~~ ~~Retinal telescreening by digital imaging of multiple different fundus areas to screen for vision threatening conditions, including imaging, interpretation and report~~ ✳

◆ **S0630** Removal of sutures; by a physician other than the physician who originally closed the wound

◆ **S0800** Laser in situ keratomileusis (LASIK)

◆ **S0810** Photorefractive keratectomy (PRK)

◆ **S0812** Phototherapeutic keratectomy (PTK)

◆ **S1001** Deluxe item, patient aware (list in addition to code for basic item)

◆ **S1002** Customized item (list in addition to code for basic item)

◆ **S1015** IV tubing extension set

◆ **S1016** Non-PVC (polyvinyl chloride) intravenous administration set, for use with drugs that are not stable in PVC e.g. paclitaxel

---

▶ New → Revised ✔ Reinstated ~~deleted~~ Deleted
⊘ Special coverage instructions ◆ Not covered or valid by Medicare ✳ Carrier discretion

◆ **S1030** Continuous noninvasive glucose monitoring device, purchase (for physician interpretation of data, use CPT code)

◆ **S1031** Continuous noninvasive glucose monitoring device, rental, including sensor, sensor replacement, and download to monitor (for physician interpretation of data, use CPT code)

◆ **S1040** Cranial remolding orthosis, pediatric, rigid, with soft interface material, custom fabricated, includes fitting and adjustment(s)

◆ **S2053** Transplantation of small intestine and liver allografts

◆ **S2054** Transplantation of multivisceral organs

◆ **S2055** Harvesting of donor multivisceral organs, with preparation and maintenance of allografts; from cadaver donor

◆ **S2060** Lobar lung transplantation

◆ **S2061** Donor lobectomy (lung) for transplantation, living donor

◆ **S2065** Simultaneous pancreas kidney transplantation

◆ **S2066** Breast reconstruction with gluteal artery perforator (GAP) flap, including harvesting of the flap, microvascular transfer, closure of donor site and shaping the flap into a breast, unilateral

◆ **S2067** Breast reconstruction of a single breast with "stacked" deep inferior epigastric perforator (DIEP) flap(s) and/or gluteal artery perforator (GAP) flap(s), including harvesting of the flap(s), microvascular transfer, closure of donor site(s) and shaping the flap into a breast, unilateral

◆ **S2068** Breast reconstruction with deep inferior epigastric perforator (DIEP) flap, or superficial inferior epigastric artery (SIEA) flap, including harvesting of the flap, microvascular transfer, closure of donor site and shaping the flap into a breast, unilateral

◆ **S2070** Cystourethroscopy, with ureteroscopy and/or pyeloscopy; with endoscopic laser treatment of ureteral calculi (includes ureteral catheterization)

◆ **S2079** Laparoscopic esophagomyotomy (Heller type)

◆ **S2080** Laser-assisted uvulopalatoplasty (LAUP)

◆ **S2083** Adjustment of gastric band diameter via subcutaneous port by injection or aspiration of saline

◆ **S2095** Transcatheter occlusion or embolization for tumor destruction, percutaneous, any method, using yttrium-90 microspheres

◆ **S2102** Islet cell tissue transplant from pancreas; allogeneic

◆ **S2103** Adrenal tissue transplant to brain

◆ **S2107** Adoptive immunotherapy i.e. development of specific anti-tumor reactivity (e.g. tumor-infiltrating lymphocyte therapy) per course of treatment

◆ **S2112** Arthroscopy, knee, surgical for harvesting of cartilage (chondrocyte cells)

◆ **S2115** Osteotomy, periacetabular, with internal fixation

◆ **S2117** Arthroereisis, subtalar

◆ **S2118** Metal-on-metal total hip resurfacing, including acetabular and femoral components

◆ **S2120** Low density lipoprotein (LDL) apheresis using heparin-induced extracorporeal LDL precipitation

◆ **S2140** Cord blood harvesting for transplantation, allogeneic

◆ **S2142** Cord blood-derived stem cell transplantation, allogeneic

◆ **S2150** Bone marrow or blood-derived stem cells (peripheral or umbilical), allogeneic or autologous, harvesting, transplantation, and related complications; including: pheresis and cell preparation/storage; marrow ablative therapy; drugs, supplies, hospitalization with outpatient follow-up; medical/surgical, diagnostic, emergency, and rehabilitative services; and the number of days of pre- and post-transplant care in the global definition

◆ **S2152** Solid organ(s), complete or segmental, single organ or combination of organs; deceased or living donor(s), procurement, transplantation, and related complications; including: drugs; supplies; hospitalization with outpatient follow-up; medical/surgical, diagnostic, emergency, and rehabilitative services, and the number of days of pre- and post-transplant care in the global definition

◆ **S2202** Echosclerotherapy

▶ New   → Revised   ✔ Reinstated   ~~deleted~~ Deleted
◯ Special coverage instructions   ◆ Not covered or valid by Medicare   ✳ Carrier discretion

◆ **S2205** Minimally invasive direct coronary artery bypass surgery involving mini-thoracotomy or mini-sternotomy surgery, performed under direct vision; using arterial graft(s), single coronary arterial graft

◆ **S2206** Minimally invasive direct coronary artery bypass surgery involving mini-thoracotomy or mini-sternotomy surgery, performed under direct vision; using arterial graft(s), two coronary arterial grafts

◆ **S2207** Minimally invasive direct coronary artery bypass surgery involving mini-thoracotomy or mini-sternotomy surgery, performed under direct vision; using venous graft only, single coronary venous graft

◆ **S2208** Minimally invasive direct coronary artery bypass surgery involving mini-thoracotomy or mini-sternotomy surgery, performed under direct vision; using single arterial and venous graft(s), single venous graft

◆ **S2209** Minimally invasive direct coronary artery bypass surgery involving mini-thoracotomy or mini-sternotomy surgery, performed under direct vision; using two arterial grafts and single venous graft

◆ **S2225** Myringotomy, laser-assisted

◆ **S2230** Implantation of magnetic component of semi-implantable hearing device on ossicles in middle ear

◆ **S2235** Implantation of auditory brain stem implant

◆ **S2260** Induced abortion, 17 to 24 weeks

◆ **S2265** Induced abortion, 25 to 28 weeks

◆ **S2266** Induced abortion, 29 to 31 weeks

◆ **S2267** Induced abortion, 32 weeks or greater

~~S2270~~ ~~Insertion of vaginal cylinder for application of radiation source or clinical brachytherapy (report separately in addition to radiation source delivery)~~ ✖

◆ **S2300** Arthroscopy, shoulder, surgical; with thermally-induced capsulorrhaphy

◆ **S2325** Hip core decompression

◆ **S2340** Chemodenervation of abductor muscle(s) of vocal cord

◆ **S2341** Chemodenervation of adductor muscle(s) of vocal cord

◆ **S2342** Nasal endoscopy for post-operative debridement following functional endoscopic sinus surgery, nasal and/or sinus cavity(s), unilateral or bilateral

~~S2344~~ ~~Nasal/sinus endoscopy, surgical; with enlargement of sinus ostium opening using inflatable device (i.e., balloon sinuplasty)~~ ✖

◆ **S2348** Decompression procedure, percutaneous, of nucleus pulpous of intervertebral disc, using radiofrequency energy, single or multiple levels, lumbar

◆ **S2350** Diskectomy, anterior, with decompression of spinal cord and/or nerve root(s), including osteophytectomy; lumbar, single interspace

◆ **S2351** Diskectomy, anterior, with decompression of spinal cord and/or nerve root(s) including osteophytectomy; lumbar, each additional interspace (list separately in addition to code for primary procedure)

◆ **S2360** Percutaneous vertebroplasty, one vertebral body, unilateral or bilateral injection; cervical

◆ **S2361** Each additional cervical vertebral body (list separately in addition to code for primary procedure)

◆ **S2400** Repair, congenital diaphragmatic hernia in the fetus using temporary tracheal occlusion, procedure performed in utero

◆ **S2401** Repair, urinary tract obstruction in the fetus, procedure performed in utero

◆ **S2402** Repair, congenital cystic adenomatoid malformation in the fetus, procedure performed in utero

◆ **S2403** Repair, extralobar pulmonary sequestration in the fetus, procedure performed in utero

◆ **S2404** Repair, myelomeningocele in the fetus, procedure performed in utero

◆ **S2405** Repair of sacrococcygeal teratoma in the fetus, procedure performed in utero

◆ **S2409** Repair, congenital malformation of fetus, procedure performed in utero, not otherwise classified

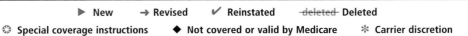

▶ New   → Revised   ✔ Reinstated   ~~deleted~~ Deleted
⊙ Special coverage instructions   ◆ Not covered or valid by Medicare   ✳ Carrier discretion

◆ **S2411** Fetoscopic laser therapy for treatment of twin-to-twin transfusion syndrome

◆ **S2900** Surgical techniques requiring use of robotic surgical system (list separately in addition to code for primary procedure)

◆ **S3000** Diabetic indicator; retinal eye exam, dilated, bilateral

◆ **S3005** Performance measurement, evaluation of patient self assessment, depression

◆ **S3600** STAT laboratory request (situations other than S3601)

◆ **S3601** Emergency STAT laboratory charge for patient who is homebound or residing in a nursing facility

◆ **S3620** Newborn metabolic screening panel, includes test kit, postage and the laboratory tests specified by the state for inclusion in this panel (e.g. galactose; hemoglobin, electrophoresis; hydroxyprogesterone, 17-D; phenylalanine (PKU); and thyroxine, total)

◆ **S3625** Maternal serum triple marker screen including alpha-fetoprotein (AFP), estriol, and human chorionic gonadotropin (HCG)

◆ **S3626** Maternal serum quadruple marker screen including alpha-fetoprotein (AFP), estriol, human chorionic gonadotropin (HCG) and inhibin a

~~S3628~~ ~~Placental alpha microglobulin-~~ ✳
~~1 rapid immunoassay for detection~~
~~of rupture of fetal membranes~~

◆ **S3630** Eosinophil count, blood, direct

◆ **S3645** HIV-1 antibody testing of oral mucosal transudate

◆ **S3650** Saliva test, hormone level; during menopause

◆ **S3652** Saliva test, hormone level; to assess preterm labor risk

◆ **S3655** Antisperm antibodies test (immunobead)

◆ **S3708** Gastrointestinal fat absorption study

◆ **S3711** Circulating tumor cell test

◆ **S3713** KRAS mutation analysis testing

▶ ◆ **S3722** Dose optimization by area under the curve (AUC) analysis, for infusional 5-fluorouracil

◆ **S3800** Genetic testing for amyotrophic lateral sclerosis (ALS)

◆ **S3818** Complete gene sequence analysis; BRCA1 gene

◆ **S3819** Complete gene sequence analysis; BRCA2 gene

◆ **S3820** Complete BRCA1 and BRCA2 gene sequence analysis for susceptibility to breast and ovarian cancer

◆ **S3822** Single mutation analysis (in individual with a known BRCA1 or BRCA2 mutation in the family) for susceptibility to breast and ovarian cancer

◆ **S3823** Three-mutation BRCA1 and BRCA2 analysis for susceptibility to breast and ovarian cancer in Ashkenazi individuals

◆ **S3828** Complete gene sequence analysis; MLH1 gene

◆ **S3829** Complete gene sequence analysis; MSH2 gene

◆ **S3830** Complete MLH and MSH2 gene sequence analysis for hereditary nonpolyposis colorectal cancer (HNPCC) genetic testing

◆ **S3831** Single-mutation analysis (in individual with a known MLH and MSH2 mutation in the family) for hereditary nonpolyposis colorectal cancer (HNPCC) genetic testing

◆ **S3833** Complete APC gene sequence analysis for susceptibility to familial adenomatous polyposis (FAP) and attenuated FAP

◆ **S3834** Single-mutation analysis (in individual with a known APC mutation in the family) for susceptibility to familial adenomatous polyposis (FAP) and attenuated FAP

◆ **S3835** Complete gene sequence analysis for cystic fibrosis genetic testing

◆ **S3837** Complete gene sequence analysis for hemochromatosis genetic testing

◆ **S3840** DNA analysis for germline mutations of the RET proto-oncogene for susceptibility to multiple endocrine neoplasia type 2

◆ **S3841** Genetic testing for retinoblastoma

◆ **S3842** Genetic testing for von Hippel-Lindau disease

◆ **S3843** DNA analysis of the F5 gene for susceptibility to Factor V Leiden thrombophilia

◆ **S3844** DNA analysis of the connexin 26 gene (GJB2) for susceptibility to congenital, profound deafness

◆ **S3845**   Genetic testing for alpha-thalassemia

◆ **S3846**   Genetic testing for hemoglobin E beta-thalassemia

◆ **S3847**   Genetic testing for Tay-Sachs disease

◆ **S3848**   Genetic testing for Gaucher disease

◆ **S3849**   Genetic testing for Niemann-Pick disease

◆ **S3850**   Genetic testing for sickle cell anemia

◆ **S3851**   Genetic testing for Canavan disease

◆ **S3852**   DNA analysis for APOE epilson 4 allele for susceptibility to Alzheimer's disease

◆ **S3853**   Genetic testing for myotonic muscular dystrophy

◆ **S3854**   Gene expression profiling panel for use in the management of breast cancer treatment

◆ **S3855**   Genetic testing for detection of mutations in the presenilin - 1 gene

◆ **S3860**   Genetic testing, comprehensive cardiac ion channel analysis, for variants in 5 major cardiac ion channel genes for individuals with high index of suspicion for familial long QT syndrome (LQTS) or related syndromes

◆ **S3861**   Genetic testing, sodium channel, voltage-gated, type V, alpha subunit (SCN5A) and variants for suspected Brugada syndrome

◆ **S3862**   Genetic testing, family-specific ion channel analysis, for blood-relatives of individuals (index case) who have previously tested positive for a genetic variant of a cardiac ion channel syndrome using either one of the above test configurations or confirmed results from another laboratory

◆ **S3865**   Comprehensive gene sequence analysis for hypertrophic cardiomyopathy

◆ **S3866**   Genetic analysis for a specific gene mutation for hypertrophic cardiomyopathy (HCM) in an individual with a known HCM mutation in the family

◆ **S3870**   Comparative genomic hybrization (CGH) microarray testing for developmental delay, autism spectrum disorder and/or mental retardation

◆ **S3890**   DNA analysis, fecal, for colorectal cancer screening

◆ **S3900**   Surface electromyography (EMG)

◆ **S3902**   Ballistrocardiogram

◆ **S3904**   Masters two step
Bill on paper. Requires a report.

S3905   Non-invasive electrodiagnostic testing with automatic computerized hand-held device to stimulate and measure neuromuscular signals in diagnosing and evaluating systemic and entrapment neuropathies ✳

◆ **S4005**   Interim labor facility global (labor occurring but not resulting in delivery)

◆ **S4011**   In vitro fertilization; including but not limited to identification and incubation of mature oocytes, fertilization with sperm, incubation of embryo(s), and subsequent visualization for determination of development

◆ **S4013**   Complete cycle, gamete intrafallopian transfer (GIFT), case rate

◆ **S4014**   Complete cycle, zygote intrafallopian transfer (ZIFT), case rate

◆ **S4015**   Complete in vitro fertilization cycle, not otherwise specified, case rate

◆ **S4016**   Frozen in vitro fertilization cycle, case rate

◆ **S4017**   Incomplete cycle, treatment cancelled prior to stimulation, case rate

◆ **S4018**   Frozen embryo transfer procedure cancelled before transfer, case rate

◆ **S4020**   In vitro fertilization procedure cancelled before aspiration, case rate

◆ **S4021**   In vitro fertilization procedure cancelled after aspiration, case rate

◆ **S4022**   Assisted oocyte fertilization, case rate

◆ **S4023**   Donor egg cycle, incomplete, case rate

◆ **S4025**   Donor services for in vitro fertilization (sperm or embryo), case rate

◆ **S4026**   Procurement of donor sperm from sperm bank

◆ **S4027**   Storage of previously frozen embryos

◆ **S4028**   Microsurgical epididymal sperm aspiration (MESA)

◆ **S4030**   Sperm procurement and cryopreservation services; initial visit

---

▶ **New**   → **Revised**   ✔ **Reinstated**   ~~deleted~~ **Deleted**
✆ **Special coverage instructions**   ◆ **Not covered or valid by Medicare**   ✳ **Carrier discretion**

◆ **S4031** Sperm procurement and cryopreservation services; subsequent visit

◆ **S4035** Stimulated intrauterine insemination (IUI), case rate

◆ **S4037** Cryopreserved embryo transfer, case rate

◆ **S4040** Monitoring and storage of cryopreserved embryos, per 30 days

◆ **S4042** Management of ovulation induction (interpretation of diagnostic tests and studies, non-face-to-face medical management of the patient), per cycle

◆ **S4981** Insertion of levonorgestrel-releasing intrauterine system

◆ **S4989** Contraceptive intrauterine device (e.g. Progestasert IUD), including implants and supplies

◆ **S4990** Nicotine patches, legend

◆ **S4991** Nicotine patches, non-legend

◆ **S4993** Contraceptive pills for birth control

Only billed by Family Planning Clinics

◆ **S4995** Smoking cessation gum

◆ **S5000** Prescription drug, generic

◆ **S5001** Prescription drug, brand name

◆ **S5010** 5% dextrose and 0.45% normal saline, **1000 ml**

◆ **S5011** 5% dextrose in lactated Ringer's, **1000 ml**

◆ **S5012** 5% dextrose with potassium chloride, **1000 ml**

◆ **S5013** 5% dextrose/0.45% normal saline with potassium chloride and magnesium sulfate, **1000 ml**

◆ **S5014** 5% dextrose/0.45% normal saline with potassium chloride and magnesium sulfate, **1500 ml**

◆ **S5035** Home infusion therapy, routine service of infusion device (e.g. pump maintenance)

◆ **S5036** Home infusion therapy, repair of infusion device (e.g. pump repair)

◆ **S5100** Day care services, adult; per 15 minutes

◆ **S5101** Day care services, adult; per half day

◆ **S5102** Day care services, adult; per diem

◆ **S5105** Day care services, center-based; services not included in program fee, per diem

◆ **S5108** Home care training to home care client, per 15 minutes

◆ **S5109** Home care training to home care client, per session

◆ **S5110** Home care training, family; per 15 minutes

◆ **S5111** Home care training, family; per session

◆ **S5115** Home care training, non-family; per 15 minutes

◆ **S5116** Home care training, non-family; per session

◆ **S5120** Chore services; per 15 minutes

◆ **S5121** Chore services; per diem

◆ **S5125** Attendant care services; per 15 minutes

◆ **S5126** Attendant care services; per diem

◆ **S5130** Homemaker service, NOS; per 15 minutes

◆ **S5131** Homemaker service, NOS; per diem

◆ **S5135** Companion care, adult (e.g. IADL/ADL); per 15 minutes

◆ **S5136** Companion care, adult (e.g. IADL/ADL); per diem

◆ **S5140** Foster care, adult; per diem

◆ **S5141** Foster care, adult; per month

◆ **S5145** Foster care, therapeutic, child; per diem

◆ **S5146** Foster care, therapeutic, child; per month

◆ **S5150** Unskilled respite care, not hospice; per 15 minutes

◆ **S5151** Unskilled respite care, not hospice; per diem

◆ **S5160** Emergency response system; installation and testing

◆ **S5161** Emergency response system; service fee, per month (excludes installation and testing)

◆ **S5162** Emergency response system; purchase only

◆ **S5165** Home modifications; per service

◆ **S5170** Home delivered meals, including preparation; per meal

◆ **S5175** Laundry service, external, professional; per order

◆ **S5180** Home health respiratory therapy, initial evaluation

◆ **S5181** Home health respiratory therapy, NOS, per diem

▶ New	→ Revised	✔ Reinstated	~~deleted~~ Deleted

☼ **Special coverage instructions**   ◆ **Not covered or valid by Medicare**   ✳ **Carrier discretion**

◆ **S5185**   Medication reminder service, non-face-to-face; per month

◆ **S5190**   Wellness assessment, performed by non-physician

◆ **S5199**   Personal care item, NOS, each

◆ **S5497**   Home infusion therapy, catheter care/ maintenance, not otherwise classified; includes administrative services, professional pharmacy services, care coordination, and all necessary supplies and equipment (drugs and nursing visits coded separately), per diem

◆ **S5498**   Home infusion therapy, catheter care/ maintenance, simple (single lumen), includes administrative services, professional pharmacy services, care coordination and all necessary supplies and equipment, (drugs and nursing visits coded separately), per diem

◆ **S5501**   Home infusion therapy, catheter care/ maintenance, complex (more than one lumen), includes administrative services, professional pharmacy services, care coordination, and all necessary supplies and equipment (drugs and nursing visits coded separately), per diem

◆ **S5502**   Home infusion therapy, catheter care/ maintenance, implanted access device, includes administrative services, professional pharmacy services, care coordination, and all necessary supplies and equipment, (drugs and nursing visits coded separately), per diem (use this code for interim maintenance of vascular access not currently in use)

◆ **S5517**   Home infusion therapy, all supplies necessary for restoration of catheter patency or declotting

◆ **S5518**   Home infusion therapy, all supplies necessary for catheter repair

◆ **S5520**   Home infusion therapy, all supplies (including catheter) necessary for a peripherally inserted central venous catheter (PICC) line insertion

Bill on paper. Requires a report.

◆ **S5521**   Home infusion therapy, all supplies (including catheter) necessary for a midline catheter insertion

◆ **S5522**   Home infusion therapy, insertion of peripherally inserted central venous catheter (PICC), nursing services only (no supplies or catheter included)

◆ **S5523**   Home infusion therapy, insertion of midline central venous catheter, nursing services only (no supplies or catheter included)

◆ **S5550**   Insulin, rapid onset, **5 units**

◆ **S5551**   Insulin, most rapid onset (Lispro or Aspart); **5 units**

◆ **S5552**   Insulin, intermediate acting (NPH or Lente); **5 units**

◆ **S5553**   Insulin, long acting; **5 units**

◆ **S5560**   Insulin delivery device, reusable pen; **1.5 ml** size

◆ **S5561**   Insulin delivery device, reusable pen; **3 ml** size

◆ **S5565**   Insulin cartridge for use in insulin delivery device other than pump; **150 units**

◆ **S5566**   Insulin cartridge for use in insulin delivery device other than pump; **300 units**

◆ **S5570**   Insulin delivery device, disposable pen (including insulin); **1.5 ml** size

◆ **S5571**   Insulin delivery device, disposable pen (including insulin); **3 ml** size

◆ **S8030**   Scleral application of tantalum ring(s) for localization of lesions for proton beam therapy

◆ **S8035**   Magnetic source imaging

◆ **S8037**   Magnetic resonance cholangiopancreatography (MRCP)

◆ **S8040**   Topographic brain mapping

◆ **S8042**   Magnetic resonance imaging (MRI), low-field

◆ **S8049**   Intraoperative radiation therapy (single administration)

◆ **S8055**   Ultrasound guidance for multifetal pregnancy reduction(s), technical component (only to be used when the physician doing the reduction procedure does not perform the ultrasound, guidance is included in the CPT code for multifetal pregnancy reduction - 59866)

◆ **S8080**   Scintimammography (radioimmunoscintigraphy of the breast), unilateral, including supply of radiopharmaceutical

◆ **S8085**   Fluorine-18 fluorodeoxyglucose (F-18 FDG) imaging using dual-head coincidence detection system (non-dedicated PET scan)

◆ **S8092**   Electron beam computed tomography (also known as ultrafast CT, cine CT)

◆ **S8096**   Portable peak flow meter

◆ **S8097** Asthma kit (including but not limited to portable peak expiratory flow meter, instructional video, brochure, and/or spacer)

◆ **S8100** Holding chamber or spacer for use with an inhaler or nebulizer; without mask

◆ **S8101** Holding chamber or spacer for use with an inhaler or nebulizer; with mask

◆ **S8110** Peak expiratory flow rate (physician services)

◆ **S8120** Oxygen contents, gaseous, 1 unit equals 1 cubic foot

◆ **S8121** Oxygen contents, liquid, 1 unit equals 1 pound

▶ ◆ **S8130** Interferential current stimulator, 2 channel

▶ ◆ **S8131** Interferential current stimulator, 4 channel

◆ **S8185** Flutter device

◆ **S8186** Swivel adaptor

◆ **S8189** Tracheostomy supply, not otherwise classified

◆ **S8210** Mucus trap

◆ **S8262** Mandibular orthopedic repositioning device, each

◆ **S8265** Haberman feeder for cleft lip/palate

◆ **S8270** Enuresis alarm, using auditory buzzer and/or vibration device

◆ **S8301** Infection control supplies, not otherwise specified

◆ **S8415** Supplies for home delivery of infant

◆ **S8420** Gradient pressure aid (sleeve and glove combination), custom made

◆ **S8421** Gradient pressure aid (sleeve and glove combination), ready made

◆ **S8422** Gradient pressure aid (sleeve), custom made, medium weight

◆ **S8423** Gradient pressure aid (sleeve), custom made, heavy weight

◆ **S8424** Gradient pressure aid (sleeve), ready made

◆ **S8425** Gradient pressure aid (glove), custom made, medium weight

◆ **S8426** Gradient pressure aid (glove), custom made, heavy weight

◆ **S8427** Gradient pressure aid (glove), ready made

◆ **S8428** Gradient pressure aid (gauntlet), ready made

◆ **S8429** Gradient pressure exterior wrap

◆ **S8430** Padding for compression bandage, roll

◆ **S8431** Compression bandage, roll

◆ **S8450** Splint, prefabricated, digit (specify digit by use of modifier)

◆ **S8451** Splint, prefabricated, wrist or ankle

◆ **S8452** Splint, prefabricated, elbow

◆ **S8460** Camisole, post-mastectomy

◆ **S8490** Insulin syringes (100 syringes, any size)

◆ **S8940** Equestrian/Hippotherapy, per session

◆ **S8948** Application of a modality (requiring constant provider attendance) to one or more areas; low-level laser; each 15 minutes

◆ **S8950** Complex lymphedema therapy, each 15 minutes

◆ **S8990** Physical or manipulative therapy performed for maintenance rather than restoration

◆ **S8999** Resuscitation bag (for use by patient on artificial respiration during power failure or other catastrophic event)

◆ **S9001** Home uterine monitor with or without associated nursing services

◆ **S9007** Ultrafiltration monitor

◆ **S9015** Automated EEG monitoring

◆ **S9024** Paranasal sinus ultrasound

◆ **S9025** Omnicardiogram/cardiointegram

◆ **S9034** Extracorporeal shockwave lithotripsy for gall stones (if performed with ERCP, use 43265)

◆ **S9055** Procuren or other growth factor preparation to promote wound healing

◆ **S9056** Coma stimulation per diem

◆ **S9061** Home administration of aerosolized drug therapy (e.g., pentamidine); administrative services, professional pharmacy services, care coordination, all necessary supplies and equipment (drugs and nursing visits coded separately), per diem

~~S9075~~ ~~Smoking cessation treatment~~ ✳

◆ **S9083** Global fee urgent care centers

◆ **S9088** Services provided in an urgent care center (list in addition to code for service)

▶ New   → Revised   ✔ Reinstated   ~~deleted~~ Deleted

○ Special coverage instructions   ◆ Not covered or valid by Medicare   ✳ Carrier discretion

◆ **S9090** Vertebral axial decompression, per session

◆ **S9097** Home visit for wound care

◆ **S9098** Home visit, phototherapy services (e.g. Bili-Lite), including equipment rental, nursing services, blood draw, supplies, and other services, per diem

◆ **S9109** Congestive heart failure telemonitoring, equipment rental, including telescale, computer system and software, telephone connections, and maintenance, per month

◆ **S9117** Back school, per visit

◆ **S9122** Home health aide or certified nurse assistant, providing care in the home; per hour

◆ **S9123** Nursing care, in the home; by registered nurse, per hour (use for general nursing care only, not to be used when CPT codes 99500-99602 can be used)

◆ **S9124** Nursing care, in the home; by licensed practical nurse, per hour

◆ **S9125** Respite care, in the home, per diem

◆ **S9126** Hospice care, in the home, per diem

◆ **S9127** Social work visit, in the home, per diem

◆ **S9128** Speech therapy, in the home, per diem

◆ **S9129** Occupational therapy, in the home, per diem

◆ **S9131** Physical therapy; in the home, per diem

◆ **S9140** Diabetic management program, follow-up visit to non-MD provider

◆ **S9141** Diabetic management program, follow-up visit to MD provider

◆ **S9145** Insulin pump initiation, instruction in initial use of pump (pump not included)

◆ **S9150** Evaluation by ocularist

◆ **S9152** Speech therapy, re-evaluation

◆ **S9208** Home management of preterm labor, including administrative services, professional pharmacy services, care coordination, and all necessary supplies or equipment (drugs and nursing visits coded separately), per diem (do not use this code with any home infusion per diem code)

◆ **S9209** Home management of preterm premature rupture of membranes (PPROM), including administrative services, professional pharmacy services, care coordination, and all necessary supplies or equipment (drugs and nursing visits coded separately), per diem (do not use this code with any home infusion per diem code)

◆ **S9211** Home management of gestational hypertension, includes administrative services, professional pharmacy services, care coordination, and all necessary supplies and equipment (drugs and nursing visits coded separately); per diem (do not use this code with any home infusion per diem code)

◆ **S9212** Home management of postpartum hypertension, includes administrative services, professional pharmacy services, care coordination, and all necessary supplies and equipment (drugs and nursing visits coded separately), per diem (do not use this code with any home infusion per diem code)

◆ **S9213** Home management of preeclampsia, includes administrative services, professional pharmacy services, care coordination, and all necessary supplies and equipment (drugs and nursing services coded separately); per diem (do not use this code with any home infusion per diem code)

◆ **S9214** Home management of gestational diabetes, includes administrative services, professional pharmacy services, care coordination, and all necessary supplies and equipment (drugs and nursing visits coded separately); per diem (do not use this code with any home infusion per diem code)

◆ **S9325** Home infusion therapy, pain management infusion; administrative services, professional pharmacy services, care coordination, and all necessary supplies and equipment, (drugs and nursing visits coded separately), per diem (do not use this code with S9326, S9327 or S9328)

◆ **S9326** Home infusion therapy, continuous (twenty-four hours or more) pain management infusion; administrative services, professional pharmacy services, care coordination, and all necessary supplies and equipment (drugs and nursing visits coded separately), per diem

◆ **S9327** Home infusion therapy, intermittent (less than twenty-four hours) pain management infusion; administrative services, professional pharmacy services, care coordination, and all necessary supplies and equipment (drugs and nursing visits coded separately), per diem

◆ **S9328** Home infusion therapy, implanted pump pain management infusion; administrative services, professional pharmacy services, care coordination, and all necessary supplies and equipment (drugs and nursing visits coded separately), per diem

◆ **S9329** Home infusion therapy, chemotherapy infusion; administrative services, professional pharmacy services, care coordination, and all necessary supplies and equipment (drugs and nursing visits coded separately), per diem (do not use this code with S9330 or S9331)

◆ **S9330** Home infusion therapy, continuous (twenty-four hours or more) chemotherapy infusion; administrative services, professional pharmacy services, care coordination, and all necessary supplies and equipment (drugs and nursing visits coded separately), per diem

◆ **S9331** Home infusion therapy, intermittent (less than twenty-four hours) chemotherapy infusion; administrative services, professional pharmacy services, care coordination, and all necessary supplies and equipment (drugs and nursing visits coded separately), per diem

◆ **S9335** Home therapy, hemodialysis; administrative services, professional pharmacy services, care coordination, and all necessary supplies and equipment (drugs and nursing services coded separately), per diem

◆ **S9336** Home infusion therapy, continuous anticoagulant infusion therapy (e.g. heparin), administrative services, professional pharmacy services, care coordination, and all necessary supplies and equipment (drugs and nursing visits coded separately), per diem

◆ **S9338** Home infusion therapy, immunotherapy, administrative services, professional pharmacy services, care coordination, and all necessary supplies and equipment (drug and nursing visits coded separately), per diem

◆ **S9339** Home therapy; peritoneal dialysis, administrative services, professional pharmacy services, care coordination and all necessary supplies and equipment (drugs and nursing visits coded separately), per diem

◆ **S9340** Home therapy; enteral nutrition; administrative services, professional pharmacy services, care coordination, and all necessary supplies and equipment (enteral formula and nursing visits coded separately), per diem

◆ **S9341** Home therapy; enteral nutrition via gravity; administrative services, professional pharmacy services, care coordination, and all necessary supplies and equipment (enteral formula and nursing visits coded separately), per diem

◆ **S9342** Home therapy; enteral nutrition via pump; administrative services, professional pharmacy services, care coordination, and all necessary supplies and equipment (enteral formula and nursing visits coded separately), per diem

◆ **S9343** Home therapy; enteral nutrition via bolus; administrative services, professional pharmacy services, care coordination, and all necessary supplies and equipment (enteral formula and nursing visits coded separately), per diem

◆ **S9345** Home infusion therapy, anti-hemophilic agent infusion therapy (e.g. Factor VIII); administrative services, professional pharmacy services, care coordination, and all necessary supplies and equipment (drugs and nursing visits coded separately), per diem

◆ **S9346** Home infusion therapy, alpha-1-proteinase inhibitor (e.g., Prolastin); administrative services, professional pharmacy services, care coordination, and all necessary supplies and equipment (drugs and nursing visits coded separately), per diem

◆ **S9347** Home infusion therapy, uninterrupted, long-term, controlled rate intravenous or subcutaneous infusion therapy (e.g. Epoprostenol); administrative services, professional pharmacy services, care coordination, and all necessary supplies and equipment (drugs and nursing visits coded separately), per diem

---

▶ New → Revised ✔ Reinstated ~~deleted~~ Deleted
☺ Special coverage instructions ◆ Not covered or valid by Medicare ✳ Carrier discretion

◆ **S9348** Home infusion therapy, sympathomimetic/inotropic agent infusion therapy (e.g., Dobutamine); administrative services, professional pharmacy services, care coordination, all necessary supplies and equipment (drugs and nursing visits coded separately), per diem

◆ **S9349** Home infusion therapy, tocolytic infusion therapy; administrative services, professional pharmacy services, care coordination, and all necessary supplies and equipment (drugs and nursing visits coded separately), per diem

◆ **S9351** Home infusion therapy, continuous or intermittent anti-emetic infusion therapy; administrative services, professional pharmacy services, care coordination, and all necessary supplies and equipment (drugs and visits coded separately), per diem

◆ **S9353** Home infusion therapy, continuous insulin infusion therapy; administrative services, professional pharmacy services, care coordination, and all necessary supplies and equipment (drugs and nursing visits coded separately), per diem

◆ **S9355** Home infusion therapy, chelation therapy; administrative services, professional pharmacy services, care coordination, and all necessary supplies and equipment (drugs and nursing visits coded separately), per diem

◆ **S9357** Home infusion therapy, enzyme replacement intravenous therapy; (e.g. Imiglucerase); administrative services, professional pharmacy services, care coordination, and all necessary supplies and equipment (drugs and nursing visits coded separately), per diem

◆ **S9359** Home infusion therapy, anti-tumor necrosis factor intravenous therapy; (e.g. Infliximab); administrative services, professional pharmacy services, care coordination, and all necessary supplies and equipment (drugs and nursing visits coded separately), per diem

◆ **S9361** Home infusion therapy, diuretic intravenous therapy; administrative services, professional pharmacy services, care coordination, and all necessary supplies and equipment (drugs and nursing visits coded separately), per diem

◆ **S9363** Home infusion therapy, anti-spasmotic therapy; administrative services, professional pharmacy services, care coordination, and all necessary supplies and equipment (drugs and nursing visits coded separately), per diem

◆ **S9364** Home infusion therapy, total parenteral nutrition (TPN); administrative services, professional pharmacy services, care coordination, and all necessary supplies and equipment including standard TPN formula (lipids, specialty amino acid formulas, drugs other than in standard formula, and nursing visits coded separately) per diem (do not use with home infusion codes S9365-S9368 using daily volume scales)

◆ **S9365** Home infusion therapy, total parenteral nutrition (TPN); one liter per day, administrative services, professional pharmacy services, care coordination, and all necessary supplies and equipment including standard TPN formula (lipids, specialty amino acid formulas, drugs other than in standard formula and nursing visits coded separately), per diem

◆ **S9366** Home infusion therapy, total parenteral nutrition (TPN); more than one liter but no more than two liters per day, administrative services, professional pharmacy services, care coordination, and all necessary supplies and equipment including standard TPN formula; (lipids, specialty amino acid formulas, drugs other than in standard formula and nursing visits coded separately), per diem

◆ **S9367** Home infusion therapy, total parenteral nutrition (TPN); more than two liters but no more than three liters per day, administrative services, professional pharmacy services, care coordination, and all necessary supplies and equipment including standard TPN formula; (lipids, specialty amino acid formulas, drugs other than in standard formula and nursing visits coded separately), per diem

◆ **S9368** Home infusion therapy, total parenteral nutrition (TPN); more than three liters per day, administrative services, professional pharmacy services, care coordination, and all necessary supplies and equipment (including standard TPN formula; lipids, specialty amino acid formulas, drugs other than in standard formula and nursing visits coded separately), per diem

▶ New   → Revised   ✔ Reinstated   deleted Deleted   ☺ Special coverage instructions   ◆ Not covered or valid by Medicare   ✳ Carrier discretion

◆ **S9538** Home transfusion of blood product(s); administrative services, professional pharmacy services, care coordination, and all necessary supplies and equipment (blood products, drugs, and nursing visits coded separately), per diem

◆ **S9542** Home injectable therapy; not otherwise classified, including administrative services, professional pharmacy services, care coordination, and all necessary supplies and equipment (drugs and nursing visits coded separately), per diem

◆ **S9558** Home injectable therapy; growth hormone, including administrative services, professional pharmacy services, care coordination, and all necessary supplies and equipment (drugs and nursing visits coded separately), per diem

◆ **S9559** Home injectable therapy; interferon, including administrative services, professional pharmacy services, care coordination, and all necessary supplies and equipment (drugs and nursing visits coded separately), per diem

◆ **S9560** Home injectable therapy; hormonal therapy (e.g., Leuprolide, Goserelin), including administrative services, professional pharmacy services, care coordination, and all necessary supplies and equipment (drugs and nursing visits coded separately), per diem

◆ **S9562** Home injectable therapy, palivizumab, including administrative services, professional pharmacy services, care coordination, and all necessary supplies and equipment (drugs and nursing visits coded separately), per diem

◆ **S9590** Home therapy, irrigation therapy (e.g. sterile irrigation of an organ or anatomical cavity); including administrative services, professional pharmacy services, care coordination, and all necessary supplies and equipment (drugs and nursing visits coded separately), per diem

◆ **S9810** Home therapy; professional pharmacy services for provision of infusion, specialty drug administration, and/or disease state management, not otherwise classified, per hour (do not use this code with any per diem code)

→ ◆ **S9900** Services by journal-listed Christian Science Practitioner for the purpose of healing, per diem

◆ **S9970** Health club membership, annual

◆ **S9975** Transplant related lodging, meals and transportation, per diem

◆ **S9976** Lodging, per diem, not otherwise classified

◆ **S9977** Meals, per diem, not otherwise specified

◆ **S9981** Medical records copying fee, administrative

◆ **S9982** Medical records copying fee, per page

◆ **S9986** Not medically necessary service (patient is aware that service not medically necessary)

◆ **S9988** Services provided as part of a Phase I clinical trial

◆ **S9989** Services provided outside of the United States of America (list in addition to code(s) for services(s))

◆ **S9990** Services provided as part of a Phase II clinical trial

◆ **S9991** Services provided as part of a Phase III clinical trial

◆ **S9992** Transportation costs to and from trial location and local transportation costs (e.g., fares for taxicab or bus) for clinical trial participant and one caregiver/companion

◆ **S9994** Lodging costs (e.g., hotel charges) for clinical trial participant and one caregiver/companion

◆ **S9996** Meals for clinical trial participant and one caregiver/companion

◆ **S9999** Sales tax

▶ New   → Revised   ✔ Reinstated   ‑deleted‑ Deleted
☼ Special coverage instructions   ◆ Not covered or valid by Medicare   ✳ Carrier discretion

TEMPORARY NATIONAL CODES ESTABLISHED BY MEDICAID (T1000-T9999)

Not Valid For Medicare

◆ **T1000** Private duty/independent nursing service(s) - licensed, up to 15 minutes

◆ **T1001** Nursing assessment/evaluation

◆ **T1002** RN services, up to 15 minutes

◆ **T1003** LPN/LVN services, up to 15 minutes

◆ **T1004** Services of a qualified nursing aide, up to 15 minutes

◆ **T1005** Respite care services, up to 15 minutes

◆ **T1006** Alcohol and/or substance abuse services, family/couple counseling

◆ **T1007** Alcohol and/or substance abuse services, treatment plan development and/or modification

◆ **T1009** Child sitting services for children of the individual receiving alcohol and/or substance abuse services

◆ **T1010** Meals for individuals receiving alcohol and/or substance abuse services (when meals not included in the program)

◆ **T1012** Alcohol and/or substance abuse services, skills development

◆ **T1013** Sign language or oral interpretive services, per 15 minutes

◆ **T1014** Telehealth transmission, per minute, professional services bill separately

◆ **T1015** Clinic visit/encounter, all-inclusive

◆ **T1016** Case Management, each 15 minutes

◆ **T1017** Targeted Case Management, each 15 minutes

◆ **T1018** School-based individualized education program (IEP) services, bundled

◆ **T1019** Personal care services, per 15 minutes, not for an inpatient or resident of a hospital, nursing facility, ICF/MR or IMD, part of the individualized plan of treatment (code may not be used to identify services provided by home health aide or certified nurse assistant)

◆ **T1020** Personal care services, per diem, not for an inpatient or resident of a hospital, nursing facility, ICF/MR or IMD, part of the individualized plan of treatment (code may not be used to identify services provided by home health aide or certified nurse assistant)

◆ **T1021** Home health aide or certified nurse assistant, per visit

◆ **T1022** Contracted home health agency services, all services provided under contract, per day

◆ **T1023** Screening to determine the appropriateness of consideration of an individual for participation in a specified program, project or treatment protocol, per encounter

◆ **T1024** Evaluation and treatment by an integrated, specialty team contracted to provide coordinated care to multiple or severely handicapped children, per encounter

◆ **T1025** Intensive, extended multidisciplinary services provided in a clinic setting to children with complex medical, physical, mental and psychosocial impairments, per diem

◆ **T1026** Intensive, extended multidisciplinary services provided in a clinic setting to children with complex medical, physical, medical and psychosocial impairments, per hour

◆ **T1027** Family training and counseling for child development, per 15 minutes

◆ **T1028** Assessment of home, physical and family environment, to determine suitability to meet patient's medical needs

◆ **T1029** Comprehensive environmental lead investigation, not including laboratory analysis, per dwelling

◆ **T1030** Nursing care, in the home, by registered nurse, per diem

◆ **T1031** Nursing care, in the home, by licensed practical nurse, per diem

◆ **T1502** Administration of oral, intramuscular and/or subcutaneous medication by health care agency/professional, per visit

◆ **T1503** Administration of medication, other than oral and/or injectable, by a health care agency/professional, per visit

▶ ◆ **T1505** Electronic medication compliance management device, includes all components and accessories, not otherwise classified

◆ **T1999** Miscellaneous therapeutic items and supplies, retail purchases, not otherwise classified; identify product in "remarks"

◆ **T2001** Non-emergency transportation; patient attendant/escort

◆ **T2002** Non-emergency transportation; per diem

◆ **T2003** Non-emergency transportation; encounter/trip

◆ **T2004** Non-emergency transport; commercial carrier, multi-pass

◆ **T2005** Non-emergency transportation: stretcher van

◆ **T2007** Transportation waiting time, air ambulance and non-emergency vehicle, one-half (1/2) hour increments

◆ **T2010** Preadmission screening and resident review (PASRR) level I identification screening, per screen

◆ **T2011** Preadmission screening and resident review (PASRR) level II evaluation, per evaluation

◆ **T2012** Habilitation, educational, waiver; per diem

◆ **T2013** Habilitation, educational, waiver; per hour

◆ **T2014** Habilitation, prevocational, waiver; per diem

◆ **T2015** Habilitation, prevocational, waiver; per hour

◆ **T2016** Habilitation, residential, waiver; per diem

◆ **T2017** Habilitation, residential, waiver; 15 minutes

◆ **T2018** Habilitation, supported employment, waiver; per diem

◆ **T2019** Habilitation, supported employment, waiver; per 15 minutes

◆ **T2020** Day habilitation, waiver; per diem

◆ **T2021** Day habilitation, waiver; per 15 minutes

◆ **T2022** Case management, per month

◆ **T2023** Targeted case management; per month

◆ **T2024** Service assessment/plan of care development, waiver

◆ **T2025** Waiver services; not otherwise specified (NOS)

◆ **T2026** Specialized childcare, waiver; per diem

◆ **T2027** Specialized childcare, waiver; per 15 minutes

◆ **T2028** Specialized supply, not otherwise specified, waiver

◆ **T2029** Specialized medical equipment, not otherwise specified, waiver

◆ **T2030** Assisted living, waiver; per month

◆ **T2031** Assisted living; waiver, per diem

◆ **T2032** Residential care, not otherwise specified (NOS), waiver; per month

◆ **T2033** Residential care, not otherwise specified (NOS), waiver; per diem

◆ **T2034** Crisis intervention, waiver; per diem

◆ **T2035** Utility services to support medical equipment and assistive technology/ devices, waiver

◆ **T2036** Therapeutic camping, overnight, waiver; each session

◆ **T2037** Therapeutic camping, day, waiver; each session

◆ **T2038** Community transition, waiver; per service

◆ **T2039** Vehicle modifications, waiver; per service

◆ **T2040** Financial management, self-directed, waiver; per 15 minutes

◆ **T2041** Supports brokerage, self-directed, waiver; per 15 minutes

◆ **T2042** Hospice routine home care; per diem

◆ **T2043** Hospice continuous home care; per hour

◆ **T2044** Hospice inpatient respite care; per diem

◆ **T2045** Hospice general inpatient care; per diem

◆ **T2046** Hospice long term care, room and board only; per diem

◆ **T2048** Behavioral health; long-term care residential (non-acute care in a residential treatment program where stay is typically longer than 30 days), with room and board, per diem

◆ **T2049** Non-emergency transportation; stretcher van, mileage; per mile

◆ **T2101** Human breast milk processing, storage and distribution only

◆ **T4521** Adult sized disposable incontinence product, brief/diaper, small, each

IOM: 100-03, 4, 280.1

▶ New → Revised ✔ Reinstated deleted Deleted
☺ Special coverage instructions ◆ Not covered or valid by Medicare ✳ Carrier discretion

◆ **T4522** Adult sized disposable incontinence product, brief/diaper, medium, each

IOM: 100-03, 4, 280.1

◆ **T4523** Adult sized disposable incontinence product, brief/diaper, large, each

IOM: 100-03, 4, 280.1

◆ **T4524** Adult sized disposable incontinence product, brief/diaper, extra large, each

IOM: 100-03, 4, 280.1

◆ **T4525** Adult sized disposable incontinence product, protective underwear/pull-on, small size, each

IOM: 100-03, 4, 280.1

◆ **T4526** Adult sized disposable incontinence product, protective underwear/pull-on, medium size, each

IOM: 100-03, 4, 280.1

◆ **T4527** Adult sized disposable incontinence product, protective underwear/pull-on, large size, each

IOM: 100-03, 4, 280.1

◆ **T4528** Adult sized disposable incontinence product, protective underwear/pull-on, extra large size, each

IOM: 100-03, 4, 280.1

◆ **T4529** Pediatric sized disposable incontinence product, brief/diaper, small/medium size, each

IOM: 100-03, 4, 280.1

◆ **T4530** Pediatric sized disposable incontinence product, brief/diaper, large size, each

IOM: 100-03, 4, 280.1

◆ **T4531** Pediatric sized disposable incontinence product, protective underwear/pull-on, small/medium size, each

IOM: 100-03, 4, 280.1

◆ **T4532** Pediatric sized disposable incontinence product, protective underwear/pull-on, large size, each

IOM: 100-03, 4, 280.1

◆ **T4533** Youth sized disposable incontinence product, brief/diaper, each

IOM: 100-03, 4, 280.1

◆ **T4534** Youth sized disposable incontinence product, protective underwear/pull-on, each

IOM: 100-03, 4, 280.1

◆ **T4535** Disposable liner/shield/guard/pad/undergarment, for incontinence, each

IOM: 100-03, 4, 280.1

◆ **T4536** Incontinence product, protective underwear/pull-on, reusable, any size, each

IOM: 100-03, 4, 280.1

◆ **T4537** Incontinence product, protective underpad, reusable, bed size, each

IOM: 100-03, 4, 280.1

◆ **T4538** Diaper service, reusable diaper, each diaper

IOM: 100-03, 4, 280.1

◆ **T4539** Incontinence product, diaper/brief, reusable, any size, each

IOM: 100-03, 4, 280.1

◆ **T4540** Incontinence product, protective underpad, reusable, chair size, each

IOM: 100-03, 4, 280.1

◆ **T4541** Incontinence product, disposable underpad, large, each

◆ **T4542** Incontinence product, disposable underpad, small size, each

◆ **T4543** Disposable incontinence product, brief/diaper, bariatric, each

IOM: 100-03, 4, 280.1

◆ **T5001** Positioning seat for persons with special orthopedic needs, supply, not otherwise specified

◆ **T5999** Supply, not otherwise specified

▶ New → Revised ✔ Reinstated deleted Deleted
☺ Special coverage instructions ◆ Not covered or valid by Medicare ✳ Carrier discretion

VISION SERVICES (V0000-V2999)

Frames

V2020-V2025: Bill DME/MAC

⊛ **V2020** Frames, purchases

Includes cost of frame/replacement and dispensing fee. One unit of service represents one frame.

IOM: 100-02, 15, 120

◆ **V2025** Deluxe frame

Not a benefit. Billing deluxe frames— submit V2020 on one line; V2025 on second line

IOM: 100-04, 1, 30.3.5

Spectacle Lenses

NOTE: If a CPT procedure code for supply of spectacles or a permanent prosthesis is reported, recode with the specific lens type listed below. For aphakic temporary spectacle correction, see CPT.

Single Vision, Glass or Plastic

❋ **V2100** Sphere, single vision, plano to plus or minus 4.00, per lens

Bill DME/MAC

❋ **V2101** Sphere, single vision, plus or minus 4.12 to plus or minus 7.00d, per lens

Bill DME/MAC

❋ **V2102** Sphere, single vision, plus or minus 7.12 to plus or minus 20.00d, per lens

Bill DME/MAC

❋ **V2103** Spherocylinder, single vision, plano to plus or minus 4.00d sphere, .12 to 2.00d cylinder, per lens

Bill DME/MAC

❋ **V2104** Spherocylinder, single vision, plano to plus or minus 4.00d sphere, 2.12 to 4.00d cylinder, per lens

Bill DME/MAC

❋ **V2105** Spherocylinder, single vision, plano to plus or minus 4.00d sphere, 4.25 to 6.00d cylinder, per lens

Bill DME/MAC

❋ **V2106** Spherocylinder, single vision, plano to plus or minus 4.00d sphere, over 6.00d cylinder, per lens

Bill DME/MAC

❋ **V2107** Spherocylinder, single vision, plus or minus 4.25 to plus or minus 7.00 sphere, .12 to 2.00d cylinder, per lens

Bill DME/MAC

❋ **V2108** Spherocylinder, single vision, plus or minus 4.25d to plus or minus 7.00d sphere, 2.12 to 4.00d cylinder, per lens

Bill DME/MAC

❋ **V2109** Spherocylinder, single vision, plus or minus 4.25 to plus or minus 7.00d sphere, 4.25 to 6.00d cylinder, per lens

Bill DME/MAC

❋ **V2110** Sperocylinder, single vision, plus or minus 4.25 to 7.00d sphere, over 6.00d cylinder, per lens

Bill DME/MAC

❋ **V2111** Spherocylinder, single vision, plus or minus 7.25 to plus or minus 12.00d sphere, .25 to 2.25d cylinder, per lens

Bill DME/MAC

❋ **V2112** Spherocylinder, single vision, plus or minus 7.25 to plus or minus 12.00d sphere, 2.25d to 4.00d cylinder, per lens

Bill DME/MAC

❋ **V2113** Spherocylinder, single vision, plus or minus 7.25 to plus or minus 12.00d sphere, 4.25 to 6.00d cylinder, per lens

Bill DME/MAC

❋ **V2114** Spherocylinder, single vision, sphere over plus or minus 12.00d, per lens

Bill DME/MAC

❋ **V2115** Lenticular, (myodisc), per lens, single vision

Bill DME/MAC

❋ **V2118** Aniseikonic lens, single vision

Bill DME/MAC

⊛ **V2121** Lenticular lens, per lens, single

Bill DME/MAC

IOM: 100-02, 15, 120; 100-04, 3, 10.4

❋ **V2199** Not otherwise classified, single vision lens

Bill DME/MAC

Bill on paper. Requires report of type of single vision lens and optical lab invoice.

Bifocal, Glass or Plastic

❋ **V2200** Sphere, bifocal, plano to plus or minus 4.00d, per lens

Bill DME/MAC

▶ New ⟶ Revised ✔ Reinstated ~~deleted~~ Deleted

⊛ Special coverage instructions ◆ Not covered or valid by Medicare ❋ Carrier discretion

* **V2201** Sphere, bifocal, plus or minus 4.12 to plus or minus 7.00d, per lens
  Bill DME/MAC

* **V2202** Sphere, bifocal, plus or minus 7.12 to plus or minus 20.00d, per lens
  Bill DME/MAC

* **V2203** Spherocylinder, bifocal, plano to plus or minus 4.00d sphere, .12 to 2.00d cylinder, per lens
  Bill DME/MAC

* **V2204** Spherocylinder, bifocal, plano to plus or minus 4.00d sphere, 2.12 to 4.00d cylinder, per lens
  Bill DME/MAC

* **V2205** Spherocylinder, bifocal, plano to plus or minus 4.00d sphere, 4.25 to 6.00d cylinder, per lens
  Bill DME/MAC

* **V2206** Spherocylinder, bifocal, plano to plus or minus 4.00d sphere, over 6.00d cylinder, per lens
  Bill DME/MAC

* **V2207** Spherocylinder, bifocal, plus or minus 4.25 to plus or minus 7.00d sphere, .12 to 2.00d cylinder, per lens
  Bill DME/MAC

* **V2208** Spherocylinder, bifocal, plus or minus 4.25 to plus or minus 7.00d sphere, 2.12 to 4.00d cylinder, per lens
  Bill DME/MAC

* **V2209** Spherocylinder, bifocal, plus or minus 4.25 to plus or minus 7.00d sphere, 4.25 to 6.00d cylinder, per lens
  Bill DME/MAC

* **V2210** Spherocylinder, bifocal, plus or minus 4.25 to plus or minus 7.00d sphere, over 6.00d cylinder, per lens
  Bill DME/MAC

* **V2211** Spherocylinder, bifocal, plus or minus 7.25 to plus or minus 12.00d sphere, .25 to 2.25d cylinder, per lens
  Bill DME/MAC

* **V2212** Spherocylinder, bifocal, plus or minus 7.25 to plus or minus 12.00d sphere, 2.25 to 4.00d cylinder, per lens
  Bill DME/MAC

* **V2213** Spherocylinder, bifocal, plus or minus 7.25 to plus or minus 12.00d sphere, 4.25 to 6.00d cylinder, per lens
  Bill DME/MAC

* **V2214** Spherocylinder, bifocal, sphere over plus or minus 12.00d, per lens
  Bill DME/MAC

* **V2215** Lenticular (myodisc), per lens, bifocal
  Bill DME/MAC

* **V2218** Aniseikonic, per lens, bifocal
  Bill DME/MAC

* **V2219** Bifocal seg width over 28mm
  Bill DME/MAC

* **V2220** Bifocal add over 3.25d
  Bill DME/MAC

© **V2221** Lenticular lens, per lens, bifocal
  Bill DME/MAC
  IOM: 100-02, 15, 120; 100-04, 3, 10.4

* **V2299** Specialty bifocal (by report)
  Bill DME/MAC

  Bill on paper. Requires report of type of specialty bifocal lens and optical lab invoice.

Trifocal, Glass or Plastic

* **V2300** Sphere, trifocal, plano to plus or minus 4.00d, per lens
  Bill DME/MAC

* **V2301** Sphere, trifocal, plus or minus 4.12 to plus or minus 7.00d per lens
  Bill DME/MAC

* **V2302** Sphere, trifocal, plus or minus 7.12 to plus or minus 20.00, per lens
  Bill DME/MAC

* **V2303** Spherocylinder, trifocal, plano to plus or minus 4.00d sphere, .12 to 2.00d cylinder, per lens
  Bill DME/MAC

* **V2304** Spherocylinder, trifocal, plano to plus or minus 4.00d sphere, 2.25-4.00d cylinder, per lens
  Bill DME/MAC

* **V2305** Spherocylinder, trifocal, plano to plus or minus 4.00d sphere, 4.25 to 6.00 cylinder, per lens
  Bill DME/MAC

* **V2306** Spherocylinder, trifocal, plano to plus or minus 4.00d sphere, over 6.00d cylinder, per lens
  Bill DME/MAC

▶ New → Revised ✔ Reinstated ~~deleted~~ Deleted
© Special coverage instructions ◆ Not covered or valid by Medicare * Carrier discretion

✳ **V2307** Spherocylinder, trifocal, plus or minus 4.25 to plus or minus 7.00d sphere, .12 to 2.00d cylinder, per lens
Bill DME/MAC

✳ **V2308** Spherocylinder, trifocal, plus or minus 4.25 to plus or minus 7.00d sphere, 2.12 to 4.00d cylinder, per lens
Bill DME/MAC

✳ **V2309** Spherocylinder, trifocal, plus or minus 4.25 to plus or minus 7.00d sphere, 4.25 to 6.00d cylinder, per lens
Bill DME/MAC

✳ **V2310** Spherocylinder, trifocal, plus or minus 4.25 to plus or minus 7.00d sphere, over 6.00d cylinder, per lens
Bill DME/MAC

✳ **V2311** Spherocylinder, trifocal, plus or minus 7.25 to plus or minus 12.00d sphere, .25 to 2.25d cylinder, per lens
Bill DME/MAC

✳ **V2312** Spherocylinder, trifocal, plus or minus 7.25 to plus or minus 12.00d sphere, 2.25 to 4.00d cylinder, per lens
Bill DME/MAC

✳ **V2313** Spherocylinder, trifocal, plus or minus 7.25 to plus or minus 12.00d sphere, 4.25 to 6.00d cylinder, per lens
Bill DME/MAC

✳ **V2314** Spherocylinder, trifocal, sphere over plus or minus 12.00d, per lens
Bill DME/MAC

✳ **V2315** Lenticular, (myodisc), per lens, trifocal
Bill DME/MAC

✳ **V2318** Aniseikonic lens, trifocal
Bill DME/MAC

✳ **V2319** Trifocal seg width over 28 mm
Bill DME/MAC

✳ **V2320** Trifocal add over 3.25d
Bill DME/MAC

⊙ **V2321** Lenticular lens, per lens, trifocal
Bill DME/MAC
IOM: 100-02, 15, 120; 100-04, 3, 10.4

✳ **V2399** Specialty trifocal (by report)
Bill DME/MAC
Bill on paper. Requires report of type of trifocal lens and optical lab invoice.

Variable Asphericity

✳ **V2410** Variable asphericity lens, single vision, full field, glass or plastic, per lens
Bill DME/MAC

✳ **V2430** Variable asphericity lens, bifocal, full field, glass or plastic, per lens
Bill DME/MAC

✳ **V2499** Variable sphericity lens, other type
Bill DME/MAC
Bill on paper. Requires report of other type of lens and optical lab invoice.

Contact Lenses

If a CPT procedure code for supply of contact lens is reported, recode with specific lens type listed below (per lens).

✳ **V2500** Contact lens, PMMA, spherical, per lens
Bill DME/MAC
Requires prior authorization for patients under age 21.

✳ **V2501** Contact lens, PMMA, toric or prism ballast, per lens
Bill DME/MAC
Requires prior authorization for clients under age 21.

✳ **V2502** Contact lens PMMA, bifocal, per lens
Bill DME/MAC
Requires prior authorization for clients under age 21. Bill on paper. Requires optical lab invoice.

✳ **V2503** Contact lens PMMA, color vision deficiency, per lens
Bill DME/MAC
Requires prior authorization for clients under age 21. Bill on paper. Requires optical lab invoice.

✳ **V2510** Contact lens, gas permeable, spherical, per lens
Bill DME/MAC
Requires prior authorization for clients under age 21.

✳ **V2511** Contact lens, gas permeable, toric, prism ballast, per lens
Bill DME/MAC
Requires prior authorization for clients under age 21.

▶ New   → Revised   ✔ Reinstated   ~~deleted~~ Deleted
⊙ Special coverage instructions   ◆ Not covered or valid by Medicare   ✳ Carrier discretion

* **V2512** Contact lens, gas permeable, bifocal, per lens

  Bill DME/MAC

  Requires prior authorization for clients under age 21.

* **V2513** Contact lens, gas permeable, extended wear, per lens

  Bill DME/MAC

  Requires prior authorization for clients under age 21.

☼ **V2520** Contact lens, hydrophilic, spherical, per lens

  If "incident to" a physician service, do not bill; otherwise, bill DME/MAC

  Requires prior authorization for clients under age 21.

  IOM: 100-03, 1, 80.1; 100-03, 1, 80.4

☼ **V2521** Contact lens, hydrophilic, toric, or prism ballast, per lens

  If "incident to" a physician's service, do not bill; otherwise, bill DME/MAC.

  Requires prior authorization for clients under age 21.

  IOM: 100-03, 1, 80.1; 100-03, 1, 80.4

☼ **V2522** Contact lens, hydrophilic, bifocal, per lens

  If "incident to" a physician's service, do not bill; otherwise, bill DME/MAC.

  Requires prior authorization for clients under age 21.

  IOM: 100-03, 1, 80.1; 100-03, 1, 80.4

☼ **V2523** Contact lens, hydrophilic, extended wear, per lens

  If "incident to" a physician's service, do not bill; otherwise, bill DME/MAC.

  Requires prior authorization for clients under age 21.

  IOM: 100-03, 1, 80.1; 100-03, 1, 80.4

* **V2530** Contact lens, scleral, gas impermeable, per lens (for contact lens modification, see 92325)

  Bill DME/MAC

  Requires prior authorization for clients under age 21.

☼ **V2531** Contact lens, scleral, gas permeable, per lens (for contact lens modification, see 92325)

  Bill DME/MAC

  DME regional carrier

  Requires prior authorization for clients under age 21. Bill on paper. Requires optical lab invoice.

  IOM: 100-03, 1, 80.5

* **V2599** Contact lens, other type

  If "incident to" a physician's service, do not bill; otherwise, bill DME/MAC.

  Requires prior authorization for clients under age 21. Bill on paper. Requires report of other type of contact lens and optical invoice.

Low Vision Aids

If a CPT procedure code for supply of low vision aid is reported, recode with specific systems listed below.

* **V2600** Hand held low vision aids and other nonspectacle mounted aids

  Bill DME/MAC

  Requires prior authorization.

* **V2610** Single lens spectacle mounted low vision aids

  Bill DME/MAC

  Requires prior authorization.

* **V2615** Telescopic and other compound lens system, including distance vision telescopic, near vision telescopes and compound microscopic lens system

  Bill DME/MAC

  Requires prior authorization. Bill on paper. Requires optical lab invoice.

Prosthetic Eye

☼ **V2623** Prosthetic eye, plastic, custom

  Bill DME/MAC

  DME regional carrier. Requires prior authorization. Bill on paper. Requires optical lab invoice.

* **V2624** Polishing/resurfacing of ocular prosthesis

  Bill DME/MAC

  Requires prior authorization. Bill on paper. Requires optical lab invoice.

▶ New   → Revised   ✔ Reinstated   deleted Deleted
☼ Special coverage instructions   ◆ Not covered or valid by Medicare   * Carrier discretion

✳ **V2625** Enlargement of ocular prosthesis

Bill DME/MAC

Requires prior authorization. Bill on paper. Requires optical lab invoice.

✳ **V2626** Reduction of ocular prosthesis

Bill DME/MAC

Requires prior authorization. Bill on paper. Requires optical lab invoice.

✿ **V2627** Scleral cover shell

Bill DME/MAC

DME regional carrier

Requires prior authorization. Bill on paper. Requires optical lab invoice.

IOM: 100-03, 4, 280.2

✳ **V2628** Fabrication and fitting of ocular conformer

Bill DME/MAC

Requires prior authorization. Bill on paper. Requires optical lab invoice.

✳ **V2629** Prosthetic eye, other type

Bill DME/MAC

Requires prior authorization. Bill on paper. Requires optical lab invoice.

Intraocular Lenses

✿ **V2630** Anterior chamber intraocular lens

Bill local carrier

IOM: 100-02, 15, 120

✿ **V2631** Iris supported intraocular lens

Bill local carrier

IOM: 100-02, 15, 120

✿ **V2632** Posterior chamber intraocular lens

Bill local carrier

IOM: 100-02, 15, 120

Miscellaneous

✳ **V2700** Balance lens, per lens

Bill DME/MAC

◆ **V2702** Deluxe lens feature

Bill DME/MAC

IOM: 100-02, 15, 120; 100-04, 3, 10.4

✳ **V2710** Slab off prism, glass or plastic, per lens

Bill DME/MAC

✳ **V2715** Prism, per lens

Bill DME/MAC

✳ **V2718** Press-on lens, Fresnel prism, per lens

Bill DME/MAC

✳ **V2730** Special base curve, glass or plastic, per lens

Bill DME/MAC

✿ **V2744** Tint, photochromatic, per lens

Bill DME/MAC

Requires prior authorization.

IOM: 100-02, 15, 120; 100-04, 3, 10.4

✿ **V2745** Addition to lens, tint, any color, solid, gradient or equal, excludes photochroatic, any lens material, per lens

Bill DME/MAC

Includes photochromatic lenses (V2744) used as sunglasses, which are prescribed in addition to regular prosthetic lenses for aphakic patient will be denied as not medically necessary.

IOM: 100-02, 15, 120; 100-04, 3, 10.4

✿ **V2750** Anti-reflective coating, per lens

Bill DME/MAC

Requires prior authorization.

IOM: 100-02, 15, 120; 100-04, 3, 10.4

✿ **V2755** U-V lens, per lens

Bill DME/MAC

IOM: 100-02, 15, 120; 100-04, 3, 10.4

✳ **V2756** Eye glass case

Bill DME/MAC

✳ **V2760** Scratch resistant coating, per lens

Bill DME/MAC

✿ **V2761** Mirror coating, any type, solid, gradient or equal, any lens material, per lens

Bill DME/MAC

IOM: 100-02, 15, 120; 100-04, 3, 10.4

✿ **V2762** Polarization, any lens material, per lens

Bill DME/MAC

IOM: 100-02, 15, 120; 100-04, 3, 10.4

✳ **V2770** Occluder lens, per lens

Bill DME/MAC

Requires prior authorization.

✳ **V2780** Oversize lens, per lens

Bill DME/MAC

Requires prior authorization.

▶ New   → Revised   ✔ Reinstated   ̶d̶e̶l̶e̶t̶e̶d̶ Deleted
✿ Special coverage instructions   ◆ Not covered or valid by Medicare   ✳ Carrier discretion

❋ **V2781** Progressive lens, per lens

Bill DME/MAC

Requires prior authorization.

❂ **V2782** Lens, index 1.54 to 1.65 plastic or 1.60 to 1.79 glass, excludes polycarbonate, per lens

Bill DME/MAC

Do not bill in addition to V2784

IOM: 100-02, 15, 120; 100-04, 3, 10.4

❂ **V2783** Lens, index greater than or equal to 1.66 plastic or greater than or equal to 1.80 glass, excludes polycarbonate, per lens

Bill DME/MAC

Do not bill in addition to V2784

IOM: 100-02, 15, 120; 100-04, 3, 10.4

❂ **V2784** Lens, polycarbonate or equal, any index, per lens

Bill DME/MAC

Covered only for patients with functional vision in one eye—in this situation, an impact-resistant material is covered for both lenses if eyeglasses are covered. Claims with V2784 that do not meet this coverage criterion will be denied as not medically necessary.

IOM: 100-02, 15, 120; 100-04, 3, 10.4

❋ **V2785** Processing, preserving and transporting corneal tissue

Bill local carrier

Bill on paper. Must attach eye bank invoice to claim.

❂ **V2786** Specialty occupational multifocal lens, per lens

Bill DME/MAC

IOM: 100-02, 15, 120; 100-04, 3, 10.4

◆ **V2787** Astigmatism correcting function of intraocular lens

Bill local carrier

Medicare Statute 1862(a)(7)

◆ **V2788** Presbyopia correcting function of intraocular lens

Bill local carrier

Medicare Statute 1862a7

❋ **V2790** Amniotic membrane for surgical reconstruction, per procedure

Bill local carrier

❋ **V2797** Vision supply, accessory and/or service component of another HCPCS vision code

Bill DME/MAC

❋ **V2799** Vision service, miscellaneous

Bill DME/MAC

Bill on paper. Requires report of miscellaneous service and optical lab invoice.

HEARING SERVICES (V5000-V5999)

NOTE: These codes are for non-physician services.

V5008-V5299: Bill local carrier

◆ **V5008** Hearing screening

IOM: 100-02, 16, 90

◆ **V5010** Assessment for hearing aid

Medicare Statute 1862a7

◆ **V5011** Fitting/orientation/checking of hearing aid

Medicare Statute 1862a7

◆ **V5014** Repair/modification of a hearing aid

Medicare Statute 1862a7

◆ **V5020** Conformity evaluation

Medicare Statute 1862a7

◆ **V5030** Hearing aid, monaural, body worn, air conduction

Medicare Statute 1862a7

◆ **V5040** Hearing aid, monaural, body worn, bone conduction

Medicare Statute 1862a7

◆ **V5050** Hearing aid, monaural, in the ear

Medicare Statute 1862a7

◆ **V5060** Hearing aid, monaural, behind the ear

Medicare Statute 1862a7

◆ **V5070** Glasses, air conduction

Medicare Statute 1862a7

◆ **V5080** Glasses, bone conduction

Medicare Statute 1862a7

◆ **V5090** Dispensing fee, unspecified hearing aid

Medicare Statute 1862a7

◆ **V5095** Semi-implantable middle ear hearing prosthesis

Medicare Statute 1862a7

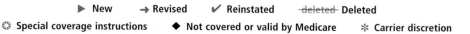

▶ New   → Revised   ✔ Reinstated   -deleted- Deleted
❂ Special coverage instructions   ◆ Not covered or valid by Medicare   ❋ Carrier discretion

◆ **V5100**   Hearing aid, bilateral, body worn
Medicare Statute 1862a7

◆ **V5110**   Dispensing fee, bilateral
Medicare Statute 1862a7

◆ **V5120**   Binaural, body
Medicare Statute 1862a7

◆ **V5130**   Binaural, in the ear
Medicare Statute 1862a7

◆ **V5140**   Binaural, behind the ear
Medicare Statute 1862a7

◆ **V5150**   Binaural, glasses
Medicare Statute 1862a7

◆ **V5160**   Dispensing fee, binaural
Medicare Statute 1862a7

◆ **V5170**   Hearing aid, CROS, in the ear
Medicare Statute 1862a7

◆ **V5180**   Hearing aid, CROS, behind the ear
Medicare Statute 1862a7

◆ **V5190**   Hearing aid, CROS, glasses
Medicare Statute 1862a7

◆ **V5200**   Dispensing fee, CROS
Medicare Statute 1862a7

◆ **V5210**   Hearing aid, BICROS, in the ear
Medicare Statute 1862a7

◆ **V5220**   Hearing aid, BICROS, behind
the ear
Medicare Statute 1862a7

◆ **V5230**   Hearing aid, BICROS, glasses
Medicare Statute 1862a7

◆ **V5240**   Dispensing fee, BICROS
Medicare Statute 1862a7

◆ **V5241**   Dispensing fee, monaural hearing
aid, any type
Medicare Statute 1862a7

◆ **V5242**   Hearing aid, analog, monaural, CIC
(completely in the ear canal)
Medicare Statute 1862a7

◆ **V5243**   Hearing aid, analog, monaural, ITC
(in the canal)
Medicare Statute 1862a9

◆ **V5244**   Hearing aid, digitally programmable
analog, monaural, CIC
Medicare Statute 1862a7

◆ **V5245**   Hearing aid, digitally programmable,
analog, monaural, ITC
Medicare Statute 1862a7

◆ **V5246**   Hearing aid, digitally programmable
analog, monaural, ITE (in the ear)
Medicare Statute 1862a7

◆ **V5247**   Hearing aid, digitally programmable
analog, monaural, BTE (behind the ear)
Medicare Statute 1862a7

◆ **V5248**   Hearing aid, analog, binaural, CIC
Medicare Statute 1862a7

◆ **V5249**   Hearing aid, analog, binaural, ITC
Medicare Statute 1862a7

◆ **V5250**   Hearing aid, digitally programmable
analog, binaural, CIC
Medicare Statute 1862a7

◆ **V5251**   Hearing aid, digitally programmable
analog, binaural, ITC
Medicare Statute 1862a7

◆ **V5252**   Hearing aid, digitally programmable,
binaural, ITE
Medicare Statute 1862a7

◆ **V5253**   Hearing aid, digitally programmable,
binaural, BTE
Medicare Statute 1862a7

◆ **V5254**   Hearing aid, digital, monaural, CIC
Medicare Statute 1862a7

◆ **V5255**   Hearing aid, digital, monaural, ITC
Medicare Statute 1862a7

◆ **V5256**   Hearing aid, digital, monaural, ITE
Medicare Statute 1862a7

◆ **V5257**   Hearing aid, digital, monaural, BTE
Medicare Statute 1862a7

◆ **V5258**   Hearing aid, digital, binaural, CIC
Medicare Statute 1862a7

◆ **V5259**   Hearing aid, digital, binaural, ITC
Medicare Statute 1862a7

◆ **V5260**   Hearing aid, digital, binaural, ITE
Medicare Statute 1862a7

◆ **V5261**   Hearing aid, digital, binaural, BTE
Medicare Statute 1862a7

◆ **V5262**   Hearing aid, disposable, any type,
monaural
Medicare Statute 1862a7

◆ **V5263**   Hearing aid, disposable, any type,
binaural
Medicare Statute 1862a7

◆ **V5264**   Ear mold/insert, not disposable,
any type
Medicare Statute 1862a7

▶ New   → Revised   ✔ Reinstated   ~~deleted~~ Deleted

✪ **Special coverage instructions**   ◆ **Not covered or valid by Medicare**   ✳ **Carrier discretion**

◆ **V5265** Ear mold/insert, disposable, any type

Medicare Statute 1862a7

◆ **V5266** Battery for use in hearing device

Medicare Statute 1862a7

◆ **V5267** Hearing aid supplies/accessories

Medicare Statute 1862a7

◆ **V5268** Assistive listening device, telephone amplifier, any type

Medicare Statute 1862a7

◆ **V5269** Assistive listening device, alerting, any type

Medicare Statute 1862a7

◆ **V5270** Assistive listening device, television amplifier, any type

Medicare Statute 1862a7

◆ **V5271** Assistive listening device, television caption decoder

Medicare Statute 1862a7

◆ **V5272** Assistive listening device, TDD

Medicare Statute 1862a7

◆ **V5273** Assistive listening device, for use with cochlear implant

Medicare Statute 1862a7

◆ **V5274** Assistive listening device, not otherwise specified

Medicare Statute 1862a7

◆ **V5275** Ear impression, each

Medicare Statute 1862a7

◆ **V5298** Hearing aid, not otherwise classified

Medicare Statute 1862a7

◌ **V5299** Hearing service, miscellaneous

IOM: 100-02, 16, 90

Speech-Language Pathology Services

NOTE: These codes are for non-physician services.

◆ **V5336** Repair/modification of augmentative communicative system or device (excludes adaptive hearing aid)

Bill DME/MAC

Medicare Statute 1862a7

◆ **V5362** Speech screening

Bill local carrier

Medicare Statute 1862a7

◆ **V5363** Language screening

Bill local carrier

Medicare Statute 1862a7

◆ **V5364** Dysphagia screening

Bill local carrier

Medicare Statute 1862a7

V5265 – V5364 HEARING SERVICES